Crises
in the
Psychotherapy
Session

Crises
in the
Psychotherapy
Session

Transforming
Critical Moments
Into Turning Points

Julian D. Ford

 AMERICAN PSYCHOLOGICAL ASSOCIATION

Published by
American Psychological Association
750 First Street, NE
Washington, DC 20002
https://www.apa.org

Order Department
https://www.apa.org/pubs/books
order@apa.org

In the U.K., Europe, Africa, and the Middle East, copies may be ordered from Eurospan
https://www.eurospanbookstore.com/apa
info@eurospangroup.com

Typeset in Charter and Interstate by Circle Graphics, Inc., Reisterstown, MD

Printer: Sheridan Books, Chelsea, MI
Cover Designer: Beth Schlenoff Design, Bethesda, MD

Library of Congress Cataloging-in-Publication Data

Names: Ford, Julian D., author.
Title: Crises in the psychotherapy session : transforming critical moments into turning points / Julian D. Ford.
Description: Washington, DC : American Psychological Association, [2021] | Includes bibliographical references and index.
Identifiers: LCCN 2020029213 (print) | LCCN 2020029214 (ebook) | ISBN 9781433832871 (paperback) | ISBN 9781433834141 (ebook)
Subjects: LCSH: Psychotherapy. | Psychotherapist and patient.
Classification: LCC RC480.5 .F66 2021 (print) | LCC RC480.5 (ebook) | DDC 616.89/14—dc23
LC record available at https://lccn.loc.gov/2020029213
LC ebook record available at https://lccn.loc.gov/2020029214

https://doi.org/10.1037/0000225-000

Printed in the United States of America

10 9 8 7 6 5 4 3 2 1

For Judy, my muse and cotherapist, and my beloved partner in life.

Contents

Acknowledgments

Many thanks to the American Psychological Association (APA) Publishing editors who have made this book not only possible but better at every stage from inception to publication: Susan Reynolds, Beth Hatch, and Laurel Vincenty.

I am deeply grateful to many invaluable mentors, teachers, and colleagues from whom I have learned so much about the practice of psychotherapy, first in the form of behavior modification at the University of Michigan and Ypsilanti State Hospital, then as cognitive behavior therapy at SUNY Stony Brook, family systems therapy at the Palo Alto VA Medical Center and the California Family Study Center, health psychology at Stanford University and UCLA, community mental health at the San Fernando Valley CMHCs, psychodynamic, self psychology, and experiential psychotherapy in private practice, trauma-focused psychotherapy at the Portland and White River Junction VA Medical Centers and the National Center for PTSD Executive Division, and child and adolescent psychotherapy at the UConn Health Center and in the State of Connecticut juvenile justice and child welfare systems and the National Child Traumatic Stress Network (NCTSN). I want to particularly thank the NCTSN and UConn Health colleagues, and the New Zenith Theatre and Looking In Theatre directors, staff, and actors, who have been instrumental in creating and sustaining the Center for the Treatment of Developmental Trauma Disorders and developing and filming the Critical Moments psychotherapy sessions that serve as the foundation for the second section of this book—especially the brilliant youth and adult actors who brought the dramatized clients so fully to life; and Drs. Rocio Chang, William Saltzman, Glenn Saxe, and Maureen Allwood for their skillful and sensitive handling of the psychotherapy crises in Chapters 7 through 10.

Finally, there is another cohort of wise and courageous women and men, boys and girls, and couples and families to whom I also owe a great debt of gratitude as my teachers and a source of inspiration—the clients whom I have been privileged to work with in psychotherapy over these past 5 decades.

Crises
in the
Psychotherapy
Session

INTRODUCTION

Transforming Crises Into Turning Points in Psychotherapy

Crises in the psychotherapy session are complex and take many forms. The most evident forms of in-session crises are blowups or outbursts involving overt suicidality, self-harm, rage, inconsolable grief, aggression (or threats), panic, flashbacks, dissociation, despair and dependency, detachment and unreachability, or regression to earlier phases of psychosocial development. Crises also may involve a client's disclosure of abuse or other severe threats to their safety. Or a client might abruptly announce a determination to end the therapy. Subtler crises can take the form of apparently involuntary self-harm, unspoken suicidality, or disorientation because of preoccupation with inner voices, visions, memories, or ruminations.

Although crises can have dire consequences, they also provide a unique opportunity for powerful breakthroughs in psychotherapy. For this reason, the term *crisis* is often defined as a critical point with the potential for either good or bad outcomes. Dictionary definitions of crisis include the following range of events or circumstances (Merriam-Webster, n.d.):

- "the turning point for better or worse in an acute disease or fever";

- "a paroxysmal attack of pain, distress, or disordered function";

https://doi.org/10.1037/0000225-001
Crises in the Psychotherapy Session: Transforming Critical Moments Into Turning Points,
by J. D. Ford

- "an emotionally significant event or radical change of status in a person's life";

- "the decisive moment";

- "an unstable or crucial time or state of affairs in which a decisive change is impending . . . especially: one with the distinct possibility of a highly undesirable outcome"; and

- "a situation that has reached a critical phase."

Each of these aspects of a crisis is essential to understanding and dealing with crises that occur in the process of psychotherapy. When a crisis occurs in a psychotherapy session, at that moment, the client is experiencing intense emotional pain, distress, and impairment that has reached a decisive point that could fundamentally change the client's life significantly for the worse. The crises that occur in psychotherapy sessions involve the imminent threat, or the actual occurrence, of violence, self-harm, loss of hope or the will to live; the decision to give up on the therapy, the therapeutic relationship, and the prospect of healing; or the decision to give in to impulses or external coercion that put the client's life at risk. Given this risk, it is not surprising that crises in psychotherapy call for the therapist to rapidly focus on taking immediate actions that reduce the client's distress and dysregulation. Optimally, a therapist will not only help the client to regain emotional regulation during a crisis but also will use the crisis to facilitate a transformative therapeutic breakthrough.

Therefore, it is the turning point aspect of crises that should be the therapist's focus when crises occur in the psychotherapy session. A *turning point* occurs when the crisis is redefined as a problem that must be, and can be, solved. To be solvable, a problem must be defined as an adverse circumstance that can be used as an opportunity for healing and transformation. The threat or danger involved in a crisis is not denied or minimized in this approach. Instead, the therapist views it as an aspect of the problem that must be addressed to achieve the safety required to achieve healing and positive transformation. The concept of transformation is crucial, because without fundamental change, the crisis will inevitably reoccur even if there is healing and what appears to be a positive resolution of the problem and the client's distress at that time.

Thus, a crisis is a moment in which a problem has become so acute and dangerous that in addition to restoring immediate safety—indeed, to genuinely restore safety—and to restore calm and begin to heal the resultant emotional wounds, a transformative change is necessary. Attempting to solve the problem(s) at the heart of a crisis by repeating reactions that leave the person's situation essentially unchanged (i.e., doing "more of the same"; Watzlawick et al., 1974) is doomed to failure. The opportunity that every crisis provides is to help the client to find a fundamental change in direction in life: a turning point.

Changing a problem into a turning point is a transformation that is difficult to achieve under any circumstances. The difficulty of achieving a turning point is drastically elevated when the problem is a crisis in which every second and every word and action make a difference between a catastrophic outcome and the restoration of safety. This book tackles that challenge by providing a conceptual and practical framework to guide therapists and their clients in transforming critical moments in the psychotherapy session into turning points in the client's life.

Knowing what to do and what to think at moments of maximum stress and uncertainty are key to transforming the crisis into a positive turning point. Yet, the guidance available to therapists is limited and generally focuses on stock techniques to help the client de-escalate and make a safety plan. What's not talked about is how the therapist resets internally to think clearly, act rapidly, and guide the client back to safety.

When a crisis occurs in a psychotherapy session, it is the therapist's responsibility to protect the safety of everyone involved, to preserve or restore the therapeutic alliance, and to enable the client to continue in and benefit from the therapy. Although there is no single formula for how to handle crises in psychotherapy sessions, strategies from a variety of sources can enable therapists to rapidly and effectively respond to in-session crises. This book takes therapists, both those in practice and those still in training, right into the critical moments that occur in crises in the psychotherapy session. For nontherapists, the book provides a unique view into the workings of both the psychotherapy process and of the mind of psychotherapists and their clients when crises occur in session.

A FRAMEWORK FOR CRISIS INTERVENTION IN THE PSYCHOTHERAPY SESSION: FREEDOM

I have been intrigued by crises because, as a psychotherapist for more than 40 years, I never felt certain that I was prepared to handle the next crisis that was going to happen, often sooner rather than later, as I have conducted therapy sessions. While generic rules of thumb for handling crises have been helpful, I've never had an explicit map or guide to draw on to prepare myself to effectively handle crises that are so sudden or complex that I've often felt like a deer frozen in the headlights. At those moments, generic tactics for de-escalating and containing a client who is in a state of overwhelming distress were at best only a partial answer.

I thought about what I learned on the fly by observing or debriefing with talented colleagues who seemed to intuitively know how to handle in-session crises adroitly. Somehow, these therapists had the presence of mind to be able to think clearly and respond reassuringly and empathically in crises with severely distressed, dysregulated, dissociated, or detached clients. The key phrase is *presence of mind*—being able to stop, think clearly, and act decisively and therapeutically while in the midst of a crisis.

Based on these observations, I realized that crises in the psychotherapy session can best be handled if the therapist engages with the client in a parallel process of coregulation that leads to the restoration of self-regulation for both. As the first six chapters in this book make clear, this conclusion is consistent with research on attachment, emotion regulation, acute and prolonged stress reactions, posttraumatic stress reactions, and crisis management theory. Guided by this principle, I developed a framework for achieving the presence of mind necessary to respond effectively to crises. I call this framework FREEDOM (Ford, 2020c), which stands for

- **F**ocusing by rapidly shifting into a state of mindful awareness, orienting to a core personal value or commitment, and self-monitoring one's level of stress and personal control

- **R**ecognizing triggers that set off the alarm (i.e., both external stimuli and contexts as well as internal physiological states) followed by reappraisal in four domains

- **E**motion awareness (including both reactive and core emotions)

- **E**valuation of both reactive and core thoughts and beliefs

- **D**efining both reactive and core goals and motivations

- **O**ptions for action (including both reactive and proactive behaviors)

- **M**aking a contribution by upholding core values and acting with self-regulation

The FREEDOM framework serves as the practical guide for the therapist's internal work to maintain or restore their own self-regulation. This enables the therapist to not just teach the client how to self-regulate but, more important, to authentically experientially serve as a role model for the client by demonstrating how it is possible to recognize dysregulation and think clearly and strategically so as to regain self-regulation. This is not to say that therapists experience the exact same degree or symptoms of dysregulation as their clients; rather, when faced with the dual challenge of helping a severely dysregulated client and managing one's own internal stress reactions (including countertransference), it is essential for therapists to pay careful attention to their own self-regulation. That is a large order, but it's what's necessary for therapists to have the presence of mind to use their psycho-therapy skills effectively in handling crises.

The FREEDOM framework has been tested as the core of a therapeutic intervention, Trauma Affect Regulation: Guide for Education and Therapy (TARGET; Ford, 2020c). TARGET was first developed and tested as a group therapy intervention for adults with psychiatric or substance abuse disorders, or both, comorbid with complex posttraumatic stress disorder (CPTSD). In a randomized controlled trial (RCT) comparing outpatient group therapy either with CPTSD psychoeducation or with TARGET, TARGET was asso-ciated with significant reductions in trauma-related beliefs and symptoms, and with sustained sobriety-related self-efficacy (Frisman et al., 2008). A second RCT compared manualized supportive group therapy versus TARGET groups with incarcerated women with CPTSD (Ford et al., 2013). TARGET was associated with significant reductions in PTSD, depression, anxiety, and anger symptoms; increased self-efficacy; and low dropout rates (< 5%). In addition, TARGET proved to be more effective than supportive therapy in increasing sense of forgiveness toward self and toward trauma perpetrators, as well as greater reductions in trauma-related beliefs about self and relationships, and increases in affect regulation capacities. Moving from adults to adolescents, two quasi-experimental studies compared TARGET groups with services as usual in a juvenile justice residential setting. Teach-ing the FREEDOM skills to these youth and the staff working with them was associated with reductions in dangerous incidents, coercive punishments (e.g., physical restraints, solitary confinement), recidivism, depression, and anxiety symptoms, and also associated with increased youth self-efficacy and engagement in rehabilitation (Ford & Hawke, 2012; Marrow et al., 2012). In the Ford and Hawke (2012) and Marrow et al. (2012) studies, TARGET also served as a total milieu intervention: All staff, teachers, and administrators were trained to use the FREEDOM skills in their interactions with youth— importantly, including in handling crises.

The FREEDOM framework also has been tested as a one-to-one psycho-therapy with both adults and youth. An RCT compared TARGET versus an evidence-based social problem-solving therapy for PTSD (present-centered therapy) with low-income mothers with complex trauma histories and severe PTSD who were caring for young children (Ford et al., 2011). TARGET was more effective than present-centered therapy in achieving sustained (at 3- and 6-month follow-up assessments) reductions in PTSD severity and enhanced affect regulation capacities, as well as in reducing anxiety and trauma-related self-cognitions and blame, and in increasing active coping and secure attachment working models. In a second RCT, TARGET was more effective than a manualized relational therapy in reducing juvenile justice–involved girls' PTSD (intrusive reexperiencing and avoidance) and anxiety symptoms, and improving posttraumatic cognitions and emotion regulation (Ford et al., 2012). A third RCT with military veterans with CPTSD (Ford, Grasso, Greene, et al., 2018) demonstrated that TARGET resulted in comparable or superior reductions in PTSD and CPTSD symptoms with substantially fewer dropouts than prolonged exposure therapy.

Based on this research evidence, the FREEDOM framework appears applicable and effective in therapeutic work with both youth and adult clients who frequently experience crises. When crises occur, the client needs a partner and a guide who is personally walking the walk and not just talking the talk. The purpose of this book is to provide psychotherapists with a practical and evidence-based approach to becoming that partner and guide. I'll show you how—with the FREEDOM framework as their guide—psychotherapists can transform crises into turning points.

WHAT'S IN THIS BOOK?

The book is organized in two parts. Part I reviews the science and clinical wisdom that inform the FREEDOM framework, and then presents the framework itself. I begin by drawing on crisis theory to unpack the core feature of a crisis, which is emotional dysregulation (Chapter 1), and then establish an attainable target for resolving crises, which is to help the client restore adaptive self-regulation (Chapter 2). I describe relevant strategies from the crisis intervention field (Chapter 3) and the psychotherapy literature (Chapter 4). Based on this background, I propose an integrative practical framework for handling crises in the psychotherapy session (Chapter 5) and apply that framework to a crucial and often missing piece in crisis resolution: the therapist's own emotion regulation when crisis occurs (Chapter 6).

Part II presents the client–therapist dialogue from six psychotherapy sessions in which crises occur to show how different therapists put the FREEDOM framework and the crisis intervention and psychotherapy strategies into practice. The cases feature

- a young woman who was sexually assaulted and is descending a downward spiral into passive withdrawal, dissociation, and the early manifestations of self-harm (Chapter 7);

- a young man struggling with depression who suddenly decides to stop therapy to hide painful secrets and a profound sense of shame, betrayal, and hopelessness (Chapter 8);

- the same young man featured in Chapter 8 who, after a halted suicide attempt, reveals a dissociative alter "personality" who shames him and commands him to kill himself (Chapter 9);

- a young woman who has been the recent victim of sexting and a victim of past childhood maltreatment, and who is seething with anger at her psychotherapist (Chapter 10);

- a mother and her preteen son and teenage daughter who have experienced family violence and abuse; in a session, the son becomes immobilized by fear and dissociation (Chapter 11); and

- the same mother and daughter featured in Chapter 11 who, in a subsequent session, simultaneously experience an escalating crisis of rage (Chapter 12).

The cases are drawn from a webinar series on the same topic developed by The National Child Traumatic Stress Network (NCTSN) Learning Center. Readers can access the webinars at no cost by going to the Learning Center's webpage (see https://learn.nctsn.org/course/index.php?categoryid=78). Alternatively, readers can go to the main website for NCTSN (see https://learn.nctsn.org), click on "Clinical Training" in the menu at the top of the page, and then click on "Identifying Critical Moments and Healing Complex Trauma." The chapters in Part II provide transcripts of the client–therapist dialogue along with my detailed comments and annotations highlighting

- the psychotherapist's unspoken thoughts and reactions,
- key take-home points for crisis management and prevention, and
- questions to engage the reader in reflection about the crisis and the therapist's choices.

Although readers can use the webinars and this book independently, they will have a richer learning experience if they use both resources in tandem. I recommend watching the webinars first and then reading the transcripts and analysis in the chapters.

A NOTE ABOUT THE CASES

To create the webinar cases, actors portrayed the "clients" to ensure privacy, confidentiality, and safety. Working with actors also made it possible to hone in on specific crises without waiting for them to occur spontaneously. However, once in role, the actors were free to improvise, so what actually occurred was not scripted in advance. The actors also were able to express a wide range of emotional and behavioral reactions while staying true to the character of the person portrayed and ensuring that a predefined crisis occurred as vividly as possible.

The therapists in the cases were real therapists who were doing therapy exactly as they would with a real client and were not simply acting. As one of the therapists, I can personally attest to the realism of the encounter. I didn't know how the actor client(s) would react to what I said or did until it actually was happening in real time. I had a forewarning and more time to prepare for the "crisis" than I would have had in an actual in-session crisis, but I never knew exactly what the actor client(s) would actually do, nor did I know what I would say and do in the moment when I had to respond immediately to clients who were in a state of crisis and looking for me to say and do the right thing to help them at that moment. The time urgency was heightened by the need to make each session brief enough so that key clinical moments and teaching points were readily observable and not lost in an overly lengthy and circuitous (or just plain boring and repetitive) interaction that ultimately went nowhere.

The therapists who conducted the critical moment sessions also represented a range of personal backgrounds, professional experiences and orientations, and psychotherapy styles, as you will see as you are introduced to them in the case examples in Part II of this book. The variation in the therapists' responses to each unique crisis and stuck point demonstrates that therapeutic crises can be understood and dealt with in the moment in a variety of ways. Clearly no one size fits all, and there is no single evidence-based approach to crisis prevention and resolution in psychotherapy sessions. However, consistent with this book's framework, a common denominator that emerged across all of the therapists, therapist–"client" pairings and varied in-session crises is the foundational approach of *modeling and restoring self-regulation,* that is, beginning with the therapist themself and extending to the client with the therapist's support and guidance. This process occurs in as many different ways as there are therapists and clients.

In debriefing each of the filmed sessions, the therapists (including me) universally said that the session felt entirely real—that from the first moment of the "session," the actors seemed in every way like real people who needed their therapist's unflinching and highly focused therapeutic attention, empathic understanding, compassion, and help in regaining hope. The actors, in postsession debriefing interviews in which they were both in and out of character, said that their crises and stuck points seemed completely real and emotionally intense, and that the therapist's presence and intervention felt crucial in helping them find an authentic way to understand and safely come through the moments of crisis and detachment. Both actor clients and therapists said that, at any given moment in the session, they felt immersed in the interaction and unsure or frankly doubtful whether the session would come to a positive conclusion. Therapists and actor clients alike said that, despite being prepared with a general outline of the crisis and how it might play out in the session, they found themselves reacting spontaneously rather than with scripted lines—and for therapists, these were some of the most gut-wrenching therapy sessions they'd ever done with clients whose suffering and despair was intense and real.

The filmed psychotherapy sessions differed from real therapy sessions in three main ways. Each session had a scripted crisis, although the exact form that those critical moments actually took and the way they played out were entirely improvised by the actors. Each session also was rehearsed and filmed several times rather than occurring only once in real time, and this enhanced rather than detracted from the spontaneity and realness of the interaction for both the actor client(s) and the therapist. And each session condensed what would have taken at least 50 minutes into 20–30 minutes, and the final film was edited down to 15–20 minutes, to zero in on the crisis and the clients' dysregulation.

WHO IS THIS BOOK FOR?

The intended audience for this book is practicing psychotherapists and counselors of all theoretical orientations and professional disciplines, as well as students, trainees, and teachers—and also clients in psychotherapy or other nonclinicians who are interested in the crises that can occur in therapy and how therapists guide their clients safely through them. This includes therapists from many professional disciplines, including clinical and counseling psychology, professional and peer counseling, marriage and family therapy, social work, psychiatry, creative arts therapy, faith-based counseling, occupational and recreational therapy, and primary care and complementary nursing and medicine. Although written from the perspective of the psychotherapist, the dilemmas and principles apply to all helping professionals and their clients.

Crises are an opportunity to help clients grapple with their most challenging emotions. If handled well, these critical moments can become turning points in the psychotherapy. Join me in unraveling the complexities that make crises so challenging and crucial to resolve. Together, we will explore many paths that can lead to the transformation of crises into turning points.

PART I

ESSENTIAL PRINCIPLES AND PRACTICES FOR RESOLVING CRISES IN THE PSYCHOTHERAPY SESSION

1 A STAGE-BASED CRISIS MODEL

A key starting point for responding effectively to in-session crises is understanding their core features. A formative definition of what constitutes a crisis was provided more than 50 years ago by a pioneer in the field, Gerald Caplan (1964): encounters with stressors that overwhelm the individual's (or group's or community's) capacity to cope effectively. More specifically, the signature feature of crises in the psychotherapy session is a breakdown of coping that results in emotional dysregulation. Understanding and knowing how to help clients recover from severe emotional dysregulation thus are the keys to resolving crises in the psychotherapy session. This is easier said than done, especially when the emotional dysregulation is accompanied by a deep sense of hopelessness—not just distress (which is the bread and butter of psychotherapy) but a profound sense on the client's part that the distress they feel is impossible to live with.

Crises often happen rapidly and involve distinct peaks of intensity However, crises don't happen just at a single moment. According to Caplan (1964), crises evolve over time in four stages:

- exposure to stressor(s) and attempts to restore homeostasis
- failure to restore homeostasis

https://doi.org/10.1037/0000225-002
Crises in the Psychotherapy Session: Transforming Critical Moments Into Turning Points, by J. D. Ford

- behavioral emergency
- breakdown of health and psychosocial functioning

This chapter describes the four stages of crisis in depth. Although Caplan's (1964) model is widely used in community, school, employment, and medical settings (Roberts, 2005), there has been limited research testing of the model. The most recent meta-analysis of research studies on crisis intervention was published 15 years ago (Roberts & Everly, 2006). Crisis intervention programs that were loosely based on Caplan's (1964) crisis model showed promise in preventing critical outcomes (e.g., suicide, posttraumatic stress disorder, family breakdown), although single-session debriefings with individuals tended to be ineffective, and multisession interventions that included preparation before crises as well as follow-up after a crisis were most consistently beneficial. As a result, psychotherapists should apply—with caution—crisis theory and the crisis intervention practices that have been developed based on it. As Roberts and Everly (2006) concluded, crisis intervention is "not a panacea" (p. 10) and must be conducted with careful attention to the specific circumstances and personal characteristics of the people in crisis in each unique case.

Caplan's (1964) four-stage model of crises provides a useful overall framework for assessing the situation and developing an individualized intervention when a crisis occurs in the psychotherapy session. In addition, the seven-step FREEDOM sequence that I use as a practical framework for intervening in crises fits nicely with crisis theory. Each of the FREEDOM steps represents an attempt to restore homeostasis (Caplan's Stage 1). When the individual in crisis is unable to focus and recognize triggers that are eliciting stress reactions (the "FR" [focusing, recognizing triggers] steps in FREEDOM), homeostasis cannot be restored (Caplan's Stage 2). When the individual continues in a state of stress reactivity, behavioral emergencies (Caplan's Stage 3) occur as a result of the escalation of reactive emotions, thoughts, goals, and behavior (the "EEDO" [emotion awareness, evaluation, defining goals, options] steps in FREEDOM). If the individual is unable to balance this reactivity with a stabilizing awareness of the core emotions, beliefs, and life goals that are the foundation for adaptive coping behavior, the resultant dysregulation can lead to a breakdown (Caplan's Stage 4) that is characterized by a sense of hopelessness, ineffectiveness, and overwhelming distress (e.g., anger, terror, grief, shame), which is the polar opposite of making a contribution (the "M" [making a contribution] step in FREEDOM).

To prepare for applying the FREEDOM framework as a guide to transforming each stage into a turning point, let's look more closely at the four stages in which crises unfold.

STAGE 1: EXPOSURE TO STRESSOR(S) AND ATTEMPTS TO RESTORE HOMEOSTASIS

According to Caplan (1964), the first stage of a crisis has two parts: (a) an encounter with a *stressor*, which is defined as a threat to the person's physical and psychological state of inner balance and wellness or safety and interpersonal connectedness (i.e., homeostasis); and (b) an adaptive attempt to restore homeostasis by using familiar coping or problem-solving strategies.

In the context of a psychotherapy session, this first stage of a crisis often begins well before the start of the session, when clients encounter stressors in their daily lives that trigger the emergence or worsening of the symptoms or the life dilemmas that have brought them into therapy in the first place. For example, clients may arrive at a therapy session while still in the throes of reacting to and attempting to cope with recent conflicts, disappointments, or losses in relationships, school or work, or important avocations. Or they may be experiencing flare-ups of physical or psychological symptoms, or the aftereffects of traumatic victimization or other life-threatening or life-altering dangers that remain unresolved. Even with empathic support from the therapist, clients who are in, or on the verge of, this first stage of a crisis in their daily life may escalate into crisis when in a psychotherapy session for several reasons. Talking in therapy about stressors and their impact can be a relief and an opportunity to feel less alone and to develop new solutions and ways of coping, but it also can be extraordinarily stressful. This is especially the case when a client has been avoiding or suppressing awareness of the feelings of distress and thoughts or memories associated with stressors. "Opening up," so to speak, can break the inner dam created by avoidance, resulting in a flood of built-up distress. Talking about stressors and distress also can be demoralizing when clients feel that they have failed in their attempts to cope or resolve the problems, leading to an upsurge in feelings of shame and hopelessness.

For other clients, their lives are such that there doesn't seem to be any desirable "normal" to get back to because the stressor(s) and the clients' familiar ways of coping have become their new normal (e.g., when trapped in abusive relationships, when suffering chronic psychiatric problems or addictions). In other cases, the stressor(s) and associated distress are so familiar and apparently inescapable that the client believes there's nothing to disclose, that it's worthless to talk with their therapist because nothing ever seems to get better, and that therapy yields no useful solutions. Returning to therapy may seem like a pointless exercise in futility and a constant reminder of their failure as a person and their powerlessness to overcome the problems in their life.

From the psychotherapist's perspective, the first stage of in-session crises often looks like a continuation of the client's chronic problems in living and the resultant symptoms. This is true, but it's not the entire story. Crises involve a paradigm shift—from coping as best one can with stressors to reaching a turning point at which the stressors and the pain and effort involved in coping have become unmanageable. This is the transition from distress to dysregulation. Distress can be coped with, but *dysregulation* is a state in which coping becomes replaced by frantic attempts to simply survive (emotionally). On the surface, dysregulation may look (and to the client, feel) like a burst of rage, hostility, guilt, remorse, splitting, or suicidality— or an implosion of dependency, dissociation, detachment, or indifference. However, the essential experience in all forms of dysregulation is terror that is driven by an intense dialectical alternation between a sense of desperate need for a solution on the one hand and utter hopelessness and despair on the other.

The driving force behind dysregulation is not the stressor(s) per se that clients are facing (or have faced in the past) but a bipartite reaction to the accumulation of stressors in their lives. One of the reactions is a profound sense of attachment insecurity, which often is enacted in the form of disorganized attempts to merge with and simultaneously reject all contact from others. The essential dilemma caused by this kind of disorganized attachment is that people tend to feel imposed on or even harassed and violated by the person's demands for attention, caring, and closeness while they also feel helpless and hurt by the messages of rejection from that person. The individual who is dysregulated thus cuts themselves off from the very sources of support that they are seeking from relationships, resulting in a sense of profound aloneness that is terrifying.

The second contributor to dysregulation is a breakdown in self-regulation. To cope with the physical strain and emotional distress that are caused by unresolved stressor(s), physiological and psychological adaptations are necessary. Those adaptations enable the body to maintain a state of homeostasis (or to regain homeostasis when it has been lost) and the person to achieve a parallel state of balance in emotions that enables the person to tolerate the distress. This combination of physiological and psychological adaptation is the essence of self-regulation. When these self-regulation adaptations are insufficient to restore physical homeostasis and emotional balance, distress becomes unmanageable and escalates into a state of dysregulation that the person experiences as a loss of the ability to control bodily functions (e.g., hyper- or hypoarousal, physical tension, pain) and emotions (e.g., panic, despair, rage, guilt, shame)—and also associated behavioral excesses (e.g., impulsivity, aggression) and deficits (e.g., isolation).

Based on this understanding of crises as episodes of dysregulation that are driven by attachment disorganization and a breakdown in self-regulation, two determining factors distinguish persistent unresolved psychosocial problems with mild to moderate (but manageable) psychiatric symptoms versus symptoms or reactions sufficiently severe to constitute crises. These factors are (a) support provided by important relationships and (b) the client's psychophysiological ability to tolerate and recover from defensive stress reactions. However, the support provided by relationships and the individual's capacity to cope with stress reactions, although necessary, are often insufficient to prevent or resolve crises. This may explain (at least in part) why supportive psychotherapy can be helpful as a source of encouragement, a model for healthy relationships, and a way of reducing the avoidance of emotions and interpersonal isolation of clients with relatively mild symptoms and impairments (Conte, 1994; Farber et al., 2018; Peluso & Freund, 2018; Tryon et al., 2018) but nevertheless consistently is less effective (especially over long-term follow-up assessments) with severely symptomatic clients than psychotherapies that teach cognitive, behavioral, or relational skills for self-regulation (Bisson et al., 2013; Hartnett et al., 2017; Higa-McMillan et al., 2016; Ijaz et al., 2018; Porter & Chambless, 2015; van der Pol et al., 2017; Wang et al., 2018). In other words, support is helpful in the short term, but helping clients develop the ability to emotionally regulate has the long-term impact.

Crises in psychotherapy sessions can be especially shocking if they emerge at a point at which a client appears to be doing well in treatment and in life. This can happen simply because stressor(s) occur that profoundly disrupt the client's sense of attachment security (e.g., breakup, loss of a primary relationship) or that are extremely threatening or shocking in nature (e.g., major life transitions, losses, life-threatening or life-altering traumatic events). The stressors may objectively seem predictable and even have been anticipated, yet the client could go into crisis if caught off guard precisely because things seemed to be going well—or because of having been in denial and wishfully believing "it can't happen to me." Or the stressors actually may come "from out of the blue" and figuratively (or literally) blindside the client. It's crucial for therapists to not assume that progress by a client in therapy creates immunity to crises. Indeed, it's often precisely at the point at which progress is occurring that crises also emerge.

Furthermore, crisis may be triggered not by an external stressor (or only in part by this) but instead by the client's reaction to something that the therapist says or does (or fails to do). This may happen right in the moment in a session or as a delayed reaction on the client's part to something the therapist has said, done, or not done in previous sessions or in their communication in between sessions. Specific nonverbal gestures or words that might seem innocuous on the surface can have profound significance for clients who are feeling understandably emotionally vulnerable in the therapeutic relationship and for whom those nonverbal or verbal messages have been hurtful or threatening in other past or present relationships. It's impossible for anyone—even the most skilled, sensitive, and experienced psychotherapist—to anticipate and prevent all of the possible triggering actions (or inaction) that could signal to a client that a criticism, devaluation, betrayal, or abandonment has occurred in the therapeutic relationship. Moreover, a therapist cannot possibly catch and mitigate or prevent every projection that could lead a client to misperceive the therapist's behavior or attitude as hurtful or threatening. Indeed, often it is when the therapist is expressing genuine empathic interest, understanding, support, and validation and nonjudgmental acceptance that a client may have an apparently paradoxical reaction of experiencing rejection, devaluation, or some other type of emotional wound. Some clients are more prone than others to these kinds of defensive reactions to actual or perceived emotional injury by other people, but this can happen to anyone in the emotionally charged context of psychotherapy. Caution is warranted when a client has shown a proclivity to be keenly aware of and distressed by subtle as well as obvious signs of emotional threat or devaluation in their interactions in and outside of therapy. However, such caution should be a basis for heightened self-awareness and empathic attention to the meaning of behaviors that have emotional significance for the client but not for any negative judgments of the client that could lead to countertransference enactments by the therapist.

The importance of tracking countertransference reactions and preventing enactments that undermine the therapeutic relationship is discussed further in Chapter 6. Crises are stressors for the psychotherapist, no matter how well they are prepared and able to handle the crisis. Although the therapist's primary focus is appropriately on the client's experience and well-being, therapists are still only human, and their (our) reactions to clients' experiences, reactions, and symptoms play a major role in their (our) ability to maintain an empathic and nonjudgmental perspective and unconditional and positive regard. The shock, anxiety, frustration, or other reactions that can occur for the psychotherapist when a client is in crisis—with the almost inevitable flare-up of symptoms or shutting down of emotions and engagement, and of conflict/contempt or dependency/desperation in relation to the therapist—is a lot to handle!

The key challenge for therapists, therefore, at the outset of a crisis is to rapidly formulate an understanding of the client's state of dysregulation while they simultaneously maintain or restore their own self-regulation. When therapists focus only on the client, leaving their own personal reactions unattended—or worse yet, suppressed, concealed, or disguised in an attempt to appear professionally "neutral," "accepting," or "unaffected"— the client inevitably becomes aware of the therapist's stress reactions on either (or both) a conscious or subconscious level. An iatrogenic contagion of mutually escalating dysregulation by the client and therapist can result. This communicates to the client that the therapist cannot handle their own stress reactions and, therefore, that the therapist cannot be relied on to help the client cope and resolve the crisis. The unintended iatrogenic effect is to escalate the client's sense of insecurity and distress—compounding rather than alleviating the client's dysregulation and the crisis itself.

However, crises can be averted or at least best managed if we, as therapists, practice what we preach and mindfully pay attention to our internal reactions to the client's early nonverbal or paraverbal signs of crisis. Therapists can "put on their own oxygen mask first" by applying basic self-regulation tactics to themselves when a crisis is imminent or emerging (e.g., silently scanning for their own physical signs of stress, frustration, confusion, distraction, avoidance, inattention). Self-calming does not interrupt or interfere with the therapist's focus on empathic attunement with the client but instead is entirely compatible with (and indeed is a prerequisite for) being fully attentive to the client. From a position of self-awareness, the therapist is in a position to clearly see, understand, and nonjudgmentally accept the client's dysregulation as the client's adaptive attempts to restore homeostasis to achieve the goals that appear to be blocked by stressors. Holding the idea that the client's reactions are purposeful and adaptive in intent (i.e., to restore homeostasis, not simply to vent or give up) can help the therapist to maintain (or regain) an essential calming, respectful, and empathic manner with the client.

STAGE 2: FAILURE TO RESTORE HOMEOSTASIS

According to Caplan (1964), in the second stage of a crisis, the person's attempts to restore homeostasis fail (at least partially—and in severe crises, often totally). This may take the form of fight and flight stress reactions (i.e., flare-ups of rage, terror, guilt, shame, grief, hopelessness, despair, addiction, dissociation; Lanius et al., 2017; Selye, 1951). Or it may occur as a breakdown of body systems and bodily health and integrity with increased susceptibility to cardiopulmonary, metabolic, immune system, or inflammatory problems as well as infections or pain (McEwen, 2017). Behaviorally, the failure to restore homeostasis may involve impulsivity, aggression, avoidance, isolation, physical collapse, or self-harm (even in the moment). Relationally, a failure to maintain or regain homeostasis is expressed as conflict, hostility, contempt, aggression, dependency/compliance, withdrawal, objectification, or vulnerability to victimization. All of these manifestations of crisis by a client can best be understood as a reaction to the inability to recover biopsychosocial homeostasis when active attempts to handle stressors fail to restore the individual's homeostasis.

Over time, chronic unsuccessful attempts to restore bodily and psychosocial homeostasis place a strain on the body, the mind, and relationships that can lead to crises as a result of the breakdown of the individual's core physical and psychological health. This has been described as *allostatic load*, the strain on the body, mind, and relationships that occurs when homeostasis is not regained despite persistent exhausting attempts, usually in response to repeated or chronic traumatic stressors that are inescapable (McEwen, 2017). Allostasis takes a serious toll, severely depleting the individual's internal capacities (i.e., bodily, emotional, and cognitive) and external resources (e.g., social support, primary relationships, access to services). The resultant state of exhaustion is often punctuated by frantic renewed attempts to restore the lost sense of balance, which, by definition, are the beginnings of crises. Allostasis also can prolong and escalate an existing crisis, depriving the individual of the energy and presence of mind to consider or try out alternative approaches to regaining homeostasis and to achieving the original goal(s). If that were not enough, allostasis increases the individual's susceptibility to other crises in the future. When allostasis is chronic, the individual lives a life on overload that compromises the achievement of key life goals and the ability to sustain (or regain) homeostasis (i.e., health and quality of life).

In many cases, allostasis is accompanied by a sense of helplessness, powerlessness, or defeat that leads to what appears to be a state of passivity or a fatalistic attitude of resignation and despair. Or there may what appears to be a complete abdication of personal responsibility, whether this takes the form of extreme agitation, paralysis, collapse, dependency, or aggression (Karatsoreos & McEwen, 2011; McEwen, 2017). This can lead therapists to mistakenly assume that they must take charge and instruct clients who are in crisis on how to take a more active role in coping, calming, or reorienting themselves. To the contrary, the challenge is to empower the client—not to take control away from them.

This challenge is captured in the biblical parable of the choice between feeding a person fish or teaching them how to fish for themselves. The second stage of a crisis is the point at which it is crucial for the therapist to carefully assess how the client is actively, but unsuccessfully, trying to restore homeostasis despite fearing (or believing) that the situation is hopeless. The therapist's goal, therefore, should not simply be to assist the client to cope or become calm but to help them to experience alternative ways of restoring homeostasis. The goal is to enable the client to regain a sense of self-efficacy and to develop alternative approaches to achieving the apparently unattainable goal and to regain a sense of calm confidence (i.e., homeostasis).

STAGE 3: BEHAVIORAL EMERGENCY

Crises emerge full blown in the third stage, when distress persists and escalates, and the person's state of mind and body, and their relationships, become radically out of balance and disorganized (James & Gilliland, 2017). At this point, the person in crisis shifts from a state of urgency to emergency in which there is a paradoxical combination of desperation to find a solution and hopelessness that this is possible. At the point of emergency, the person in crisis shifts into survival mode, resorting to coping tactics that are impulsive, aggressive, avoidant, or a combination of these; disorganized; and ultimately exhausting and ineffective—and therefore more likely to exacerbate rather than resolve the dilemmas posed by the stressor(s).

The issues involved when a crisis reaches the stage of a behavioral emergency are well illustrated by comments from psychotherapy patients who were interviewed after seeking crisis assistance because of suicidality, acute psychosis, anxiety, or depression, or "ill defined complaints" (Skodol et al., 1979, p. 586) at a psychiatric emergency unit. These patients described feeling abandoned by their therapists and desperately alone in the face of danger, confusion, and despair. Although they did not want their therapists to dictate to them what they should do or exactly how to solve their problems, they wanted guidance about how to feel less overwhelmed and wanted support in a manner that communicated an understanding by their therapist of the legitimacy of their feelings, seriousness of the problems, and validity of their goals. They also wanted permission—and ideally, a clear invitation—to express rather than conceal any doubts or concerns they had about the therapist's willingness or ability to understand and support them.

This suggests that, as emergencies develop in the psychotherapy session, it is prudent for therapists to be open to the possibility that they may have overlooked, misinterpreted, or even criticized important feelings or concerns of their client—or may have been perceived by the client as having done so.

Even a flawlessly nonjudgmental, accepting, and empathically attuned therapist will make mistakes, and whether missteps actually occurred "objectively" or not, expressing willingness to learn more or be corrected by the client conveys a message of humility, respect, and confidence in the therapeutic process and in the client. That, in turn, can open the door to communication and understanding while also being extremely reassuring to the client in crisis.

The therapist who acknowledges imperfection and demonstrates a willingness to both learn from and collaboratively work with a client to better understand the client—and to translate that understanding into useful practical assistance to a client in crisis—is a role model for both self-understanding and effective problem-solving. Given Skodol et al.'s (1979) finding that clients in crisis were more likely to have wanted help in achieving self-understanding than their therapists appeared to recognize (or were able to communicate to their client), demonstrating interest in better understanding the client's feelings, thoughts, problems, and goals may be important in restoring ruptures in the therapeutic alliance that can lead to or exacerbate crises. When a client is encouraged to communicate, this sharing can reduce the sense of isolation, abandonment, betrayal, or worthlessness that often is at the core of the stress reactions that may result in or exacerbate crises. Sharing also can help the client experience the therapist as a trusted partner in working together to understand and solve the problems that are fueling an emerging crisis.

As is evident from Skodol et al.'s (1979) results, clients in psychotherapy also may be deeply concerned about their therapist's expertise and character, even though they may express this concern at either end of the spectrum from positive reactions sometimes based on transference (e.g., admiration) to negative (e.g., devaluation). A therapist's authentic admission of not fully understanding the client's feelings, concerns, and goals—in combination with a clear statement of being dedicated to achieving that understanding— is often enough to help the client shift from idealization or hypercriticism to reality-based appraisal. This action on the therapist's part can also reduce a client's distrust of or fear of negative reactions or of alienating, or of being inadequate in the eyes of (and, as a result, potentially being abandoned by) the therapist—the transference reactions that Skodol and colleagues identified as often being unrecognized or misread by the therapists whose clients were in crisis. With an enhanced sense of security and support in the therapeutic relationship, the client who is in, or who is approaching, a crisis is psychologically far better equipped to engage in productive reflection and problem-solving rather than in further escalation.

Another potential common denominator across diverse cases of psychiatric emergencies (Skodol et al., 1979) is behavior on the part of the therapist that reflects countertransference enactments (see Chapter 6). Whether a client accurately perceived or inaccurately misinterpreted, the therapist's intent and evaluation is important to clarify in ongoing psychotherapy, and it may be the case that the client misunderstood or misinterpreted the therapist's actions (or inaction). However, in crises, the therapist should first authentically acknowledge any actions that were potentially hurtful, disrespectful, devaluing, or neglectful, or were criticisms from the client's point of view. This acknowledgment communicates nonjudgmental acceptance and a genuine interest in supporting the client's feelings, hopes, and well-being—as well as the humility and strength necessary to take responsibility for making and correcting mistakes without taking on blame, which is a role model that often has been missing in many clients' lives.

The importance of the therapist's willingness to take responsibility for actions that may be inadvertently hurtful to their client has several implications for handling crises that have risen to the level of behavioral emergencies in the psychotherapy session. Most immediately, therapists should be prepared to do a rapid internal inventory of potential actions on their part that may have conveyed frustration, impatience, criticism, disinterest, disbelief, pessimism, or even more extreme negative reactions (e.g., fear, disgust, contempt, hopelessness) to the client. Recognizing the early warning signs of these stress reactions can enable the therapist to proactively take constructive steps to prevent actions that iatrogenically escalate a crisis (e.g., refocusing on an empathic and respectful understanding of the client's strengths as well as the risks to the client's safety and well-being).

Skodol et al.'s (1979) results provided several examples of therapist's actions that could inadvertently escalate an emergency, from apparently minor disruptions of the therapeutic alliance (e.g., when the therapist interrupts the client, insists on their own point of view, starts sessions late and cuts them short) to major boundary violations (e.g., "nasty comments to patients, revealing personal information about themselves, and touching patients"; p. 591). A key theme was that patients who sought crisis assistance reported perceiving their therapist as "overly controlling, domineering, and intrusive in session," whereas their therapists reported "significant feelings of frustration, anger, and pessimism directed at [these] patient[s]" (p. 591). Thus, although it is important for therapists to focus on helping the client who is in crisis to cope adaptively with external stressors that are causing distress or impeding their achievement of important goals, it appears equally if not more important for the therapist to constructively and empathically address conflicts or gaps in the client–therapist alliance and relationship when a behavioral emergency develops. Whether or not "an unusual degree of instability in the therapeutic relationship that . . . outweigh[s] life's problems in determining [when] crises [occur]" (p. 592), the therapeutic relationship is the foundation for clients' trust and hope. Therefore, reaffirming (and, when necessary, restoring) a client's security and sense of confidence and trust in the therapist is a crucial foundation for safely resolving behavioral emergencies without a major breakdown.

STAGE 4: BREAKDOWN OF HEALTH AND PSYCHOSOCIAL FUNCTIONING

The ultimate stage of a crisis involves a breakdown in the client's psychosocial functioning, physical health, or both. This is the point at which the client or others are in imminent danger when a client's actions (or inaction) are directly or indirectly harmful, threatening, or severely disorganized. When health and psychosocial functioning have broken down, mortal safety can be at risk (e.g., resulting from nonsuicidal self-injury; suicidality—ideation, planning and preparation, and attempts; homicidality or violent acts or intentions toward the therapist or others). Breakdown also may take the form of emotional outbursts, dissociative fugue states, blackouts, flashbacks, paralysis, conversion reactions, disrobing, or other attempts to shock the therapist or to indicate availability or desire for sexual contact. From a psychiatric perspective, breakdown can take the form of fragmentation of the self, episodes of psychosis or mania, relapse into addiction, inconsolable grief, panic, incapacitating anxiety or depression, abrupt terminations, or extreme regression or psychological detachment (including physical collapse and catatonia).

Such explosive or implosive breakdowns are not simply technical challenges and emotionally distressing for the therapist but are shocking, terrifying, confusing emotionally (even if they are completely understandable objectively), and potentially severely demoralizing for the therapist. Breakdowns by a client can evoke in the therapist a wide range of feelings, including anxiety, guilt, shame, anger, grief, and horror, and a sense of inadequacy, defeat, hopelessness, and numbness that parallel the distress and despair experienced by their client.

Crisis theory (Caplan, 1964) and common sense dictate that, if the ultimate stage of crisis is reached, the first priority is for the therapist to take immediate steps to ensure the safety of the client, significant others, and the therapist themself. To prevent imminent suicide, homicide, permanently damaging injury, and abuse and neglect, psychotherapists typically are mandated to make a report to legal authorities and to take practical steps to prevent the client from acting in a manner that could lead to those adverse outcomes. However, there is a great deal of variability in the legal requirements and professional standards for psychotherapists and other health care professionals regarding when and how to intervene to prevent or mitigate the potential harm of danger to self or others (Herendeen et al., 2014; Johnson et al., 2014; Kapoor & Zonana, 2010; Levi & Crowell, 2011; Roth & Meisel, 1977; Steinberg et al., 1997; van der Feltz-Cornelis et al., 2011; Watson & Levine, 1989).

Moreover, such urgent steps to prevent a lethal outcome do not address a crucial source of harm reduction that is of particular importance when a life-threatening breakdown occurs or is imminent in a psychotherapy session: the strengthening or restoration of the therapeutic alliance (Bryan et al., 2019; Plakun, 2019). The key role of the therapeutic alliance in fostering enhanced attachment security and self-regulation by clients has been well demonstrated empirically (Flückiger et al., 2018; Friedlander et al., 2018; Nienhuis et al., 2018; Slade & Holmes, 2019). What's more, when therapists intentionally identify and take action to repair "ruptures" to the therapeutic alliance, there is empirical evidence that clients are more likely to experience symptom improvement and to fully complete psychotherapy of varied approaches and treatment lengths (Eubanks, Muran, & Safran, 2018). The sense of attachment security and the enhanced capacity for emotional and behavioral self-regulation that are fostered by a sustained or repaired therapeutic alliance would seem to be exactly what is needed not only by the client but also by the therapist when a client in crisis experiences a breakdown.

For example, communicating empathic and nonjudgmental understanding of the client's concerns has been found to be associated with a reduction in the severity of distressed clients' suicidality (Perry et al., 2013). Focusing on a shared commitment to mutual respect, trust, and partnering as a team in service of the client's life goals—and acknowledging and taking responsibility both for having caused the client distress because of empathic failures or mistakes and for regaining the client's trust and confidence by making adjustments to prevent any future repetition—can shift the context fundamentally from the client's feeling desperate and threatened or abandoned by the therapist to the client's experiencing a renewed sense of trust, security, hope, and self-esteem. Even small increases in a suicidal client's sense of security and ability to emotionally regulate can alter the client's trajectory from escalating breakdown to renewed efforts to cope and trust the therapist. From the crisis theory perspective, this is a shift from being in the breakdown or behavioral emergency stage to regaining Stage 1 homeostasis (i.e., feeling secure in the therapeutic relationship and being able to emotionally regulate) and thereby resuming the Stage 1 attempt to overcome the barriers to achieving important life goals.

An added complication posed by the breakdown stage of crisis has been described by crisis theorists James and Gilliland (2017) as a "transcrisis state" (p. 12). In a *transcrisis state*, severe impairment becomes a way of life rather than a singular or occasional episodic problem, and people in crisis tend to redefine themselves and the stressors that are causing distress or appearing to make important life goals unattainable, or both, as hopeless and permanently irresolvable. This leads to a chronic sense of failure, defeat, and resignation that, whether loudly voiced or denied, minimized, hidden, or unrecognized by the person in crisis, tends to be accompanied by intense feelings of hostility, shame, and guilt. When a psychotherapy client has recurrent meltdowns or explosive episodes in and outside of psychotherapy, this can be understood as a manifestation of the individual's having become mired in a transcrisis state and a chaotic, unregulated, and unmanageable life. There is additional risk when a client enters this transcrisis state. Both clients and therapists can become paradoxically desensitized and inured to actual or potentially serious crises when the client has daily crises or relatively predictable "crisis of the week or month." Stage 4 breakdown crises can become just as "routine" as the less dangerous and intense earlier stage crises. Therapists as well as clients can become lulled into a fatalistic sense that the client simply has to survive by "coping" with a never-ending and often chronically deteriorating series of breakdowns in their functioning and health. This makes it is important that the therapist not trivialize or normalize repeated behavioral emergencies, especially when they accumulate and can escalate into severe breakdowns.

On the other hand, from a strengths-based perspective, the client who seems mired in a perpetual transcrisis state actually may be highly resilient (Cicchetti, 2010; Masten, 2019; Musicaro et al., 2019; Ungar, 2015). It requires courage and determination to cope with constant or apparently endlessly recurring crises. Typically, people living in a transcrisis state have a limited or negatively biased sense of their own capabilities, having long struggled with a multitude of stressors, chaos, barriers, and unrealized hopes and goals. Often, they have had to cope with ongoing emotional invalidation or abuse; physical, sexual, or interpersonal violence or victimization, or a combination thereof; neglect; and significant losses of, or separations from, or exploitation in formative relationships with caregivers and (if they have not become chronically isolated) intimate partners. Or, they may have been hit with a series of misfortunes and losses over which they had little or no control, which is both exhausting and demoralizing. Frequently, they also have faced stigma, harassment, bullying, poverty and lack of resources, and rejection in their families, neighborhoods, schools, and workplaces, and from society. Many appear to (and feel that they have) given up on themselves and their support systems, and feel forced to accept the role of a victim or a failure as their identity. In the midst of this myriad of difficulties, what too often gets lost—and can go unnoticed or unappreciated by even an experienced therapist—are the intelligence, resourcefulness, creativity, determination, and other talents and abilities that have allowed these individuals to persevere as well as the successes they actually have achieved.

Acknowledging the specific ways in which a client at the point of breakdown has shown resilience (e.g., courage, determination, perseverance, honesty, compassion, loyalty) can be a crucial first step not only in resolving the immediate crisis but in helping that person to make changes that can transform their life from a chronic transcrisis state to a life worth living.

Accessing strengths may seem counterintuitive when working with a desperate or despondent client who is in severe crisis and breaking down. However, this shift is consistent with the definition of a crisis as a reaction to failing to attain important life goals: Regardless of the actual attainability of the goals, it is the self-perception of powerlessness and failure as a person and the sense that others are rejecting, exploiting, or abandoning oneself that drives and escalates crises to the point of a breakdown. Therefore, assistance in (re)gaining a sense of self-confidence and reassurance that others recognize one's worth and abilities (and do not view one as powerless or a failure) can provide a calming and adaptively reorienting effect on a person in severe crisis.

The individual in crisis, especially at or beyond the point of breakdown, by definition does not immediately have the presence of mind or cognitive and emotional bandwidth needed to calmly learn new problem-solving, executive functioning, stress management, emotion regulation, or interpersonal communication/assertiveness skills. This does not mean that they are unintelligent or incompetent—only that under the current conditions of extreme stress, they are unable to access and use those abilities. The psychotherapist can serve as a "surrogate prefrontal cortex" (i.e., the brain site involving the ability to assess, understand, judge, solve, and act effectively) and model these skills for the client on a short-term basis. However, this must be done only on a temporary basis and with the goal of helping the person regain access to and effectively use their own abilities in the longer term. Otherwise, the therapist has become a rescuer and enabler rather than a guide and bridge assisting the client to resume control of their own life. The therapist as permanent rescuer only adds to the stigma and invalidation that the client in crisis often is experiencing, and has the further unintended negative effect of fostering dependency and further diminishing the client's self-confidence and motivation to actively prevent or resolve future crises. Consistent with this cautionary view, Skodol et al.'s (1979) study reported that a key dissatisfaction voiced by patients in the survey who had been in psychiatric crisis was experiencing the psychotherapist as controlling and domineering.

However, if the psychotherapist intervenes by not only validating the difficulty and distressing nature of the stressors that the client is experiencing but also by expressing confidence in the client based on their resilience and capabilities, and offering guidance affirming and helping the client to recognize and access those strengths, this can avoid those pitfalls. As a result, a client in crisis can become able to see themselves as a person who is respected and capable of handling difficult challenges. This approach can counteract the breakdown in the client's psychosocial functioning by promoting hope (Frank, 1968), morale (i.e., self-efficacy and self-esteem; Frank, 1974), and security and trust in the therapist and the therapeutic alliance (Eubanks, Burckell, & Goldfried, 2018; Eubanks, Muran, & Safran, 2018; Slade & Holmes, 2019).

Identifying and showing respect for a client's competence and resilience can seem illogical at a point at which a client seems to be (and feels) helpless, hopeless, and broken. It also can backfire if the therapist is insincere or ambivalent, offering reassurance in a superficial attempt to bolster the client's self-esteem—which amounts to "damning with faint praise." However, when a client's worth, abilities, and achievements are acknowledged with genuine respect, doing so can enable the client to recall specific memories from their own life that were hard-earned successes based on the client's courage, integrity, perseverance, skill, and compassion. Accessing and reappraising those memories as a true measure of the client's personal worth and competence—with the genuine respect and appreciation of the therapist as a relational context—can begin to simultaneously restore the client's capacity for self-regulation and the client's sense of security and trust in a primary relationship. This is only a beginning and must be extended to other parts of the client's life and other primary relationships, but the seeds of restored self-regulation and attachment security can be planted in the depths of a crisis—even (and perhaps most crucially) at the extreme point at which a crisis has become a breakdown.

CONCLUSION

Think back to the crises that you have encountered or learned of in psychotherapy sessions. The acute and potentially dangerous episodes of aggressive, impulsive, dissociative, detached, and avoidant behavior that occur in such crises are vivid examples of Stages 3 and 4 emergencies or breakdowns. The client's loss of control or attempts to coerce and take control away from the therapist in these crises can trigger a reflexive response on the part of the therapist that is more complicated—and potentially problematic—than the evident need to restore safety and a mutually respectful client–therapist dialogue. In extreme crises, a therapist can find themselves feeling a desperate need to take control back from, and to assert control over, a client who seems to be out of control. Control definitely is important, but when a therapist feels driven to unilaterally take control away from a client, this is a recipe for escalating rather than resolving the crisis. The client is likely to react either by going into a state of collapse and dependency (or even emergent or worsened suicidality) or an escalation of aggression and impulsivity to prevent or reduce the vulnerability that occurs when under the control of another person, no matter whether that other person expresses kind intentions (which many clients have experienced as a thinly veiled cover for entrapment and exploitation).

On the other hand, if the therapist has the presence of mind to mentally walk back the acute emergency or breakdown and rapidly think through the earlier stages of the crisis, they can focus on the stressors that have thrown the client out of balance (i.e., loss of homeostasis) and the core goals that the client has been blocked from attaining as a result of those stressors. The client's apparent loss of control, or apparent attempts to coercively monopolize control, in interaction with the therapist then can be reframed and understood as desperate efforts to counteract the effects of the stressors and to achieve the core goals that are getting lost in the turmoil and chaos (or the emptiness and hopelessness) of the crisis. This is a major shift in perspective that cannot be done de novo without some careful proactive preparation. Because most crises, even if they are generally predictable based on a client's past behavior, cannot be precisely anticipated in their timing or exact form. Even if a crisis is foreseen, the immediate impact of the emotional and behavioral explosion or implosion can be sufficiently jarring to throw off even the best prepared and most calm and confident psychotherapist.

Therefore, although it is tempting to try to create a specific formula for handling each of the varied forms that crises can take in a psychotherapy session, the course that we as psychotherapists take in this book is to prepare with an overarching—but still very practical and specific—framework for the psychological unpacking of any crisis that might occur in a psychotherapy session. The starting point for this in-session psychotherapy crisis management framework is the basic insight from classic crisis theory: Every crisis begins with exposure to stressor(s) that block the attainment of core personal goals and result in a loss of psychobiological homeostasis, and the reactive behavior that makes crises problematic and potentially dangerous is an attempt to eliminate or overcome the effects of the stressor(s) and to achieve the core personal goals. This may seem obvious, but the implications are profound. From the perspective of crisis theory, resolving any crisis that occurs in a psychotherapy session requires the therapist to shift from focusing only on the breakdown and the emergency (while always making immediate safety and prevention or treatment of injuries a priority) to understanding the stressor(s) and helping the client to regain hope that they—with the therapist's help—can handle those stressors, achieve core goals, and have homeostasis (i.e., a sense of calm, confidence, and hope) restored.

Why this is so difficult to do, and how it can be done, is the focus of the rest of this book.

2 EMOTIONAL DYSREGULATION AND ADAPTIVE SELF-REGULATION

As we discussed in Chapter 1, emotional dysregulation is the central feature in crises that occur in the psychotherapy session, and it begins to emerge in Stage 1 of a crisis. Explosive, impulsive, and overtly avoidant, withdrawal, and shutdown behaviors are the most obvious manifestations of emotional dysregulation. In addition, emotional dysregulation may take the form of reflexive nonverbal expressions of tension—for example, in the form of tics, repetitive or spastic movements of the extremities, or sweating and hyperventilation or verbalizations—or in the form of behavioral attempts to reduce tension (e.g., self-harm, self-soothing, addiction, compulsive rituals; Brereton & McGlinchey, 2020). Emotional dysregulation also can involve acts or threats of violence or other reactive aggression directed verbally or behaviorally toward others (including the therapist), the self, or objects—including threats or predictions of engaging in acts likely to cause harm to oneself (e.g., reckless, self-endangering, addictive behavior). Such aggression may take the form of blame and accusations or demands for more time or availability from the therapist; or a reduction in fees; or disputation of

https://doi.org/10.1037/0000225-003
Crises in the Psychotherapy Session: Transforming Critical Moments Into Turning Points, by J. D. Ford

the therapist's credentials, expertise, ethics, or compassion; or many other forms. Emotional dysregulation also may be expressed by avoidant behavior, such as suddenly deciding to end therapy or simply getting up and running for the door to get out of the room or building. More subtle forms of escape or avoidance may occur, such as superficial compliance combined with passive detachment or the disavowal of any further need for help (Freud's, 1937/1964, so-called flight into health). Or there may be an apparent indifference or obliviousness to an evident threat or harm to themselves or others.

Whereas the previous chapter presented the stages of crisis, this chapter explores the mechanisms by which people move from one stage to the next. In particular, it explores what happens to the body and mind—especially the stress response—when a client is emotionally dysregulated and attempts to regain homeostasis; these attempts can be adaptive (Stage 1 of a crisis) or maladaptive (leading to Stage 2). Emotional dysregulation, if unchecked, subsequently escalates and leads to behavioral emergencies (Stage 3) and long-term functional deficits (Stage 4 transcrisis states).

While the chapter focuses on how clients may become dysregulated, it also considers what happens when therapists become dysregulated. Therapists are not immune to emotional dysregulation, especially in the midst of a crisis. Professional training and standards (and often parallel influences in formative life experiences and relationships long before embarking on training and a career in psychotherapy) tend to make therapists very good at masking the more obvious manifestations of stress reactions. However, subtler signs (e.g., physical tension or exhaustion; overprotectiveness; nonverbal expressions of worry, impatience, frustration) are difficult, if not impossible, to hide—and clients often are exquisitely tuned into those signs because of needing to navigate complex and difficult relationships much of their lives. In psychotherapy, everything is personal for the client (as it should be), so even when a therapist is experiencing emotional dysregulation that is only obliquely related to the client, it nevertheless is often experienced by clients as a statement about them. The message may then be processed through the filter of the client's own dysregulation, and a chain reaction of mutually escalating stress reactions can culminate in extreme dysregulation and a crisis.

Emotional dysregulation is daunting to deal with when it occurs, but it helps to recall that it is just a variation of the classic freeze-fight–flight stress response. To handle (and prevent) in-session crises by assisting the client in recovering from severe emotional dysregulation, it's important to understand how the stress response can lead to dysregulation.

THE ACUTE STRESS RESPONSE

The *acute stress response* is a reflexive and relatively automatic mobilization of the body's protective resources to achieve a state of alertness. Being alert enables the person to identify problems or opportunities and to act in a timely and effective manner to achieve optimal outcomes. Hans Selye's model of medical and psychosomatic illness, the general adaptation syndrome, describes the stress response as an adaptive adjustment by the body, brain, and mind (Selye, 1951). In contrast to a traditional emphasis on pathology (i.e., deficits, regression, injury), Selye viewed psychological and physical symptoms or illness the result of adaptive biopsychosocial reactions when stressors exceed a person's biological or psychological capacities. Note the close similarity to Caplan's (1964) definition of a crisis as a failure to regain homeostasis. Substantial research has confirmed Selye's (1951) postulated relationship between acute stress and psychopathology (e.g., depression, anxiety disorders; Fang et al., 2020; Hanna et al., 2018; McLaughlin et al., 2015) and medical illnesses (e.g., cardiovascular and respiratory conditions; Cohen et al., 1991, 2002, 2007; Feldman et al., 1999; Marsland et al., 2002; Moran et al., 2019; Thayer et al., 2010). Elevations in the body's defensive inflammatory response associated with acute stress (Marsland et al., 2002, 2017; Szabo et al., in press) and interference with working memory and other executive functions and with emotion regulation (Andreotti et al., 2013; Feldman et al., 1999; Shields, 2017) may mediate the relationship between life stress and both psychological disorders and both acute and chronic medical illness.

The classic depiction of the stress response is the fight-or-flight response. However, stress reactions are more nuanced than that. To protect themselves, people respond to stress in four well-known ways (Bracha, 2004; de Kleine et al., 2018): freeze, fight, flight, and immobility. And an additional stress reaction is based on reaching out to give and receive social support and seek social affiliation (i.e., bonding, nurturance, connection, companionship): tend and befriend (Taylor et al., 2000).

Freeze

Freeze reactions (Bracha, 2004) in response to acute stressors involve a rapid orienting response to scan the environment for stressors and for doorways to solutions or paths to escape. In the freeze response, the body appears to become very still (i.e., the "deer in the headlights" phenomenon) while it simultaneously mobilizes physiologically for action (i.e., heart pounding, muscles tensing, rapid respiration, and release of stress hormones). For example, a client might suddenly become very still and seem almost "frozen" in the midst of describing an extremely frightening experience or in reaction to a statement by the therapist that (whether intended or not) the client experiences as a criticism or a challenge. The combination of vigilance, delayed action, and physiological arousal, all of which occur almost simultaneously and without the client's conscious intention, can prevent the kinds of impulsive or pressured actions that exacerbate and prolong stressors. However, freeze reaction also can delay timely responding to stressors, potentially leaving the person paralyzed, overwhelmed, and vulnerable.

If the opportunity for preparation provided by freezing does not prevent or resolve the challenges posed by a stressor, freeze reactions can become a chronic state rather than a temporary adaptation. Persistent freeze reactions tend to fuel or escalate—rather than prevent—crises. When stuck in a chronic freeze state, emotional dysregulation often occurs: difficulty recovering from states of intense fear, anger, grief, guilt, or shame. Thinking (cognition) becomes confused and dysfunctional; for example, the client is preoccupied with distress; ruminates about problems, or even breaks down into a state of dissociation. With emotions and thinking out of balance, the person in a chronic state of freezing tends to resort to erratic or desperate behaviors (e.g., self-harm or addictions as an attempt to contain physical, emotional, or existential pain) and dysfunctional relationships (e.g., social isolation or detachment; enmeshed conflictual relationships; victimization by unscrupulous or manipulative people). Ultimately, chronic freeze reactions can deform or degrade the individual's core sense of self, leaving them with a toxic and stigmatized view of themselves as damaged, deficient, dependent, ugly, incompetent, or blameworthy.

Fight

Fight reactions are defensive actions designed to counteract stressors by taking control of the situation or people involved. Fight reactions involve a surge in bodily arousal initiated by the brain's innate alarm system (Lanius et al., 2017) and forceful actions directed to overcome, ward off, or gain control over stressors. The classic fight reaction is an attempt to overcome adversaries by aggressively repelling or even attacking them. However, fight reactions do not necessarily involve action against adversaries through the use of violence or aggression. Thus, verbal or behavioral protests, arguments, challenges, resistance, or defiance are forms of the fight reaction that can be nonviolent and nonaggressive ways of pushing back against a threat.

In psychotherapy, the fight response can take the form of threats of or even overt acts of physical violence, although fortunately threats and violence by a client are rare occurrences. Verbal or nonverbal attacks, dismissal, or invalidation in the form of accusations, insults, criticism, sarcasm, or demands are far more common in psychotherapy. Verbal or nonverbal fight reactions may constitute crises in and of themselves, and they also may lead to crises as a result of a chain of stress reactions that begin with nonaggressive challenges or disagreements and escalate into aggression or violence. When a client is experiencing a fight reaction in response to perceiving actions (or inaction) by the therapist as an annoyance or disappointment, or as a more serious emotional injury (e.g., criticism, rejection, abandonment, exploitation), a crisis is likely to ensue if the therapist interprets this reaction as uncalled for and emotionally injurious ("I'm only trying to help, and this is what I get in appreciation!"). The therapist may then freeze (i.e., feel stunned, shaken, and at a loss for what to say or do) and have their own fight reaction (e.g., giving the client a lecture on gratitude, making a critical interpretation of the client's motives or behavior). This can set in motion an unintended mutual escalation of stress responses by both client and therapist.

Fight reactions on the part of a client, however, can be understood as adaptive attempts at self-assertion and self-protection. From that perspective, the question for the therapist is not "Why is this client behaving in a manner that I find troublesome?" but "What goal is this client articulating, or what hurt or harm is this client trying to protect against, and how can I help them achieve that goal or remedy that hurt—including considering how my actions might be failing to support the adaptive aspects of that goal or contributing to that hurt?" Inherent in every fight reaction is an adaptive determination to achieve a goal or solve a problem. Fight reactions can represent taking a stand on behalf of values, principles, truths, rights, or responsibilities that have been negated, violated, or neglected. As such, identifying the principled core of a client's fight reactions often is a key to transforming crises in therapy into positive turning points.

Flight

Flight reactions (Bracha, 2004) are attempts to escape or avoid stressors that cannot be resolved or overcome either by careful assessment and delay in impulsive action (i.e., freezing) or by an aggressive change in the environment or ability to overcome a source of problems (i.e., fighting). For example, it is not uncommon for a highly anxious or extremely angry client to jump out of their chair and walk or even run away in the middle of a session. Or, a subtler form of flight can take the form of defensive avoidance or denial (see Chapter 3, this volume, for examples). Flight reactions involve an escalation of physical arousal (see Chapter 5) similar to fight reactions, but, behaviorally, they differ substantially. Flight involves mobilization to escape, avoid, or move away from or reduce exposure to problems or threats that cannot be overcome or eliminated with direct action. Flight reactions therefore tend to occur after bodily resources and strength have already been depleted by the freeze and fight responses. As such, flight responses often require intense bursts of energy that cannot be sustained for long periods without severely reducing the individual's biological and psychological reserves, and compromising bodily and psychological health (e.g., stress-related medical illnesses or behavioral health problems). Flight reactions also tend to leave the stressor(s) and the agent(s) responsible for the stressor(s) unchanged, resulting in vicious cycles in which attempts to escape or avoid can paradoxically intensify rather than ameliorate distress. For example, avoidance can lead escalating anxiety, depression, and vulnerability, thus increasing the risk of a crisis.

A number of flight reactions are involved in crises in psychotherapy. Attempting to avoid feeling distress, clients often suppress, deny, or minimize deeply troubling feelings, thoughts, or impulses. This is an expectable challenge in any psychotherapy but can lead to a buildup of distress by the client that can lead to an emotional meltdown or explosion. Avoidance also can take the form of self-medication via addictive behaviors, which can result in the client coming into a session acutely intoxicated or feeling an overwhelming sense of shame, powerlessness, or desperation that can lead to a sense of detachment from the therapist and intense emotional and behavioral volatility. Extreme forms of flight, such as dissociation, self–harm, fugue states, or suicidality, represent an intensification of the flight state into an all-out emergency or breakdown. Extreme flight reactions are primarily involuntary, although, importantly, they tend to involve warning signs or behaviors that can be anticipated and intentionally modified.

Flight reactions have a biological (e.g., analgesia, anesthesia) and psychological (e.g., alexithymia, numbing, distraction) basis, providing a temporary sense of relief and reduced vulnerability (often imagined rather than real) that can be highly reinforcing despite the longer term cost of a likely rebound of intensified distress. Flight is adaptive when it provides a genuine respite from hurt or harm, or a pause for reflection and renewal. Flight can provide an opportunity for a creative pause to assess and plan while withdrawing from immediate pressures and withholding impulsive action until a situation is better understood, necessary resources are obtained, and action is likely to achieve positive outcomes. Flight also can recruit protection or resources from others who can provide social, emotional, or material support if the individual is able to ask for and use that support.

The positive features of the flight response offer therapists several portals through which they can join with clients and constructively transform crises driven by avoidance into positive turning points. When a client is withdrawn or detached, or avoids self-disclosure, self-reflection, or even attending psychotherapy sessions, the question is not "What's lacking in the client's motivation or commitment to the therapy?" but, instead, "What hurt, harm, or fear is this client trying to escape or prevent—and what can I do to help them to regain a genuine sense of safety, including by looking carefully at how my actions may be posing or contributing to the sense of threat, hurt, or harm?"

Exhaustion and Immobility

Another way that people may respond to acute stress is an involuntary state of physical and psychological exhaustion that has been described as *tonic immobility* (TI; Volchan et al., 2011), which refers to a persistent (i.e., tonic) paralysis (i.e., immobility) that can take the form of physical collapse or psychological dissociation, or both. TI is experienced by the individual as a combination of extreme physical exhaustion and depletion; of behavioral helplessness, defeat, and capitulation; and of psychological despair and submission.

TI has been observed in research primarily as a final response when stressors are life threatening, including during or after a single incident of intentional interpersonal injury that is inescapable and irreparably harmful (e.g., violent sexual assault, torture, kidnapping; Kalaf et al., 2015). TI is less common than freeze, fight, or flight—except when severe interpersonal trauma results in complex posttraumatic stress disorder (CPTSD): More than 75% of a sample of adults in treatment for CPTSD reported experiencing TI during or soon after past traumatic experiences, and most of those individuals (72% overall) reported experiencing TI currently during episodes of intrusive reexperiencing of trauma memories (de Kleine et al., 2018).

However, TI can occur even when there is no actual immediate threat of death or severe physical injury. To understand how this can be the case, it's important to step back and examine how the body's nervous system is activated when a stress response occurs. We're all familiar with the colloquial expression that stress can trigger an "adrenaline rush." What actually happens when the body responds to a stressor with a flood of adrenaline is that portions of the body's nervous system are activated that run from the lower portions of the brain through the spinal cord and then throughout most of the body. This is called the *autonomic nervous system* because it seems to have a life of its own (i.e., to be autonomous) and reacts on automatic pilot to mobilize the body when a stressor is detected. The autonomic nervous system has two subsystems. The first is the *sympathetic branch,* which is activated in the freeze, fight, and flight stress responses—the body's accelerator, so to speak. The second is the *parasympathetic branch,* which balances this physiological mobilization by regulating breathing, heart rate, vision, smell, speech, and digestion, thus enabling the body to rest and digest. It also can serve as a brake when fight–flight mobilization becomes more extreme than the body can tolerate or sustain.

The autonomic nervous system is regulated by a nerve that extends from the brain to the abdomen: the vagus nerve. The vagus nerve is not a single fiber but instead has a complex infrastructure with three distinct subsystems that Porges (2009) described in his polyvagal theory. A first, and most primitive vagal subsystem activates the parasympathetic branch to enable natural functions that require relaxation, such as digestion and sex. This primitive vagal nerve system however also can trigger the body to slow down its metabolic (energy-producing) functions and, when faced with an extreme threat, to shut down (i.e., TI). A second vagal subsystem activates the sympathetic branch of the autonomic nervous system to trigger a fight–flight response, which gives the body a wider repertoire of stress responses than the extreme response of TI. A third and most nuanced vagal subsystem (found only in mammals) facilitates social engagement as a stress response.

Thus, if an individual perceives a severe threat that seems inescapable and they feel cut off from or unable to count on primary relationships for protection and support (and that those relationships may actually be harmful), this perception can trigger an extreme reaction from the parasympathetic branch that creates a state of immobilization. Porges (2007) demonstrated that a state of immobility occurs when the parasympathetic branch of the autonomic nervous system is hyperactivated by the primitive vagal subsystem in response to an intense and unsustainable activation of the sympathetic branch of the autonomic nervous system. This immobilization can occur whether or not a threat is objectively present and severe enough to be life threatening if the individual's perceptions and emotions lead to an appraisal of the situation as sufficiently threatening to trigger a massive primitive survival response by the parasympathetic brake. Then the parasympathetic branch does not regulate the body's activation but, instead, shuts it down almost completely. Porges (2007) called this a state of feigned death because the individual appears to be completely paralyzed and to have virtually stopped breathing. Thus, the TI response can occur at any point if a person's perception of threat, emotional distress, and isolation from supportive relationships become so extreme that the body compensates by shutting down. Therefore, TI can be understood as the physiological basis of the final crisis stage of breakdown.

TI thus may be a factor in crises in psychotherapy in which clients feel overwhelming distress to the point of severe helplessness and hopelessness. At those times, the client may become involuntarily physically and psychologically immobilized as a result of living extremely distressing or traumatic events in the form of rumination (i.e., repetitive intrusive memories), reenactments (i.e., transference reactions), or complete dissociative immersion (i.e., flashbacks). Evidence suggests that at high levels of emotional intensity, the primary motive of emotion regulation is to diminish awareness by disengaging from the immediate situation (Sheppes et al., 2014). For individuals experiencing persistent or repeated episodes of high-intensity emotional distress (e.g., because of psychiatric disorders), disengagement may be important to tolerate their inner state (Gross et al., 2019). However, when attempts to disengage from distressing emotions fail and distress escalates and becomes increasingly inescapable, a psychological variation of TI may emerge as an extreme form of disengagement: *dissociation*, which is the full or partial loss of awareness of self or the present circumstances. Dissociation can be understood as a maladaptive form of involuntary and automatic emotion regulation in which awareness becomes fragmented and confusing with a complex intermixture of past and present experiences and alternative states of self (Ford, 2009a).

What can a therapist do at that point of utter physiological and psychological breakdown? The answer is complex, but one possibility is that the therapist can help the client to activate the alternative vagal system for social engagement to counterbalance the extreme activation of the primitive feigned death vagal system that is creating TI. This would involve helping the client to recognize that they can rely on the therapist to help in restoring safety and achieving core goals. Although TI may be maladaptive, it may serve an adaptive function as an innate defense (Bracha, 2004; Marx et al., 2008) by enabling the individual to conserve a small bolus of physical and psychological resources in case escape becomes possible—that is, to live to fight (or take flight) another day. From this perspective, clients who are physically or psychologically immobilized need supportive social engagement to shift from primitive survival mode (i.e., TI) to active coping and reengagement in the therapy. To do so, therapists need to be able to communicate an understanding that the client is trapped—not fundamentally by external circumstances (although this may warrant attention) but by a sense of being alone and facing what feels like a threat to their very survival.

Social Support and Affiliation: Tend and Befriend

The *tend and befriend* acute response to experiencing stressors was coined 20 years ago by Taylor et al. (2000) to describe a protective caregiving (tend) and affiliative (befriend) response that is distinctly different from the defensive fight–flight–freeze stress response. The fight–flight–freeze defensive response to stressors involves distancing from or even attacking other individuals who are perceived as threatening or hurtful, or alternately seeking aid and comfort from other people who are perceived as rescuers or sources of caregiving. In contrast, the tend and befriend response to stress involves seeking closeness and togetherness with others for the purpose of giving as well as receiving care and emotional support.

Who is most likely to show a tend and befriend response to acute stressors, and under what conditions, has been the subject of numerous research studies. On the neurohormonal level, in laboratory studies, higher baseline levels or infusions of either oxytocin (Cardoso et al., 2013; Steinbeis et al., 2015) or cortisol (Zhang et al., 2019) have been shown to increase the sense of trust in and desire to get social support from others, and with fewer punitive responses to perceived rejection. Oxytocin is associated with maternal nurturing behaviors, and cortisol is associated with the body's attempt to restore homeostasis when in high states of arousal. However, the actual reactions that were interpreted as indicating a tend and befriend response in those studies may have been based more on seeking protection and comfort (i.e., befriending for the purpose of defensive affiliation or avoiding provocation) than providing care to others (i.e., tending).

Furthermore, in terms of gender role stereotypes, to tend and befriend in the face of stressors is associated with a feminine tendency to be empathic and nurturing versus a masculine proclivity toward competition and dominance—and indeed, a study with infants found that only girls sought comfort from their mothers when their mother appeared to be angry (David & Lyons-Ruth, 2005). However, a study with young adults found that an increase in the tend and befriend response was more evident among men who had relatively strong cortisol reactions and a low level of empathic concern for others but not as evident as might be expected among women or those with higher levels of empathic concern (Zhang et al., 2019). One possible explanation for these findings that appear inconsistent with the benevolent and affiliative nature of the proposed tend and befriend response is that high levels of stress-related anxiety or negative affect may diminish the tendency to adopt a nurturing and affiliative response toward others.

Although research evidence for a tend and befriend response to stressors is inconclusive, the concept provides a basis for the potentially trans-formational possibility that stress reactions may enable people to tap into what Abraham Lincoln (1861) called "the better angels of our nature" (last sentence of inaugural address). In research with violence-exposed toddlers, Lieberman et al. (2005) advanced the related concept of angels in the nursery. In this formulation, early life experiences with supportive and protective caregivers can not only mitigate the adverse consequences of traumatic exposure to violence but also may serve as the basis for the each generation to provide a sense of security to the next generation that can result in the multigenerational transmission of caring in the face of stress (Cooke et al., 2019). That possibility remains to be confirmed, but it provides a model for the transformation of crises in psychotherapy by therapists who respond to clients' crises by providing a clear message based on core values of caring, trustworthiness, and unconditional valuing of the client as a person.

When Stress Reactivity Becomes Emotional Dysregulation: Trapped in Survival Mode

When the freeze, fight, flight, or immobility phases of stress reactivity become a way of life rather than an acute reaction to individual stressors, the individual is trapped in a state of chronic stress reactivity that often cycles repeatedly through all four phases. Each phase of stress reactivity is an attempt to defend against some form of harm (actual or anticipated) as well as an effort to achieve some personal goal(s). Over time, when stress reactivity becomes habitual, the harm reduction aspect becomes dominant and the goal attainment aspect recedes into the background or becomes lost. Thus, when stress reactivity is the norm, the individual is largely focused on the most basic of all goals: survival. *Survival mode* is a state of desperate hypervigilance in which the individual attempts to minimize awareness of emotional distress to be prepared to defend against and survive further harm or injury (Ford, 2020a).

Survival mode is not a sophisticated and well-thought-out strategy; instead, it is a reflexive, automatic, and impulsive reaction to achieve what has been described as *reactive avoidance*, an attempt to tolerate and preserve the capacity to function at least minimally in the face of extreme distress by relying on distress reduction behaviors (DRBs) as a means of coping (Briere, 2019). Survival mode is an instinctual impulse and imperative, not a carefully formulated and planned choice. According to the reactive avoidance model, "DRBs and other forms of problem behavior [notably, dissociation and addictive behaviors] are not freely chosen actions, but rather arise from triggered trauma- or attachment-related emotional states that are potentially overwhelming in the absence of sufficient emotional regulation" (Briere, 2019, p. 48; see also Spinazzola et al., 2018).

The theorized involuntary self-protective nature of survival-oriented reactive avoidance is consistent with Porges's (2007) description of the automatic reactions to extreme stressors that are triggered by the vagal nerve (i.e., the sympathetic branch's fight–flight reaction and the primitive parasympathetic branch's TI reaction). And it also is consistent with the alterations in the connectivity among key centers in the brain that are found with survivors of childhood maltreatment and CPTSD, which have been described as a shift from a learning brain to a survival brain (Ford, 2009b, 2020a). The body "keeps the score" (van der Kolk, 2014, p. 1) and reacts self-protectively in a crisis well before the conscious mind is aware of and able to make a choice about how to respond. The question for psychotherapists, then, is how best to help a client who has experienced an involuntary shift into survival mode—and is unknowingly trapped in a state of fight, flight, or TI—to regain the ability to make choices based on their own best interest rather than continuing (and escalating the crisis) in survival mode.

Survival mode enables a person in an emergency or at the point of breakdown to carry on, but at a terrible price. To reduce awareness of distress and an often overwhelming sense of being trapped and incapacitated by distressing emotions (whether these are consciously recognized or felt as a vague but intense physical or psychological sense of "something is wrong"), people in survival mode become the prisoners and victims of their own attempts to cope. DRBs can temporarily diminish the impact, or even the awareness, of distress, but the distress does not go away and most often builds up rather than recedes. DRBs can provide a transient sense of increased personal control, but that rapidly deteriorates into a sense of frustration, anger, shame, failure, or helplessness that can escalate into suicidality, self-harm, addictive and other risky behaviors, or aggression (Briere, 2019). Emotions that are troubling become chaotic, complex, and severely distressing, or numbed and dissociated. In other words, DRBs tend to devolve into stress reactions that can rapidly escalate into a state of emotional dysregulation. Thus, crises can be understood as emergencies or breakdowns that begin with stress reactions and escalate into survival mode, which involves reliance on DRBs and a resultant state of emotional dysregulation.

When an individual goes into survival mode and relies on DRBs, their (unstated and often unconscious) goal is to regulate emotions that, as a result of extreme stress reactions, have become intolerable. Common statements made to describe being in survival mode express the dilemma (e.g., "I feel out of control," "I'm so angry that I lose it," "I can't stand feeling that way; it's killing me"), as well as the objective of finding a way to regulate the distressing emotions, either explicitly (e.g., "I'll do anything to make those feelings go away," "I have to stuff the anger and pretend it doesn't matter," "I vent so I can get rid of the feelings," "I make the feelings go away by cutting") or implicitly (e.g., "I shut down," "I lash out so someone else is the target and not me," "I distract myself with work," "I get high"). Therefore, a cross-cutting theme in all therapeutic modalities for DRB-related problems is the importance of restoring and enhancing the client's capacities for emotion regulation. This includes both directly supporting and enhancing the client's internal emotion regulation skills (Ford, 2017b) and repairing ruptures to the therapeutic alliance (i.e., the client's experience of the therapist as trustworthy and a source of meaningful support, guidance, and security) to indirectly support the client's emotion regulation (Anderson et al., 2019; Eubanks, Muran, & Safran, 2018; Flückiger et al., 2018).

At times and usually only briefly and less reliably over time, DRBs provide a temporary sense of relief; however, the ultimate result is the opposite of the intent. Instead of regulating the emotions that are causing distress, DRBs have the effect of escalating the intensity of those emotions and amplifying the overriding sense of distress to the point at which the person is unable to cope, and some form of crisis ensues. The crisis is a combination of the threat to the safety of self or others posed by the DRBs (e.g., severe physical injury, illness, death) and the disorganized thinking and behavior that results from the incapacitating state of emotional distress (which may take the form of out-of-control impulsivity, compulsions, dependency, aggression, addictions, hopelessness, mania, grief, guilt, shame, isolation, dissociation, or psychoses).

Despite the complexity and apparent intractability of these downstream effects of going into survival mode and relying on DRBs, they all can be traced back to a single source: difficulty in regulating the emotions driving the distress. This results in emotions that are chaotic, unmanageable, disorganized, confused and confusing, and intolerably intense—which is precisely the definition of emotional dysregulation. In a desperate attempt to avert overwhelming distress by preventing emotions from becoming out of control, going into survival mode and relying on DRBs ironically and paradoxically creates the very problem they are intended to prevent.

Emotional dysregulation often begins with confusion about what one is feeling and what those feelings mean, which can lead to or amplify a sense of diffuse distress: "Something's not right, I don't feel right, and I don't know what it is or why I'm feeling this way"; or "I think I know what's wrong, but I don't know what to do to make it right"; or "I don't know what to do to not feel so terrible (or to stop feeling nothing at all)." When the nature or origins of emotions, or what to do to make intolerable emotional states once again tolerable, are unclear, the resultant state of diffuse distress is a hallmark of dysregulation. In reaction to intense distress, people can find themselves acting without thinking or acting in ways that are inconsistent with their knowledge of how to handle situations effectively and in line with their core beliefs, values, and regard for themselves and their relationships. Impulses and ruminative thoughts can seem to dominate the person's thinking and behavior rather than the person's being able to exert self-control over impulses with clear thinking and rational and responsible choices. Emotional dysregulation thus is characterized by impulsive reactivity and perseverative rumination that contradict and severely undermine the person's sense of self-esteem and self-control as well as threaten the safety and integrity of key relationships and potential accomplishments (e.g., in school, at work).

In this state of distress and reactivity, the dysregulated individual understandably is going to have difficulty in setting and achieving goals—yet another cardinal feature of dysregulation. It is very difficult to develop meaningful goals or to calmly and effectively pursue them when the only goal that seems to matter is to make the intolerable emotional state (or absence of emotion) go away. As a result, the main, or only, goal for a person experiencing dysregulation can become this: Eliminate the emotions that seem intolerable. But this is an unwinnable inner battle because the attempt to suppress, repress, or vanquish emotions has the paradoxical effect of heightening the person's awareness of the very emotions that they view as the enemy. Thus, dysregulation often is associated with hyperawareness of emotions rather than nonawareness, leading to a vicious cycle of attempted rejection of emotion that results in the escalation of that very emotion or, on the other side of the coin, an amplified sense of intolerable emotional emptiness, or both. This often is compounded by intense self-criticism and self-blame both for having the intolerable emotions and for not being able to somehow get rid of or "fix" them.

At the very point at which it is crucial to be able to find a safe and effective exit from the maze created by intolerable emotions, self-defeating impulsivity, demoralizing rumination, and self-blame, the dysregulated person is least likely to be able to remember and act on the conscious choice to use adaptive emotion regulation strategies (Daros & Williams, 2019). Even if they recall adaptive emotion regulation strategies, at moments of extreme distress and reactivity, it is correspondingly difficult to summon up the presence of mind and the physical and psychological energy necessary to shift from powerfully habitual impulsive reactions to mindful ways of thinking and adaptive actions. Precisely when mindfulness and intentionality are most needed, dysregulation's complex web of distress and self-protective (although ultimately self-defeating) reactions are most likely to override any attempts to mobilize those adaptive states of mind.

In a crisis, therefore, the key problem is not simply the negative emotions and sense of distress but the inability to regulate the nature and intensity of the emotions—including the ability to access positive emotions as well as to modulate negative emotions. Whereas emotional states are the "dashboard," it is our ability to drive the "vehicle" (i.e., the body and mind) by regulating the intensity of emotional states that determines our state of body and mind, as well as our behavior and relationships. This raises an apparently obvious but actually quite complex question: What distinguishes adaptive emotion regulation from emotional dysregulation? If psychotherapists are to promote adaptive emotion regulation, they need to know exactly what distinguishes maladaptive from adaptive emotion regulation.

THE VORTEX OF MALADAPTIVE EMOTIONAL DYSREGULATION

Maladaptive emotional dysregulation involves attempts to regulate emotions that are rapid, habitual, or automatic and therefore require less mental effort (but also involve proportionately less mental flexibility and judgment, and less adaptive learning from experience) than emotion regulation that is based on forward thinking and decision making (Redish et al., 2008). For example, research shows that people with bipolar disorders do not "generally have deficits in using adaptive strategies" but tend to use them less often than maladaptive strategies (Dodd et al., 2019, p. 262). In survival mode, emotion regulation strategies that mimic defensive stress reactions—freeze, fight, flight, and withdraw—deploy automatically and autonomically.

Several emotion regulation strategies have consistently been found to result in maladaptive outcomes (e.g., compromised safety, illness, conflict;

Compas et al., 2017; Contreras et al., 2019; Dingemans et al., 2017; Dodd et al., 2019; Dryman & Heimberg, 2018; Golombek et al., 2019; Hallion et al., 2018; Koechlin et al., 2018; Ludwig et al., 2019; Oldershaw et al., 2015; Parmentier et al., 2019; Sauer et al., 2016; Schäfer et al., 2017; Sloan et al., 2017; Villalta et al., 2018; Visted et al., 2018):

- rumination
- worry
- experiential avoidance (i.e., attempting to ignore or be unaware of feelings or perceptions)
- behavioral avoidance
- submissiveness/dependency/compliance
- negative external/social comparisons
- suppression/repression
- self-blame
- externalized blame
- venting
- catastrophizing

Several common denominators can be discerned among these maladaptive strategies. All are based on fear or anxiety, whether of an external threat (e.g., physical harm, social rejection or embarrassment, failure to attain a goal), or internal (e.g., being overwhelmed by or unable to tolerate one's own emotions or thoughts). They represent attempts to protect oneself or others by anticipating some form of harm (and not being caught off guard) and either escaping from or placating (e.g., by submission or by demeaning oneself) the presumed perpetrator of that attack or injury. They also are largely automatic and require little forethought. Essentially, therefore, they represent variations on the classic innate defensive stress reactions.

Perhaps because of their utility as rapid defensive reactions, maladaptive emotion regulation strategies tend to stick with a people who are experiencing chronic states of distress in the form of persistent habits, that is, DRBs (Briere, 2019). Research shows that adults who recover from major depression tend to continue to experience emotional dysregulation (Visted et al., 2018) and that adaptive emotion regulation strategies only weakly mitigate the severity of psychiatric or psychological symptoms (Aldao et al., 2010). One possible explanation for the persistent nature of emotional dysregulation is that it often involves *perseveration*, an inflexible reliance on ways of thinking and behavior that amplify rather than reduce emotional dysregulation (Bailey et al., 2019; Clancy et al., 2016; Davey & Meeten, 2016; Meeten & Davey, 2011; Trick et al., 2016). Although we tend to think of perseveration as a symptom of obsessive-compulsive disorder (Liggett & Sellbom, 2018; Liggett et al., 2017), perseverative dysphoric rumination actually is a central feature of most mood, anxiety, substance use, eating, and sleep disorders (Clancy et al., 2016; Harrison et al., 2012; March-Llanes et al., 2017; Meeten & Davey, 2011; Studer et al., 2019; Trick et al., 2016).

Perseverative rumination is a hallmark of the stress-related physiological reactivity that can lead to emotional dysregulation as well as to health problems (e.g., blood pressure, heart rate, and cortisol levels; lower heart rate variability; Okur Güney et al., 2019) and to unhealthy coping (e.g., smoking, over- or undereating, substance use; Birk et al., 2019; Clancy et al., 2016; Kocsel et al., 2019; Ottaviani et al., 2016). The role of rumination in crises can be seen from research findings showing that it is

> likely to be deployed when individuals feel that they have not reached a satisfactory level of confidence in their judgement and this is similar to the worrier's striving to feel adequately prepared, to have considered every possible negative outcome/detect all potential danger, and to be sure that they will successfully cope with perceived future problems. (Dash et al., 2013, p. 1041)

Rumination involves heightened activation of the amygdala and input from the amygdala to the locus coeruleus (triggering bodily stress reactions) and the prefrontal cortex (interfering with problem-solving and emotion regulation) "in order to feel prepared for future threat" (Meeten et al., 2016, p. 553).

Although rumination is only one of many "maladaptive" emotion regulation strategies, it is closely linked to, and could be a final common pathway for, most other maladaptive strategies. When anxiety leads to persistent worry and catastrophizing, or dysphoria leads to negative views of self (i.e., negative external/social comparisons) and self-blame, rumination can provide an apparent escape from or way of attempting to gain some control over demoralizing thoughts when they evoke emotional distress that becomes intolerable. Rumination involves perseverative attempts to find an explanation ("Why did this happen?") and solution ("What do I need to do differently to make it stop or never happen again?"; Meeten et al., 2016), and can seem to provide a way to survive intolerable distress by shifting attention off away from distressing thoughts and feelings (i.e., experiential avoidance, suppression/repression) while simultaneously delaying action (i.e., behavioral avoidance, passivity, submissiveness).

All of this can lead to emotion regulation in the form of "worry bouts" that are self-perpetuating episodes of escalating distress (Davey & Meeten, 2016; Meeten et al., 2016). *Worry bouts* are characterized by a belief that worry can solve problems but also by the contradictory belief that problems can never really be solved and the best solution is to anticipate and prepare for as many possible threats and negative outcomes as possible (the "what if . . ." and "as many as can" rules of dysphoric perseveration; Davey & Meeten, 2016, p. 233, and Meeten et al., 2016, p. 553, respectively). Thus, rumination leads to and amplifies many other maladaptive emotion regulation strategies (e.g., catastrophizing, self-blame and self-diminishing, avoidance, submissiveness).

Although not every crisis involves obvious rumination, many crises can be understood as self-perpetuating and hyperescalating bouts of rumination. The extreme hopelessness underlying paralyzing depression or suicidality is based on a profound existential worry that life may be an endless purgatory of emotional (or physical) pain, disappointment, and failure. Self-harm tends to be an expression of fear and worry, whether consciously acknowledged or not, that there is no way to contain emotional distress and somehow make that distress tolerable or manageable. Outbursts or meltdowns of anger, although often triggered by some sort of "final straw," tend to be the product of a buildup of frustrations, indignities, injustices, or outright injuries and violations that an individual has attempted to withstand, tolerate, or resolve by perseverating. Thus, rumination can be understood as a form of the fight stress response in which worry is used to combat distress with the unfortunate result of amplifying negative emotions.

Thus, helping a client in crisis draw on adaptive emotion regulation strategies may help but cannot reliably counteract the self-perpetuating perseveration on threat and hopelessness that are hallmarks of crises. To understand why this is the case and what can be done about it, let's first look at the conventional list of adaptive emotion regulation strategies. Let's then take a deeper look at the processes of self-regulation that are more than a simple strategy and are necessary to escape the trap of self-perpetuating rumination and emotional dysregulation.

ADAPTIVE EMOTION REGULATION STRATEGIES

Psychotherapists have an extensive array of emotion regulation strategies to draw on that have been shown to be associated with adaptive functioning. These are the emotion regulation skills that research evidence supports as most likely to be adaptive (Allen & Windsor, 2019; Greenberg & Pascual-Leone, 2006; Gross, 2013; Liu & Thompson, 2017; Radkovsky et al., 2014; Sagui-Henson et al., 2018; Tortella-Feliu et al., 2014; Visted et al., 2018):

- using cognitive reappraisal of the situation (e.g., controllability, outcomes, reality, history)

- using cognitive reappraisal of the self (e.g., worth, efficacy, competence)
- using cognitive reappraisal of relationships (e.g., trustworthiness, valence, expectations)
- using cognitive reappraisal of reactions (e.g., bodily and affective feelings)
- facilitating an experiential acceptance stance
- savoring/appreciating
- applying mindful self-awareness
- seeking and accepting social support
- setting goals
- taking goal-directed action
- inhibiting impulsive actions
- focusing attention on positive emotions
- engaging in problem-solving
- planning
- monitoring outcomes

Two strategies generally have mixed, and neither entirely positive nor negative, effects:

- distraction
- dampening of emotions

One answer to the question of why people fail to use adaptive emotion regulation skills despite having the ability to do so is that it takes presence of mind, effort, patience, and persistence to put adaptive strategies into practice. Maladaptive strategies tend to be more automatic and more readily available when stress reactions occur. In a crisis, it can be incredibly difficult to hold back on the impulse to react automatically, let alone to think sufficiently calmly and clearly to be able to set and pursue goals that are more complex than fight or flight with an attitude of calm acceptance, confidence, optimism, and appreciation or gratitude. Automatic modes of information processing are a central feature of maladaptive emotion regulation strategies (e.g., avoidance, biases, rumination), but despite being maladaptive in the long run, reflexive and essentially mindless reactions tend to be the first-line defense when stress reactions occur (Ellenbogen et al., 2010) because they are more rapid and require less effort than mindful reflection and problem-solving. Automatic information processing also is especially likely to occur when strong emotions are elicited and an individual feels insecure in primary relationships (Donges et al., 2015), which is precisely the situation in many, if not most, crises that occur in psychotherapy sessions.

If simply knowing what to do to effectively manage one's emotions is not sufficient to overcome a habitual pattern of reacting to distress impulsively or avoidantly, then it makes sense that simply being aware of emotions also is not sufficient to prevent or counteract emotional dysregulation. Although it clearly is more difficult to be accurately aware of one's own emotions when using maladaptive strategies in an attempt to put emotions aside and react based on impulse and habit, in most cases, this does not eliminate awareness of emotions but only creates the illusion of feeling no distress or having no feelings at all. Even when people seem for all intents and purposes to actually be feeling nothing (e.g., dissociative depersonalization, fugue, alexithymia), emotions still show up (often powerfully) in indirect fashions through bodily reactions (e.g., pain, stress-related or somatoform illness) and nonverbal behavior (e.g., facial expressions, posture, proximity, relationship and attachment style). Emotions are indelible and can be obscured but not totally banished from awareness. Maladaptive attempts to suppress or avoid emotions, whether conscious or unconscious, thus may elicit physiological or behavioral reactions that paradoxically increase the person's awareness of distressing emotions—but in a manner that the person experiences as being trapped or tortured by aversive emotions, not in the form of emotions that, even if distressing, are experienced as tolerable and manageable.

An important corollary of this line of reasoning is that facilitating emotional awareness may not prevent or promote recovery from emotional dysregulation unless awareness is accompanied by active use of adaptive emotion regulation strategies (e.g., reflection on the meaning of emotions, translation of emotions into adaptive goals and actions designed to reduce the intensity or persistence of negative emotions and enhance positive emotional states).

Similarly, knowledge of and ability to execute adaptive emotion regulation strategies—including reflective self-awareness and acceptance of one's own emotions—are important but not the complete antidote to crises involving emotional dysregulation. Research with adults with major depressive disorder reveals that they "show intact abilities to implement many ER [emotion regulation] strategies when instructed to do so" but become dysregulated as a result of "unskillful selection . . . and habitual use of . . . ER strategies" (Liu & Thompson, 2017, p. 183). In other words, a person who is struggling with depression often can implement adaptive emotion regulation strategies in a neutral and nonthreatening context, but when stressors occur or symptoms flare up, that same person is likely to fall back on more automatic and habitual (and maladaptive) ways of coping out of a sense of urgency, desperation, and confusion. Simply knowing how to regulate emotions adaptively is necessary but not sufficient to prevent and manage crises. Helping the person who is in or on the verge of crisis to think clearly enough to choose adaptive rather than maladaptive emotion regulation strategies thus is key to crisis prevention and resolution.

People in crisis often want to use adaptive emotion regulation strategies but feel too dysregulated to remember how to do so. Or they may attempt to use strategies, such as distraction or active problem-solving or reappraisal, but find that a strategy just "doesn't cut it"—that is, doesn't provide the sense of security, efficacy, or hope they need to feel sufficiently less distressed and less hopeless so that they no longer feel overwhelmed and are able to think clearly enough to come up with viable solutions and take effective action. This dilemma is epitomized by the myth of "the power of positive thinking." That slogan, created by influential Christian minister and self-help guru Norman Vincent Peale (1952), led people to believe that they could think their way out of poverty, violence, and other severe adversities by maintaining a doggedly positive outlook. The problem is, what does one do when all the positive thinking—or other ostensibly adaptive approaches to emotion regulation—leave you still in a state of crisis?

The pioneering developers of cognitive behavior therapy early on realized what research has subsequently confirmed: Although psychotherapy can enhance a client's ability to experience positive emotions (Boumparis et al., 2016), it's not an absence of positive thinking that drives psychiatric and psychosocial problems but an excess of negative thoughts, beliefs, and emotions—that is, emotional dysregulation (Davey & Meeten, 2016; Mason et al., 2019; Mor & Winquist, 2002). Understanding and therapeutically reworking the persistently negative and maladaptive aspects of human experience are the keys to overcoming those debilitating problems in living. Positive thoughts (and emotions) are a crucial benefit of that reworking, but there is limited evidence that positive psychology interventions along those lines result in more than small changes in psychiatric or substance use disorder symptoms, and there is no evidence of fundamental changes in emotional dysregulation or maladaptive emotion regulation (Chakhssi et al., 2018; Krentzman, 2013).

SOMETIMES "MALADAPTIVE" EMOTION REGULATION STRATEGIES *DO* WORK

On the other side of the coin, emotion regulation strategies that are generally maladaptive can, under certain circumstances, actually work (Kobylińska & Kusev, 2019; Sheppes et al., 2014). Although the motive underlying emotion regulation often is hedonic—that is, to feel better—emotion regulation also may serve instrumental goals—that is, to achieve an external outcome by facilitating new learning or change in behavior (Tamir, 2016). For example, rumination could serve an adaptive function by enabling an individual to rehearse and prepare for handling a complex interpersonal scenario or technical task. Suppression of negative valence emotions could reduce the intensity of distress sufficiently to enable an individual to realistically reappraise and revise catastrophic or self-blaming beliefs. Catastrophizing could enable an individual to experience sufficient emotional activation to take seriously and pay attention to aspects of a legitimately dangerous or problematic situation that they previously ignored or avoided. Negative social comparisons could serve as a motivator for engaging in assertive behavior in key relationships. Submissiveness could de-escalate conflict in a relationship and signal a willingness to respect other persons' priorities, decisions, and feelings.

Of course, in each of these cases, the putatively maladaptive emotion regulation strategy could be applied in a way that undermines or defeats the individual's adaptive intention. However, the examples illustrate the crucial point that any emotion regulation strategy could—if selected and used in a manner that fits the context (Lopes et al., 2011; Sheppes & Gross, 2011; Suri et al., 2018)—yield adaptive benefits. This will prove important in dealing with in-session crises because it provides psychotherapists with a way to understand why (and how) a client's use of even the most apparently maladaptive emotion regulation tactics—such as DRBs—not only may be based on an adaptive goal that should be acknowledged and supported but also may serve as the starting point for a shift from survival mode into a constructive approach to resolving the crisis. This is the *utilization principle*: Even maladaptive psychological processes at times can be used therapeutically as a starting point for adaptive change (Erickson, 1959).

DEFINITION AND DEVELOPMENT OF CORE SELF-REGULATION CAPACITIES

The therapeutic treatment and management of clients who are struggling with emotional dysregulation has been addressed from a variety of theoretical and clinical perspectives in several comprehensive sourcebooks for psychotherapists (Beck, 2005; Benjamin, 2003; Briere, 2019; Brodsky, 2011; Geltner, 2013; Linehan, 1993; O'Hanlon, 2003). Although it is possible to extrapolate from the guidance provided in those texts to the handling of in-session crises, this still leaves psychotherapists with the question of what exactly are the best options at the peak moment of crisis when every word counts and immediate action is necessary. At those moments of crisis in the session, therapists need a ready-at-hand framework for safely and effectively helping the client to shift from survival mode and reliance on DRBs that leads to dysregulation to being able to think clearly and take actions to (re)gain a tolerable state of emotion and a sense of being in control. Facilitating adaptive self-regulation can serve as that framework.

Self-regulation involves several adaptive processes that are the foundation for adaptive emotion regulation but that extend beyond emotion regulation per se. Self-regulation requires (a) *attentional flexibility*, the ability to disengage, shift, and reengage with a new focus of attention (Calcott & Berkman, 2014, 2015); (b) *inhibitory control*, the ability to withhold or reduce nonoptimal behavior or cognition (Cassotti et al., 2016); (c) *effortful control*, the ability to intentionally focus attention and engage in goal-directed problem-solving, planning, and behavior (Pallini et al., 2018); (d) *working memory*, the ability to hold new information available while drawing conclusions and making decisions as well as to form long-term memories and retrieve them when needed (Yaple & Arsalidou, 2018); (e) *emotion regulation*, the ability to recognize emotions, modulate their intensity (i.e., arousal level) and valence (i.e., perceived positivity–negativity), and engage actively in attributing meaning to them and (when negative valence) coping or reparative behavior (Webb et al., 2012); and, (f) *mindfulness*, the ability to be aware of internal physiological, emotional, and mental states with nonjudgmental acceptance (Kaunhoven & Dorjee, 2017; Marusak et al., 2018). Self-regulation in childhood provides a foundation for the evolution of additional adaptive capacities over the life span (Loizzo, 2009; Mullen & Hall, 2015). This, facilitates achieving personal and relational goals by enabling the acquisition of resources to support and implement effective sustained action while also preserving personal and relational safety and health by detecting danger (Harkness et al., 2014).

The capacities underlying self-regulation emerge in early childhood from "scaffolded interactions" in which caregivers physically (e.g., by holding or feeding) and behaviorally (e.g., facial and vocal expressiveness) model self-regulation and engage the infant in coregulation (McClelland & Cameron, 2011, p. 31). Self-regulation then develops in three levels, each of which is guided and organized by a distinctive network within the brain.

Self-Regulation Level 1: Arousal Modulation and Attentional Flexibility

Level 1 self-regulation centers on the brain stem, which integrates sensory inputs from the body and environment and regulates bodily arousal states via the body's autonomic and vagal nervous systems, and the corticosteroids produced in the hypothalamic–pituitary–adrenal axis (Geva & Feldman, 2008). Arousal modulation provides the infant with the ability to achieve a first level of self-regulation: attentional flexibility. To be able to shift attention flexibly in response to outer and inner stimuli, the child must be able to maintain a level of physiological and brain arousal that is sufficient to mobilize attention but not so intense that attention becomes interrupted or confused. If arousal modulation is not well established by 4 months of age, the infant tends to be too reactive to internal arousal states to be able to regulate attention (Geva & Feldman, 2008). Children whose parents are emotionally supportive and consistent, and whose families have socio-economic advantages, tend to develop both a strong foundation of arousal modulation and good attentional flexibility by age 4 years (Berthelsen et al., 2017). The toddler develops increasing brain stem integrity and connections between the brain stem and higher level brain systems as well as more complex sensory integration and arousal modulation capacities. This is the foundation for several early forms of other key self-regulation capacities (i.e., inhibitory control, effortful control, working memory, and emotion coregulation with primary caregivers) in the first 3 years postpartum (Geva & Feldman, 2008).

Self-Regulation Level 2: Attentional Flexibility and Emergent Self-Control

The second level of self-regulation centers on the midbrain, which is located just above the brain stem in the center of the brain. In infancy and toddlerhood, midbrain centers associated with vigilance (the basal ganglia) and selective focusing of attention (the superior colliculus in concert with the parietal cortex) become selectively sensitive or insensitive to (and activated or deactivated by) change in environmental circumstances (Coubard, 2015). This extends the child's capacities for attentional flexibility, particularly if caregivers are available, physically and emotionally, to provide a base of safety and security. Caregivers also model and support the balancing of automatic attentional vigilance capacities with the self-directed intentional deployment of attention, enabling the child to be actively immersed in learning (Bosmans et al., 2007). This is the emergence of the learning brain (Ford, 2020a) as the child becomes able to selectively attend to stimuli of interest rather than simply "going with the flow" of external and internal events. Intentional shifting of attention provides the foundation for the development of inhibitory control (i.e., the ability to choose not to think or act) and effortful control (i.e., the ability to choose what to think and how to act). Working memory also begins to emerge in toddlerhood as the midbrain neurons and pathways are increasingly interconnected in integrated centers (e.g., the hippocampus) that can be activated to set and achieve goals (rather than reflexively react to inner and outer stimuli). During this early childhood epoch, the relative influence of the environment (i.e., learning) on children's inhibitory control capacities also increases dramatically compared with that of inborn maturation (i.e., genetics). Learning accounts for 94% of the variability in inhibitory control by age 3 years, half again as much as it did at age 2 (Gagne & Saudino, 2016). So, by age 3, self-regulation is mostly learned and not just inborn.

Between the ages of 2 and 4 years old, children learn to inhibit reactions by self-distraction and self-calming. The importance of this development of learned inhibitory control capacities is illustrated by findings in a study of children from economically disadvantaged backgrounds in which toddlers who developed self-distraction capacities were able to handle frustration without problematic anger by age 4 years old and had low levels of externalizing behavior problems at age 5 years old (Bendezú et al., 2018). Moreover, the children whose parents modeled ways to use language in their interactions with the child were best able to achieve inhibitory control and positive behavioral outcomes (Bendezú et al., 2018). By school age, children can use inhibitory control to tolerate frustration and disappointment with peers and with adults who request compliance and set limits (Blair & Raver, 2015). Inhibitory control also is a foundation for creativity across the life span (Cassotti et al., 2016).

Infants and toddlers also develop a repertoire of primitive emotion regulation skills, initially through coregulation with primary caregivers in Years 2 and 3 postpartum, and with increasing autonomy thereafter. By age 3 years, toddlers are able to engage in a number of tactics to delay reflexive reactions when frustrated or disappointed, including engaging in self-soothing, seeking soothing from caregiver(s), calmly seeking information, or engaging in distraction by either shifting attention elsewhere temporarily or becoming immersed in an alternative activity (Cole et al., 2017). By age 5 years, children develop emotion regulation skills involving assertive engagement in problem-solving when confronted with frustration or disappointment. By the early elementary school years, this cognitive approach to emotion regulation enhances the child's active engagement in learning (Berthelsen et al., 2017) and social competence (Penela et al., 2015). This is especially important for children who are temperamentally shy, inhibited, and dysphoric as toddlers (Penela et al., 2015) or those who have a propensity for impulsivity and dysphoria (Cole et al., 2017). As a result,

> by school age children are usually able to tolerate the difficulties of learning new material, to delay and inhibit selfish responses in order to get along with others, to comply with adult directions and prohibitions even if they conflict with their goals, and to control impulsive action even if frustrated or disappointed. (Cole et al., 2017, p. 685)

Self-regulation capacities for intentional attention shifting, inhibitory control, working memory, and effortful control thus enable school-age children to recover from emotional dysregulation as well as to develop greater self-control.

However, if caregiver protection, modeling, and coregulation are not consistently available in early childhood and the child is exposed to traumatic stressors (Copeland et al., 2007), the child's attention will become selectively focused on threat rather than on creative opportunities and interests (i.e., the survival brain). As a result, the development of other self-regulation capacities, such as inhibitory and effortful control, working memory, and emotion regulation, becomes organized around the avoidance of harm rather than on achievement, enjoyment, relatedness, and identity formation. A fundamental attentional bias toward threat developed in early life can make the survival brain dominant rather than coequal with the learning brain, placing the child on a trajectory (Briggs-Gowan et al., 2012) that can lead to lifelong problems with traumatic stress reactions (Fani et al., 2012; Felmingham et al., 2011; Iacoviello et al., 2014).

Self-Regulation Level 3: Attentional Control, Effortful Control, and Emotion Regulation

The third level of self-regulation is guided by brain networks that have their primary centers in the outer layers of the brain: the cortex. Although the brain's cortex is growing both in size and interconnections throughout early and middle childhood, a key transitional period occurs late in preadolescence and in early adolescence, when neuronal growth decelerates and the number of neurons in the brain's cortex declines (i.e., reduced volume and thickness) compared with earlier in life (Foulkes & Blakemore, 2018). The adolescent brain continues to develop connective paths linking brain centers (i.e., white matter), but within the cortical and hippocampal areas associated with effortful control and emotion regulation, hormonal changes related to puberty (Sisk, 2017) result in neurons and their interconnections being pruned, sculpted, and sealed over (myelinated; Tamnes et al., 2018;

Wierenga et al., 2014). Inhibitory control and working memory, which were intertwined before age 10, can be used by adolescents separately when and as needed (Shing et al., 2010). Thus, the youth can restrain impulsive reactions even when working memory (i.e., the ability to hold and use past learning along with new information) is not available and can draw on working memory as a guide to thoughtful action when having difficulty in inhibiting reactive impulses.

As brain networks involving the cortex develop, children and teens increasingly are able to intentionally pay attention to and use abstract concepts (e.g., self-relevant memories, mental imagery) as well as concrete sensory phenomena (e.g., environmental stimuli, bodily sensations) and thus to reflect on and remember the personal relevance and meaning of life experiences (Lückmann et al., 2014). The ability to learn from experience by recalling not only the events but also one's own personal commitments and goals enables the youth to use memory to plan for the future (i.e., prospective memory; Cona et al., 2015) and exert self-control rather than react without a plan and depend solely on the control of external rules and influences. As a result, working memory becomes more abstract, episodic memory becomes a more coherent self-focused narrative, and thinking and emotion processing/regulation become based on a more integrated understanding of self in relation to the external world (Harding et al., 2015). These capacities support preadolescents' mindfulness—nonjudgmental awareness and acceptance of one's own and other persons' thoughts, emotions, and ways of thinking and feeling (Kaunhoven & Dorjee, 2017; Marchand, 2014; Marusak et al., 2018).

In adolescence, several brain centers are still growing and maturing rather than slimming down and becoming highly efficient, including areas associated with attention (i.e., basal ganglia) and stress reactivity (i.e., amygdala), which continue to increase in volume and thickness through adolescence into early adulthood (Foulkes & Blakemore, 2018; Wierenga et al., 2014). Compared with adults, adolescents tend to be more driven by immediate rewards, the influence of peers, and fears of social exclusion, and thus are correspondingly less able to recognize and use other people's informational and emotional input when making decisions (Morris et al., 2018; Mueller et al., 2017). Youth have higher levels of brain activation than adults in response to actual or anticipated rewards in subcortical areas (e.g., striatum, insula) associated with impulsivity and emotionally driven behavior but lower levels of activation in areas involved in executive functions and emotion regulation (i.e., frontal and parietal cortices; Casey et al., 2008; Silverman et al., 2015). In response to situations eliciting disappointment or regret, teens also show less activation than young adults in brain areas associated with felt emotion (i.e., insula), appraisal of one's own and others' emotions and intentions, and inhibition (Hansen et al., 2018) of risky (e.g., sexual; Rodrigo et al., 2018) behavior. Youth, in comparison with adults, also show more impulsive (i.e., amygdala) yet affectively blunted (i.e., striatum) responses to negative emotional experiences in social contexts as well as increased connectivity between the striatum and prefrontal cortex (which may represent an attempt to inhibit impulsivity and increase relational connection; Fareri et al., 2015).

Thus, although adolescents' effortful control and emotion regulation capacities are growing stronger, more flexible, and more differentiated (i.e., more available to be deployed separately to handle complex relational, learning, and performance challenges), they continue to be challenged when attempting to deploy emotion regulation and mindfulness. Overall, childhood and adolescence are periods of notable immaturity and maturation by the brain and body, which provide a foundation for experience-dependent learning that leads to major increases in the complexity and effectiveness of the youth's self-regulation abilities. The child's learning brain develops progressively more sophisticated and interconnected centers and systems to support several emerging capacities for self-regulation: flexibly shifting and focusing attention (i.e., attentional control), inhibiting impulsive reactions (i.e., inhibitory control), planning and carrying out goal-directed actions (i.e., effortful control), integrating new information with prior learning (i.e., working memory), and maintaining emotional balance (i.e., emotion regulation). These capacities of the learning brain enable the adolescent to enter adulthood with a strong base of knowledge, psychological and physical health and resilience, a coherent and realistic sense of self and identity, and interpersonal connectedness and support.

CONCLUSION

When the adaptive attempts to regulate emotions become co-opted by the survival imperative, three fundamental changes occur that are the core of crises. First, social engagement (the sophisticated vagal system) is replaced by freeze, fight, flight, or TI (the primitive defensive vagal systems). When a person is focused exclusively on detecting and defending against threats, relationships are at best a distraction that decreases the ability to maintain vigilance or creates a burden that increases the vulnerability to harm. At worst, people are not experienced as sources of security (i.e., caring, safety, protection, friendship, companionship, and partnership) but instead are distrusted, feared or retaliated against. Survival mode thus involves a sense of isolation that can escalate stress reactions into a state of crisis. Common statements from patients reflecting this change include the following:

- "When bad things happen, I can't trust anyone to be there for me and cover my back."

- "People just get in the way, or make things worse, when there's an emergency."

- "When I feel violated, everyone looks like an abuser, even the people I love the most."

- "I just shut down. I'm in a zone where I'm all alone, and I just have to get through it."

- "I can't let myself be vulnerable because when I let down my guard, I get hurt."

- "It's like laser vision: I can only see what I have to do until the problem's solved."

- "When I'm trying to run through a minefield, I can't be concerned about anyone else, and I'm better off just being all alone; otherwise, I will take a false step and it's all over."

- "I forget about everything else, even my own safety, when I have to do whatever it takes to protect someone who can't protect themselves."

- "Don't get in my way when I'm fighting for my life. I'll just run right over you even if you're my best friend because I can't let anyone or anything stop me or slow me down."

The second fundamental change when survival mode becomes ascendant is emotional dysregulation: maladaptive variants of the fight–flight stress response in the form of attempts to combat (e.g., rumination, aggression) or avoid (e.g., detachment, impulsivity) affective distress. Common statements from patients reflecting this change include these:

- "I'm so upset that I can't think straight."
- "It's like my mind is either a whirlwind or totally blank."
- "My head feels like it's exploding, and my heart just aches."
- "Even the simplest decision is too much, so I just give up."
- "I'm too scared to do anything. I just freeze."
- "I'm so mad that I can't think of anything except getting revenge."

The third fundamental change that occurs in extreme survival mode is an extreme state of mobilization (fight–flight) or immobilization (TI) that may take the form of hopelessness and suicidality, extreme dependency, psychological or somatic dissociation, or withdrawal. Common statements from patients reflecting this change include the following:

- "Somebody has to tell me what to do. I am totally confused and helpless."
- "I can't control myself. I just lose it and go on automatic pilot."
- "I give up on myself and don't care what happens to me anymore."
- "I'm at the end of my rope and can't go on."
- "I want to die. It's the only escape from this endless suffering."
- "I go way deep into myself—so far that I'm not sure even I can find me."
- "I am done with hoping and done with getting help from anyone else."
- "I just want to stop trying. Nothing ever gets better or makes any difference."

How, then, can a psychotherapist reach a client in crisis who is trapped in survival mode? The key goals, based on this analysis of the three features of survival mode, seem to be (a) reinstating social engagement (e.g., with empathic understanding, collaborative partnership, affirmation of the client's core values, goals, resilience), (b) modeling and supporting the client's emotion regulation (i.e., coregulation), and (c) restoring the client's sense of personal control and self-efficacy. In short, this means helping the client to access, restore, and strengthen their core capacities for self-regulation. In the next chapter we examine how the field of crisis intervention has developed a portfolio of tactics for achieving these key goals.

3 ESSENTIAL ELEMENTS OF CRISIS INTERVENTION

Strategies for crisis intervention have evolved for more than 75 years (Schwartz, 1971) and were first formally tested more than 50 years ago (Auerbach & Kilmann, 1977). Despite the voluminous clinical literature that has evolved in the crisis intervention field, the question of how to understand and handle crises that occur in the psychotherapy sessions has received scant attention compared with information available for handling crises in crisis clinics, in emergency departments, or on crisis hotlines. Although general guidance is available for crisis intervention workers on how to respond to psychotherapy patients who are experiencing a crisis outside of their psychotherapy sessions (Skodol et al., 1979), by comparison, limited guidance is available for psychotherapists on how to handle crises that occur in a therapy session per se.

In this chapter, we examine the core principles and best practices of major models of crisis intervention as a framework for handling crises in the psychotherapy session. Intervention models developed for crisis intervention specialists who assist people in crises in their day-to-day lives require careful adaptation to the unique context of a crises that occurs within a

https://doi.org/10.1037/0000225-004
Crises in the Psychotherapy Session: Transforming Critical Moments Into Turning Points,
by J. D. Ford

psychotherapy session. However, the field of crisis intervention studies provides many useful lessons learned and best practice guidelines that psychotherapists can draw on when preparing for, and actually handling, crises that occur in the psychotherapy session (Robbins, 1978).

This chapter reviews crisis intervention models that are not specifically geared toward the psychotherapy context, and the next chapter considers how to adapt principles from these general models into the specific psychotherapy context. As you'll see, crisis intervention models typically target safety and stabilization first, followed by the provision of assistance in practical problem solving and access to resources. Although this approach makes sense, based on what we know about the stages of crisis development, there is a crucial intermediate step linking the initial protection phase and the problem resolution phase of crisis intervention that tends to be overlooked or taken for granted: restoring adaptive emotion regulation. As discussed in Chapter 2, a hallmark of crises is the experiencing of extreme emotional dysregulation. In crises, people attempt to restore homeostasis by trying to regain emotion regulation, but as crises worsen, they do so in increasingly maladaptive ways (e.g., avoidance, denial, worry and rumination, hypervigilance, aggression toward self or others). The classic crisis intervention techniques described in this chapter emphasize safety and stabilization and problem solving and resourcing techniques but only indirectly address emotion regulation.

As we review the classic approaches to crisis intervention, keep in mind that alongside those techniques, it is important to also systematically use strategies for facilitating adaptive emotion regulation when crisis occur in the psychotherapy session. In Chapter 4, the focus is on how a psychotherapeutic approach to emotion regulation provides additional tools and options that are consistent with, but extend beyond, the classic models of crisis intervention. First, however, let's examine the empirical evidence that supports the efficacy of crisis intervention followed by a review of several classic models of crisis intervention techniques.

EVIDENCE BASE FOR CRISIS INTERVENTION

Crisis intervention has a long history in the human/social services fields (James & Gilliland, 2017). The focus of most publications, practice guides, and research on crisis intervention has been on the response to community, school, and hospital emergencies and disasters by crisis intervention teams or by individual frontline staff and volunteers as well as professionals in the public safety (e.g., law enforcement), military (e.g., combat- or deployment-related traumas), health care (e.g., emergency medicine and nursing), disaster services (e.g., International Red Cross and Red Crescent Movement), rape and domestic violence crisis services, and broader human/social services fields (Caplan, 1989; Compton et al., 2008; Cross et al., 2014; Flannery & Everly, 2000; Kohrt et al., 2015; Lating & Bono, 2008; Simpson, 2019).

Despite the long history, outcome research on crisis intervention is quite sparse; no peer-reviewed systematic reviews or meta-analyses of research on crisis intervention efficacy or effectiveness with adults or children have been published since the first definitive review 40 years ago (Auerbach & Kilmann, 1977). A review identified only 12 studies of crisis intervention outcomes in hospital emergency departments, none of which was a randomized clinical trial. Altogether, these studies yielded insufficient data for a meta-analysis of intervention efficacy (M. P. Hamm et al., 2010). Similarly, a review of published research on crisis intervention team programs conducted by law enforcement personnel identified no studies that reported a formal empirical assessment of recipient outcomes (Compton et al., 2008).

Crisis intervention usually is conducted by workers (often volunteers) on telephone hotlines (Flannery & Everly, 2000; T. Hunt et al., 2018; Mishara et al., 2007; Stein & Lambert, 1984). Here, too, the most recent review of outcome research on telephone hotline crisis services was published 35 years ago (Stein & Lambert, 1984); its authors found very limited evidence of efficacy with the possible exception of reduced suicide rates among White girls and women. An ambitious and more recent study of more than 1,000 suicidal callers to hotlines in the United States (Gould et al., 2007) and more than 1,600 nonsuicidal callers (Kalafat et al., 2007) was able to follow up on fewer than 50% of the callers 1 year later. Among those surveyed at follow-up, hopelessness and psychological pain were reported to decrease in the weeks following the crisis call, and the caller's intent to die (or lack thereof) at the end of the call was the strongest predictor of subsequent suicidality. However, whether the crises were actually resolved safely, whether the call specifically (as opposed to other events or services) was responsible for positive outcomes, and what tactics or strategies were associated with reductions in the caller's intent to die or with improvement in the caller's safety and well-being were not determined. Thus, telephonic crisis intervention remains largely a black box that is widely used and potentially of great benefit but has largely anecdotal and improvised protocols.

More formalized crisis intervention models have been developed for people at high risk for suicide or self-harm because of serious mental illness (Murphy et al., 2015; Noyce, 2016; Ruchlewska et al., 2016) and personality disorders (Berrino et al., 2011; Koweszko et al., 2017). Nevertheless, a systematic review of randomized clinical trial studies comparing crisis intervention with standard care for adults hospitalized for crises related to chronic severe mental illness identified only eight small studies (Murphy et al., 2015). One study's promising results indicated that crisis intervention was associated with fewer repeat hospital crisis admissions in the following 6 months. However, other studies showed no evidence that crisis intervention yielded benefits on measures of family burden or the patient's mental state, overall functioning, and quality of life at follow-up assessment 3 to 6 months following hospitalization. The specific crisis intervention practices that were associated with a positive immediate or longer term response by people with serious mental illness also have not been formally described or tested.

In addition, postcrisis debriefing procedures also have been developed to assist crisis workers in mitigating the often intense emotional impact of caring for people in crisis (e.g., critical incident stress management [CISM]; Everly & Mitchell, 2000). A review identified eight outcome studies with a large overall positive effect on measures of crisis workers' perceived distress and resilience after receiving CISM—although there were no randomized clinical trial comparisons of CISM with control conditions or interventions (Everly et al., 2002). Despite these promising findings and a well-articulated protocol for delivering CISM (Everly & Mitchell, 2000), the benefits (and risks) of postcrisis debriefing and stress management for crisis responders remain uncertain, and specific practices for delivering the CISM protocol safely and effectively have not been standardized (e.g., how much and what types of self-disclosure should be encouraged and modeled by the peer and professional coleaders in debriefing sessions).

Workers with many different professional and nonprofessional backgrounds in a wide variety of settings have widely disseminated and used crisis intervention techniques with people who are experiencing numerous different types of crises. Although crisis intervention generally is associated with positive outcomes, whether these outcomes are the direct result of the crisis intervention protocol per se—and what components or practices in different crisis intervention protocols are specifically associated with positive outcomes—has not been empirically tested. Potential adverse effects of different crisis intervention practices and tactics for recipients who are experiencing different types of crises and differing life circumstances, and when delivered by interventionists with different types and levels of expertise and experience, have not been documented. Thus, with these limitations and the sparse empirical support for crisis intervention protocols that vary widely in approach, the core principles and best practices for crisis intervention that have been identified to date (James & Gilliland, 2017) should be adopted cautiously and with careful consideration of their risks and benefits in actual practice.

Nevertheless, taken cautiously and with healthy skepticism based on the limited actual evidence of effectiveness of any specific crisis intervention practice, the most widely disseminated crisis intervention principles and practices may provide useful preliminary guidance for therapists on how to approach crises in the psychotherapy session. With this understanding, we turn next to an overview of the core principles and best practices that have been formulated for crisis intervention over the past several decades.

ORIGINS OF CRISIS INTERVENTION MODELS

In the mental health field, the origins of a systematic approach to crisis intervention can be traced back to the pioneering work of two psychiatrists in the 1940s: Gerald Caplan and Eric Lindemann. Lindemann was a member of a team of mental health professionals at Massachusetts General Hospital that provided treatment to community members who were survivors or had lost loved ones in a deadly fire in a crowded private dining club, the Coconut Grove. Almost 500 people died in that horrific disaster. Based on 101 cases of acutely bereaved adults from that disaster and relatives of deceased military personnel, Lindemann (1944) identified a consistent pattern of "acute grief reactions" (p. 141). Two key features of acute grief reactions were waves of physical and emotional distress, tension, or pain as well as an overwhelming sense of physical exhaustion (Lindemann, 1944). Lindemann identified several tasks that appeared to be necessary for recovery from acute bereavement. Facilitating the completion of these recovery tasks thus essentially represents the first set of crisis intervention best practices. The tasks focus on helping the person in crisis to recognize and contain their emotional pain while sustaining their sense of relational connection to their lost loved one(s) and engaging social support:

- understand and accept the emotional pain
- review the relationship with the lost loved one
- recognize changes in emotions and their discharge or release
- express sorrow and a sense of loss in words and nonverbally
- develop a way of internally continuing the relationship with the lost loved one
- verbalize feelings of guilt
- identify people who can serve as role models and sources of support

Gerald Caplan collaborated with Lindemann and over the next 2 decades developed a community-based mental health program for crisis recovery. Caplan (1964) expanded the focus of crisis intervention from Lindemann's (1944) emphasis on facilitating adaptive grieving and coping with loss to managing a variety of forms of distress when confronted with crisis situations or problems. Caplan (1964, p. 18) identified seven characteristics of effective postcrisis coping:

- actively searching for information about the facts of what happened
- expressing both positive and negative feelings, and tolerating frustration
- actively invoking help from others
- breaking problems into manageable parts and working through them one at a time
- pacing coping efforts to manage fatigue and maintain control of as many areas of functioning as possible
- mastering feelings by being flexible and willing to change
- trusting self and others, and staying optimistic about the outcome

Caplan (1964) emphasized the importance of agency that is the individual's active assertion of self-determination, confidence, and mastery of the factual, emotional, and interpersonal dilemmas involved in the stressor and acquisition of both internal and external coping resources.

On the basis of these two sets of tasks for coping with a crisis, Caplan (1964) distilled the process of providing crisis intervention assistance into three essential phases (Kanel, 2018):

1. Develop a collaborative helping alliance with the individual in crisis with open-ended questions and reflective paraphrasing, and validating of core emotions and goals.

2. Explore and clarify the individual's perceptions of the crisis situation, event(s), or problem(s) and related beliefs, emotions, and effects on daily living and relationships.

3. Develop and support active ways of coping with distress that enable the individual to develop and put into action effective approaches to resolving the problem(s).

This three-phase approach to crisis intervention continues to be the gold standard. It concisely describes the essential tasks that enable helpers to guide people (and also larger systems, such as families, organizations, communities, and societies) to navigate crises safely and successfully. Several additional frameworks for crisis intervention have elaborated on Caplan's and Lindemann's early insights, and identify nuances that provide crisis interventionists with more specific subtasks and practical tools—but always within this core three-phase framework.

PSYCHOLOGICAL FIRST AID

Psychological first aid was introduced a decade after Lindemann's (1944) seminal article as a framework for health care providers in their attempts to assist members of communities impacted in the wake of mass disaster (Drayer et al., 1954). Psychological first aid involves several competencies and requires systematic training (Everly & Flynn, 2006; Parker et al., 2006). Based on the available earlier writings and best practices, The National Child Traumatic Stress Network and National Center for PTSD created a *Psychological First Aid: Field Operations Guide* (Brymer et al., 2006), which identifies a sequential set of eight core actions for postdisaster crisis intervention:

1. Contact/engagement: Develop an initial personal rapport.
2. Safety/comfort: Prevent or mitigate the impact of current risks/danger.
3. Stabilization: Calm extreme emotions.
4. Information gathering: Determine current context, goals, and needs.
5. Practical assistance: Provide advice and assist in problem solving.
6. Connection to social supports: Facilitate engagement in important relationships.
7. Information on stress reactions and coping: Provide psychoeducation about stress and coping.
8. Linkage to collaborative services: Make warm handoffs to other providers/ services.

INTEGRATIVE MODELS OF CRISIS INTERVENTION

Subsequently, crisis intervention process models have been proposed to elaborate on some of the key elements or phases identified in the pioneering formulations.

SAFER-R

The SAFER-R model was formulated based on the CISM approach to postcrisis debriefing to provide a structured sequence for intervening during as well as in the aftermath of crises (Flannery & Everly, 2000). This model expands the three-phase model by identifying five phases of crisis resolution:

1. **S**tabilization: Establish rapport, meet basic needs, and mitigate acute stressors.

2. **A**cknowledgment: Recognize what happened (the event) and the expectable reactions.

3. **F**acilitation: Promote understanding and normalize reactions to prevent self-blame or attributions of personal weakness.

4. **E**ncouragement: Encourage effective coping, including time management, nutrition, relaxation skills, physical exercise, catharsis, and external coping resources and supports.

5. **R**ecovery or **R**eferral: Assist with access to continuing care.

Assessment, Crisis Intervention, and Trauma Treatment

The assessment, crisis intervention, and trauma treatment (ACT) model further extends the phases of crises intervention by identifying seven stages, each of which corresponds to a crucial intervention by the helper (Roberts, 2002):

1. Conduct a biopsychosocial assessment, prioritizing lethality, resilience, and protective factors.
2. Establish rapport.
3. Identify problems, including crisis precipitants, strengths and resources, and coping skills.
4. Explore emotions (e.g., active listening, validation).
5. Explore alternatives (e.g., untapped resources, coping skills, solution-focused options).
6. Develop an action plan.
7. Follow up.

Within the ACT framework, Roberts (2002, p. 17) also proposed a 10-step sequence of acute stress management. This 10-step sequence essentially unpacks and expands on the first four stages of the ACT crisis intervention model, providing a foundation for the solution-focused stages of ACT (i.e., Stages 5–7). The first five steps are subtasks of Stage 1, conducting a biopsychosocial assessment. The most immediate priority (Step 1) is assessing for immediate danger to ensure the safety of the person in crisis and of any other person who may be directly or indirectly involved in the crisis. The next immediate priorities (Stages 2–4) are to assess and provide emergency care for injuries or medical needs. A third, and novel, immediate priority is to observe and identify "signs of traumatic stress" (e.g., flashbacks, stress reactions to reminders of traumatic aspects of the stressor experience or experiences, avoidance of reminders, hypervigilance). Thus, the first five steps in this extended ACT framework are essentially doing an immediate triage assessment for medical or psychological injuries that require rapid treatment.

The remaining five stages in the 10-stage ACT framework are the classic stages articulated by all crisis intervention models: Develop a relationship, help the person to tell their "story," provide support with active empathic listening, provide validation and education, and engage in proactive problem solving to develop a plan for the immediate situation and the future.

Hybrid Crisis Intervention Model

Ultimately, James and Gilliland (2017) proposed an integrative hybrid model of crisis intervention. Drawing on all other crisis intervention models, this hybrid describes seven sequential tasks that begin with making contact and extend past the current moment and crisis to provide the individual in crisis with ongoing support over time.

Task 1: Predisposition/Engage/Initiate Contact

From the first moment of contact, the interventionist builds an alliance by (a) establishing a psychological connection with an emphasis on support for problem solving and by communicating a clear intention to help the client maintain or regain control of the situation; and (b) clarifying the intervener's intentions—to listen, understand the client's concerns accurately from the client's perspective, and ensure the client's safety and to keep them safe from further harm (including from the helper—i.e., do no harm).

Task 2: Explore the Problem

Rather than assuming any predetermined (or paternalistic) view of the problem and the client's goals, it is essential to listen carefully and help the client define the crisis from their point of view. This is an exploration rather than an interrogation, and the intervener's responsibility is to assist the client in focusing on specific immediate precipitating events and relevant situational and relational factors that are contributing to—or that could be helpful in resolving—the immediate problem of concern to the client. The historical backdrop and future concerns that are relevant to understanding the nature and significance of the current problem to the client are useful as a context for the current problem but should not become a distraction from or barrier to defining an immediate problem that also can be addressed with immediate action (preceded by appropriate planning and deliberation). Of note, when the emergency takes place in the context of therapy, the therapist may have the advantage of background knowledge and a solid enough relational foundation with the client to put the crisis in context and to more rapidly understand and stabilize the client. Of course, the therapist should not assume to know and should check out this background knowledge with the client as to whether it is pertinent to the particular crisis.

Task 3: Provide Support

People in crisis tend to feel alone, even abandoned, regardless of the apparent objective availability of supportive relationships and resources. Therefore, rather than assuming that the client will be aware of what might seem to the intervener to be an obvious intent to provide support ("Why would I be helping this person if not as a show of support?") and that the client will automatically feel supported by the intervener's actions, it is essential to demonstrate support for the client in an explicit manner. This can take the form of psychological support (e.g., communicating a willingness to unconditionally "accept and value the person no one else is willing to accept"; James & Gilliland, 2017, p. 52). It often takes the form of offering logistical support or assistance in accessing sources of tangible assistance (e.g., "concrete assistance from church members"; James & Gilliland, 2017, p. 53), or informational support (e.g., provision of guidance concerning "where, how, who, and what resources clients can access to get out of the predicament"; James & Gilliland, 2017, p. 53).

Task 4: Examine Alternatives

Given that the client's current strategies and tactics for coping with or handling the problem may have been overwhelmed to the point of paralysis or have not produced the results that the client is seeking, in the spirit of effective problem solving (D'Zurilla & Goldfried, 1971; Schwartz, 1971), it is important to assist the client in considering alternative courses of action. This task may include identifying "situational supports" (i.e., people who care and can help, practical resources the interventionist can help to access, and "coping mechanisms" based on "positive and constructive thinking patterns"; James & Gilliland, 2017, p. 54).

Task 5: Plan to Reestablish Control

The ultimate resolution of a crisis is not just solving the immediate problem but developing a plan that restores to the person a meaningful sense of control (within the limits of external circumstances and constraints that are beyond any one person's ability to control). Planning involves defining specific action steps that maintain or increase the client's autonomy and meaningful control in the face of the current or potential future problem(s) and stressor(s). Having a meaningful degree of control in one's life does not mean being able to rewrite history or change what cannot be changed, but it does mean having a plan that provides options giving one the ability to achieve core personal goals that make life worthwhile and sustain an acceptable (to the person) quality of life. Control also is not synonymous with having only positive experiences and eliminating all distressing emotions, but, rather, it means having a plan for dealing with negative experiences and distressing emotions while also cultivating and mindfully appreciating positive experiences and emotions.

Task 6: Obtain Commitment

Resolving crises requires a psychological shift from a state of helplessness and desperation to a mindset of determination to achieve a solution to the current problem(s). Intention alone without action, however, is ineffective and potentially iatrogenic. Therefore, the goal at this point in crisis intervention is to help the client to make a definite statement of intention to follow through with the collaboratively developed action plan. When clients balk at making this commitment, if often because one or more of the prior steps in the intervention have not been fully completed. Rather than inadvertently pressuring the client to commit to a plan that is not fully formed, hesitation or reluctance to commit should be taken as a cue to revisit the discussion of the nature of the problem, sources of available helpful support, potential alternative courses of action, and practical steps in the action plan—with a goal of identifying gaps, whether actual or perceived, that require revision or further development for the client to feel sufficiently confident to genuinely commit to take action.

Task 7: Follow Up

Ideally, crisis intervention is not a one-off procedure in which the client has no further contact with the intervener. Within the limits of logistical constraints (e.g., caseload, host organization policies and procedures) and professional or paraprofessional boundaries (i.e., maintaining a position as helper and not a friend or ersatz family member), following up with clients after the immediate contact and initial resolution of the problem(s) is important for the client to sustain a sense of support and collaborative partnership as well as to identify unresolved or overlooked aspects of the problem(s) that require further exploration, planning, support, and action (James & Gilliland, 2017, pp. 49–57).

The overarching goal of the hybrid model of crisis intervention (James & Gilliland, 2017) thus matches Caplan's (1964) definition of crises: to shift the person in crisis from a being in a state of desperation and demoralization due to distress, immobility, disorganization, isolation, and helplessness, to being in a state of readiness to take realistic and meaningful action.

TACTICS FOR CRISIS INTERVENTION

To accomplish the goal of each of the sequential stages or phases of crisis intervention, a number of practical tactics are required. A focus on tactics of crisis intervention enables interveners to move from a "20,000-foot view" of the stages of crisis intervention to an "on-the-ground-level" description of what helpers need to do in their actual moment-to-moment interactions with a person in crisis. A set of universal tactics for crisis intervention was defined several decades ago (Butcher et al., 1983), and these tactics can be divided into two subgroups corresponding to the two essential goals of classic crisis intervention. Tactics for facilitating safety and stabilizing the person or people in crisis include the following:

- Offer emotional support by expressing concern, compassion, and positive regard.

- Communicate encouragement and acceptance of the expression of intense emotions (i.e., catharsis).

- Communicate empathic validation of the individual's emotions and point of view.

- Develop a collaborative agreement with the individual for how to work together.

- Listen carefully and commenting selectively on potentially helpful insights.

- Provide factual information and clearing up misconceptions when necessary.

Tactics to engage the person or people in crisis in productive problem solving and assisting in the accessing of supportive resources include these:

- Focus on and develop a clear definition of the problem and the situation.
- Communicate concisely and stick to the immediate matters at hand.
- Predict problematic future consequences of the individual's present course of action.
- Clarify and reinforce the individual's adaptive abilities and strengths.
- Follow up with the individual to assess progress after the crisis encounter and maintain ongoing contact as necessary.

Myer and James (2005) identified nine tactics for crisis intervention that overlap several of those described by Butcher et al. (1983); however, they provided additional approaches that can contribute to successful crisis resolution. To address the goals of immediate safety and stabilization, Myer and James added tactics designed to help the person or people in crisis become aware of their state of emotional dysregulation (i.e., the creating awareness tactic), although they did not describe tactics for assisting the person or people to regain a state of adaptive emotion regulation (i.e., moving from awareness to restoring regulation):

- Allow catharsis by providing safety and acceptance.
- Create awareness of denied and repressed emotions, behaviors, and thoughts.
- Provide emotional (and when appropriate and possible, tangible) support.

Myer and James (2005) also expanded the on the tactics for problem solving by providing a more detailed breakdown of the steps required to ensure that solutions are feasible and that the person or people in crisis have a plan for taking action to put the solution(s) into practice:

- Expand perspectives by offering a reframing of the problem or situation that suggests alternative possible solutions.

- Focus on specific, feasible, manageable choices that the individual can make.

- Provide proactive guidance that offers the individual practical directions for action.

- Engage in behavioral activation by encouraging the individual to define and take actions that can alter the situation or their state of mind, and that could contribute to solving the problem.

- Define, organize, and prioritize challenges and goals.

- Ensure physical and emotional safety by accessing social support and other resources.

TECHNIQUES FOR CRISIS INTERVENTION

Moving a step further toward behaviorally specific actions that the helper can take when intervening in a crisis—in addition to the broader crisis intervention stages and tactics—James and Gilliland (2017, pp. 73–91) described a number of specific crisis intervention techniques. These techniques are based largely on the clinical experience of crisis interventionists and not (as revealed in the preceding review of research) on scientific evidence. However, these techniques have been widely used to assist people in crisis across many settings (e.g., hospital, school, crisis hotline, child protective services, family preservation programs; Roberts & Everly, 2006). Interestingly, many of these classic crisis intervention techniques as follows are adapted from the client-centered (Rogers, 1957) and psychodynamic (Weiner, 1975) models of psychotherapy that the next chapter describes in more detail:

- Open-ended questions are used to communicate interest in and respect for the client's perspectives to help the client shift from a reflexive/reactive position to a position of reflective processing, and to gather information about the client's current concerns.

- Restatement is used to communicate attention to the client's statements and to check for the accuracy of the interventionist's hearing and understanding of those statements.

- Owning of feelings involves the interventionist's acknowledging their emotional reactions to the client's statements and situation with an emphasis on expressing authentic concern and mirroring the client's sense of distress.

- Facilitative listening involves encouraging the client to express their perceptions, emotions, thoughts, and goals to facilitate an open dialogue in which the interventionist can understand and support the client's perspective and priorities.

- Communication of empathy involves demonstrating verbally and non-verbally an interest in and respect for the client's unique perspective and the validity of the client's emotions.

- Communication of genuineness or authenticity involves demonstrating consistency between the nonverbal and verbal messages conveyed to the client, and a sincere interest in being of help to the client while not intruding on the client's privacy or diminishing the client's freedom and ability to make and follow through on autonomous decisions and choices.

- Communication of unconditional positive regard and acceptance involves demonstrating both nonverbally and verbally a caring for and valuing of the client regardless of the client's decisions, actions, beliefs, and personal or relational difficulties.

- Collaborative counseling involves developing and sustaining a partnership with the client in which both parties work as a team in defining and solving the problems facing the client and in supporting the client in achieving both immediate and long-term goals.

- Nondirective counseling involves providing the client with support and guidance but not explicitly or implicitly prescribing any decisions or actions, such that the client can make choices and take actions fully autonomously.

Notably missing from the preceding list of crisis intervention techniques is the technique of providing directive guidance. All of the crisis intervention models include the provision of directive guidance as an essential crisis intervention practice to help the client to identify actions that either are necessary for immediate safety or that should be avoided because they could potentially escalate problems or compromise the safety of self or others. However, as noted previously, providing explicit directions can undercut the client's sense of autonomy and confidence as well as foster a sense of devaluation and dependency. Therefore, directives concerning what (or what not) to do (or think) must be used cautiously and sparingly, and only to support the client in establishing safety and in making sound personal decisions. This fits with the fundamental principle of guiding but not attempting to direct or control a client in psychotherapy in any way that could be construed as coercion or devaluation by the client.

CONCLUSION

The crisis intervention models, strategies, and tactics described in this chapter target safety and stabilization first and problem solving and accessing resources second. This approach is consistent with the four stages Caplan (1964) described in the development of crises (see Chapter 1). When people face a challenge but cannot resolve it (Stage 1), their inability to resolve the problem leads to (or exacerbates existing) threats to their safety and results in a state of instability in which they have become emotionally dysregulated (Stage 2). This, in turn, leads to escalating negative outcomes constituting and emergency (Stage 3) and, ultimately, a breakdown (Stage 4). Restoring safety and stability, and then developing potential solutions and resources to address the original problem(s) is a commonsense approach to restoring the original homeostasis that has been lost as a result of the unsolved problem(s).

However, when problem(s) intensify into a crisis, the immediate challenge facing the interventionist actually is not the original problem(s). It is the escalating stress response that has developed as a result of the distress, desperation, and hopelessness that results from being unable to resolve the initial problem(s). In crises, the freeze phase of the stress response can become a state of emotional paralysis and perseverative worry (see Chapter 2). The fight phase can become unbridled anger and verbal or physical aggression toward oneself or others. The flight phase can become severe anxiety, isolation, distrust, and impulsive self-medication. And the tonic immobility phase can become a state of profound depression, dissociation, or even psychosis (see Chapter 2). In other words, the key problem facing the interventionist in a crisis is helping the person or people in crisis to escape a downward spiral of instability, emergency, and breakdown that occurs when emotional dysregulation has overtaken their ability to think clearly and make adaptive choices.

Crisis intervention in the context of psychotherapy thus often involves helping people who are stuck on autopilot using maladaptive coping strategies to reset their bodily and psychological stress response and regain the ability to self-regulate that makes it possible to engage in thoughtful, reflective problem solving. Thus, the crisis intervention approaches in this chapter provide a useful beginning (i.e., restoring safety and emotional stabilization) and conclusion (i.e., solving problems and accessing resources) for the resolution of crises—but a crucial intermediate phase (which begins while safety and stability are the focus) is needed: the restoration of emotion regulation. This is implicit in classic crisis intervention models but needs to be made explicit for crises to be fully and safely resolved in the context of the psychotherapy session.

The restoration of emotion regulation is the hallmark of all approaches to psychotherapy. This is particularly important because of one key difference between general crises and crises in the psychotherapy session: General crisis intervention typically occurs with no prior or subsequent relationship between the person in crisis and the helper, whereas in psychotherapy, the client and therapist have a preexisting relationship (even if relatively newly established) that ideally will extend beyond the crisis. Because of this ongoing relationship, clients in psychotherapy disclose deeply personal information that can be invaluable in resolving crises. However, this is a double-edged sword. The intensely personal relationship in psychotherapy places clients in a position of exquisite emotional vulnerability in relation to the therapist. This can lead to intense attachment insecurity and emotional dysregulation if a crisis occurs that threatens the trust they've placed in their therapist and in the therapy process. Thus, therapists have more to work with, on two levels, than acute crisis interventionists when assisting a client crisis—on one level, this can be for better (i.e., a greater depth of knowledge of the client and emotional connection with the client); but on another, it can be for worse (i.e., a greater intensity of emotional dysregulation and attachment insecurity or disorganization on the client's part). The next chapter explores the essential principles and practices of psychotherapy that directly address this crucial additional aspect of crisis intervention: the restoration of emotion regulation.

4 ESSENTIAL PSYCHOTHERAPY PRINCIPLES AND PRACTICES

Psychotherapy is an interpersonal process in which one person communicates to another that he understands him, respects him, and wants to be of help to him. . . . [Thus,] psychotherapy is unique in that the therapist strives to communicate his understanding of the patient's difficulties and to help him share in this . . . person-related understanding.

—Irving B. Weiner (1975, p. 3)

As discussed in the previous chapter, the context of psychotherapy differs significantly from other contexts in which crises can occur. Thus, although acute crisis intervention models are applicable to psychotherapy sessions, it is important to consider adaptations that account for the unique context of the psychotherapy session. This chapter begins with a brief discussion of the features that make psychotherapy unique. Next, I describe three foundational principles of psychotherapy and their implications for resolving in-session crises: supporting autonomy and security; modifying maladaptive behavioral and psychodynamic patterns; and modifying modes of relating,

https://doi.org/10.1037/0000225-005
Crises in the Psychotherapy Session: Transforming Critical Moments Into Turning Points, by J. D. Ford

communicating, and coping. These essential principles of psychotherapy across its many theoretical and technical models can provide a valuable guide for therapists in a crisis.

UNIQUE FEATURES OF THE PSYCHOTHERAPY CONTEXT

Psychotherapy is a process of self-directed and therapist-guided reflection on the nature and personal significance for the client of their perceptual, physiological, affective, cognitive, behavioral, motivational, and relational experiences. Although done in varied ways depending on the therapeutic model(s) used, all approaches to psychotherapy involve

- development of a client–therapist alliance and therapeutic relationship based on shared commitment to ensure the client's safety, well-being, autonomy, privacy, and trust

- review of stressful past and present experiences and related emotions and beliefs

- mindfulness-based facilitation of immediate experiential awareness and acceptance

- systematic problem-solving, motivational enhancement, and solution identification

- in-session and in vivo behavioral and interpersonal rehearsal of potential solutions

- discovery of personal meaning in life experiences that provides hope and empowerment

Ultimately, psychotherapy aims to enable clients to shift from being in a state of emotional dysregulation and insecure attachment to adaptive self-regulation and earned attachment security (Ford & Courtois, 2020). Crises thus are a special case of the general challenge that is addressed by psychotherapy. As the repository and agent to whom the client can turn both for answers and guidance in matters of deep personal significance (and typically also pain), the therapist is an emotional lightning rod who cannot help but draw the client's highly charged personal distress, wishes, and needs—that is, transference reactions that reflect the client's core conflictual relationship themes (CCRTs; Luborsky & Crits-Christoph, 1989). When crises emerge in psychotherapy, the crucial focus for the psycho-therapist is on how the client is experiencing either a relational need or wish in relation to the psychotherapist (e.g., to be loved, valued, cared for, rescued, dominated) or a rupture, failure, or threat in their relationship (e.g., rejection, loss, abandonment, exploitation, aggression, devaluation). Drawing on attachment theory (Cassidy et al., 2013; Levy, 2013; Spiegel, 2016), psychodynamic (Gunderson et al., 2007; Kernberg, 1979; Luborsky & Crits-Christoph, 1989; Winnicott, 1945) and self-psychology (Kohut & Wolf, 1978; Wolf, 1976, 1979) theories, and cognitive therapy (Beck, 2005; Leahy, 2001; Linehan, 1993), the core dilemmas that can lead to crises in therapy result from clients' self-protective attempts to prevent harm or restore a sense of security in the therapeutic relationship. The commonsense solution that psychotherapists typically learn for handling crises in session is as follows: Get the client to calm down and orient sufficiently to recognize that they are safe and that they can trust and rely on you to help them find a solution and feel better again. There are many practical tips and techniques for de-escalating clients in crisis by restoring the client's active engagement in problem-solving (Erickson, 1959, 1964; O'Hanlon, 2003; Roes, 2002; Satten, 2002) and by "grounding" the client who is intensely distressed, dissociated, self-harming, or suicidal (Chefetz, 2017; Fisher, 2020; Loewenstein, 2006; Myrick et al., 2015; Steele & van der Hart, 2020). In brief, de-escalation includes these techniques:

- Speak calmly.

- Minimize extraneous stimulation and avoid intruding on the client's personal space.

- Maintain eye contact and an alert but open and relaxed body posture.

- Engage the client in coregulation by encouraging them to pay attention to the natural rhythm of their breathing and to what they are feeling in their body.

- Encourage the client to observe thoughts and emotions nonjudgmentally, and to orient themselves to where they are and whom they're with—and that they are safe right now.

- Remind the client of your presence and that you're there to help.

- Define an immediate positive goal of the client's that you can help the client to achieve.

All of these techniques are good. But what if the client is too distressed or dissociated to pay attention and hear, let alone follow the de-escalation guidance offered? And what if the therapist is too stunned or shocked or confused or fearful or angry to remember to use the de-escalation tactics and to be able to select and provide one(s) that match this particular client's ways of thinking and feeling in a way that seems calm and is genuine (rather than pressured or anxious or annoyed)?

These are the "deer in the headlights" or "Oh my god, what do I do now" moments that every therapist dreads. There is no way to be fully prepared for crises, but being able to handle them calmly, wisely, and therapeutically can alter (or end) the psychotherapy and a client's life. Yet, few training or continuing education programs give crises the attention they deserve by ensuring that therapists understand what is happening in in-session crises and what they need to do to resolve such crises safely, effectively, and therapeutically when they occur.

Regardless of the specific problem(s) or approach to therapy, the focal issue of any crisis in psychotherapy sessions is a conflict, rupture, loss, or failure in the relationship between the provider and the client (Barber, 1995; Boesky, 2005; Friedlander et al., 2014; Gumz et al., 2012; M. Hunt et al., 2018; Kelly et al., 2009; Newman, 2002; Plutchik et al., 1994; Rubin, 2001; Shimoji & Miyakawa, 2000; Teckchandani & Barad, 2017; Vilhelmsson et al., 2013). Although in-session crises often involve and are at least partially precipitated by events or circumstances outside the therapeutic relationship, in-session crises center on the personal meaning for the client of the therapist's actions (or omissions) as well as what the client expects concerning the therapist's intent and likely future actions. This is the double-edged sword of therapy: By taking on the responsibility of guiding a client, therapists unavoidably assume a role of great emotional importance in the client's life that brings with it great hazard. What follows are three essential principles of psychotherapy and their implications for resolving in-session crises.

Support Autonomy and Security

A first principle of psychotherapy is that the process must consistently support the client in achieving a balance between, on the one hand, autonomous self-reflection, decision making, and action (which promote growth and healing but often are associated with emotional distress; Kohut, 1965; Ulberg et al., 2009), and on the other hand, trust in and rely on the therapist as a guide and source of support (Nienhuis et al., 2018; Norcross & Lambert, 2018). This principle is the reason that client-centered and attachment-based approaches to psychotherapy constitute the essential first step in resolving (or preventing) crises and impasses in psychotherapy sessions (Nienhuis et al., 2018; Rogers, 1957).

Client-Centered Psychotherapy

The essential practices required to put this principle into action are both a matter of common sense and a technical rule: Listen, learn, and ask questions with an open mind before jumping to conclusions or offering answers or advice (including therapeutic interpretations or prescriptions; Weiner, 1975, p. 53). This is an essential feature of client-centered psychotherapy in that it shows respect for and nonjudgmental acceptance of the client's authority as an expert on their own life as well as facilitates the development by the therapist of an empathic understanding (i.e., from the client's point of view) of the dilemmas and choices that the client is dealing with in the current crisis or stuck point.

In this vein, it also is essential, especially (but not only) early in therapy—and especially in crises—for the therapist "not to demonstrate his brilliance in picking up subtle clues to the patient's underlying thoughts and feelings, but rather to cement the patient's involvement in the treatment process" (Weiner, 1975, p. 99). The therapist as all-knowing expert, mind reader, or magician–sorcerer is a stance that encourages clients to be passively dependent on the therapist and to devalue themselves and idealize the therapist. Engaging the client's involvement in the treatment process can only occur if the therapist emphasizes the value of the client's active participation as a full partner in a search for understanding and solutions. This must be based on the knowledge that the client has of their own life, self, and circumstances as well as the therapist's complementary knowledge of how to fully and accurately access that knowledge through nonjudgmental self-reflection and a therapeutic dialogue and partnership. Learning that the therapist does not have all the answers but can be a guide and partner in the process of finding answers that provide new options can provide the client with a working model of attachment security that is crucial for adaptive emotion regulation—"I'm not alone with this problem; I can count on this therapist to support me, stand by me, help me see and understand things more clearly, and ultimately respect what I believe and choose."

Client-centered psychotherapy provides an essential foundation for the psychotherapy process and is a crucial starting point for therapists when a client is in crisis. Empathy, positive regard, and genuineness were proposed as the essential facilitative conditions of psychotherapy more than 75 years ago (Rogers, 1957). Subsequently, substantial research has demonstrated the consistent association between therapist empathy (Elliott et al., 2018), positive regard (Farber et al., 2018), and genuineness (Kolden et al., 2018) with positive therapeutic outcomes across a wide range of psychotherapy modalities. By engaging with clients in a caring, empathic, and authentic manner, therapists are able to establish a collaborative partnership (Tryon et al., 2018) dedicated to achieving changes that enhance the client's adaptive capacities, well-being, and quality of life (Flückiger et al., 2018; Friedlander et al., 2014, 2018; Karver et al., 2018). In principle, the client-centered concepts of empathy, unconditional positive regard, and genuine respect are familiar to most if not all psychotherapists, but, in practice, they require intense concentration and rigorous observation and self-reflection by the therapist, especially in situations of crisis and risk that demand timely response.

Empathy is an active form of psychological reflection and communication aimed at demonstrating understanding of another person's emotions, thoughts, and goals from the other person's unique frame of reference. Three subprocesses of empathy have been identified: emotional mirroring (i.e., resonance with the other person's nonverbal/bodily expressions of emotion), cognitive perspective-taking (i.e., formulating core assumptions and conclusions based on the other person's way of thinking and seeing things), and compassion (i.e., providing caring and support to help the other person cope with distress and feel soothed and secure; Elliott et al., 2018). Empathy involves communicating a willingness to join with the client and figuratively stand in their shoes to establish trust, respect, rapport, and attunement. In that sense, empathy conveys to the client that they have a steadfast ally who will stand with them and consistently support them while facing the challenges, obstacles, and dangers that are involved. This is not, however, blind or unthinking support because empathy also involves helping the client to self-reflect on and see more clearly what they do actually feel, know, value, and aspire to achieve, all of which often is obscured from view because of emotional dysregulation.

Unconditional positive regard is an attitude of nonjudgmental acceptance, affirmation, and nonpossessive warmth—a view of others as "persons of worth" (Rogers, 1951, p. 20). Feeling a sense of not only respect but also liking for the other person, appreciating and feeling "drawn toward" them, and viewing them as having all the rights of a "free individual," are aspects of positive regard (Farber et al., 2018, p. 412). Positive regard is communicated in several ways, including emotional warmth, friendliness, supportiveness, appreciation, and involvement. Careful choice of words to neither state nor imply criticism, dislike, or devaluation is an essential aspect of demonstrating positive regard. However, nonverbal communication (i.e., body language, eye contact, proximity, voice modulation and tone, vocalizations, gestures) are of equal or greater importance in communicating positive regard as the therapist's spoken words and therefore are important for the therapist to attend to.

Genuineness is the expression of authentic respect for and interest in without deception, dissembling, or contrivance. Also described as *congruence,* this attitude and communication of sincerity requires therapists act and speak in a manner that is fully consistent with their true feelings and beliefs without artifice or attempts at pretense. Genuineness requires a combination of rigorous and mindful self-reflection by the therapist as well as attunement with the client. Although not synonymous with genuineness, both authentic self-disclosure and a willingness to be fully present to the client and oneself are closely related to genuineness and are associated with positive therapeutic outcomes (Hill et al., 2018). This transparency and forthrightness in expressing the therapist's experience of interacting with the client must be carefully balanced with respect for and an attentive awareness of the client as a person (i.e., in a context of empathy and unconditional positive regard; Kolden et al., 2018). Self-disclosure must always be done within the boundaries of a professional relationship that is truly client centered (i.e., limited to information that is solely for the benefit of the client and does not burden or impose on the client or in any way violate the client's values or culture).

Attachment-Based Psychotherapy

Attachment-based psychotherapy extends the client-centered principles and practices by providing the client with reassurance that the therapist is emotionally available, responsive, and willing and able to partner with the client in resolving the crisis so that the client does not have to cope with the additional stressor and burden of feeling profoundly alone while in crisis. Based on John Bowlby's (1982) seminal work and subsequent research on attachment working models (Main, 2000; Miljkovitch et al., 2015), attachment-based therapy emphasizes the therapist's attunement and supportive responsiveness to the client's verbal and nonverbal expressions of security and insecurity in the therapy relationship and in historical and current relationships in the client's personal life (Dales & Jerry, 2008; Holmes, 1993; Lieberman & Zeanah, 1999; Sable, 2004; Slade & Holmes, 2019; Spiegel, 2016; Stern et al., 2001).

From an attachment perspective, the psychotherapist is viewed as providing a secure base (i.e., a relationship in which the person feels fundamentally safe enough and sufficiently cared for and valued to be able to face life's stressors and challenges proactively and with self-confidence and trust in core relationships; Talia et al., 2020; Waters & Waters, 2006). In infancy and childhood, attachment security is developed—or under nonoptimal or traumatic conditions, fails to develop—in relationship to adult primary caregivers, prototypically the child's mother (Main, 2000) but also with other caregivers, including fathers (Madigan et al., 2011). When a primary caregiver is emotionally dysregulated—for example, fearful, helpless, unresponsive, or confused and unresolved in their attachment working models (Lyons-Ruth & Spielman, 2004; Madigan et al., 2007)—the child is at risk for developing a disorganized working model of attachment that involves alternating states of intense dependency, fearful avoidance, and angry ambivalence and attack that can persist and affect close relationships for decades across the life span (Granqvist et al., 2017). Across the wide range of psychological, behavioral, and emotional problems for which people seek psychotherapy, attachment insecurity and disorganization consistently are found to play a major role (Mikulincer & Shaver, 2012; van Hoof et al., 2019).

On the other hand, attachment security is a fundamental foundation for adaptive emotion regulation and self-regulation, also beginning in infancy and extending across the life span (Zimmermann, 1999). Infants who experience secure attachment with their primary caregiver develop the earliest forms of emotion regulation by coregulating with their caregiver (Evans & Porter, 2009). Coregulation involves the caregiver modeling and joining the child in actions that enhance positive states of emotion and help the infant to recover from states of emotional dysregulation. Across cultures, coregulation can occur in many ways, although some form of shared nonverbal contact (e.g., expressive facial communication, soothing music and singing) tends to be a consistent feature (Lavelli et al., 2019).

Therefore, focusing immediately on signs of attachment insecurity or disorganization, and providing a clear nonverbal message of calm, confidence, and responsive attention to the client and the distress and stressor(s)—including the therapist's own behavior (Wolf, 1993)—can both reduce the emotional turmoil associated with compromised attachment security and begin a reparative process of coregulation through which the psychotherapist can join with the client in modeling and facilitating adaptive emotion regulation (Holmes, 2017; Slade, 2009; Slade & Holmes, 2019). Although no research studies as yet have tested this hypothesis, research showing evidence of enhanced attachment security following both psychodynamic and cognitive behavior therapies suggests that psychotherapists can have a positive influence on their clients' (often initially insecure or disorganized) attachment working models (Daniel et al., 2016; Marmarosh, 2014; Maxwell et al., 2018; Strauß et al., 2018). In a crisis or at a stuck point in psychotherapy, a client-centered focus on modeling emotion regulation and attending empathically, nonjudgmentally, respectfully, and collaboratively to the client's sense of insecurity or emotional confusion functions to provide that crucial secure base.

Modify Maladaptive Behavioral and Psychodynamic Patterns

A second principle of psychotherapy is that much, if not most, of the distress that brings clients into psychotherapy results from emotions, beliefs, and patterns of behavior that are unrecognized or confusing and not fully understood by the client (Kramer et al., 2013; Perry & Bond, 2012). Even when clients forcefully state what they perceive to be "the problem" (i.e., an unattainable goal or unresolvable conflict), there are aspects that they find puzzling and hope a therapist can help to clarify (e.g., "Why do I get so angry or feel so hopeless?" "Why would he treat me like that?" "Why doesn't she see it my way?"). Therefore, psychotherapy aims to help clients recognize and understand feelings, beliefs, and associated patterns of behavior in a new and fuller way to enable them to have new choices that can help them to handle previously unsolved problems. To achieve this aim, therapists must develop not just a diagnostic formulation but what Weiner (1975) called a *dynamic formulation* (pp. 56–60), a description of how the client's distress is caused or exacerbated by what the client "is not understanding" (or is incompletely understanding) about their life situation, their personality and behavior patterns, and their relationships (Perry & Bond, 2012; Petraglia et al., 2015).

In practice, applying the dynamic formulation principle requires the therapist to conduct psychotherapy in a manner that is suitable for each individual client based on their motivations, their willingness and ability to engage in self-reflection—what Weiner (1975) called their "personality integration" (p. 59). *Personality integration* (Kohut, 1965) is the client's ability to self-regulate, that is, to experience emotions and impulses without becoming dysregulated (e.g., enraged, suicidal, overwhelmed by grief or shame, terrified and panicked, dissociative, detached and isolative; Courtois & Ford, 2013). Psychotherapy thus enables clients to gain hope and make changes by engaging them in a process of guided self-reflection (Carcione et al., 2011; Fonagy & Campbell, 2017; Ford, 2018; J. A. Hamm & Lysaker, 2018) that involves understanding their personal limitations (i.e., their personality dynamics) while simultaneously recognizing, drawing on, and enhancing their personal strengths and capacities for self-regulation (Ford, 2013; Ford et al., 2005), and their personality integration (Kohut, 1965). Although originally stated in the context of psychodynamic psychotherapy, this principle is at the heart of theoretical orientations to psychotherapy that span the full spectrum from behavioral to metacognitive to psychodynamic approaches to psychotherapy (Frank, 1971).

Behavioral Psychotherapy and Cognitive Behavior Therapy

Applied behavior analysis (Follette et al., 2009) and cognitive behavior therapy (Jackson et al., 2020) address the dynamics of behavior and cognition in psychotherapy. The goal is to develop a *functional analysis* that takes the form of a "chain" describing the sequential connections (hence the term "chain") that link A, B, and C:

- **A**ntecedents (i.e., events or changes in the external environment or in the client's internal bodily, affective, or cognitive experience)

- **B**ehavior (i.e., actual or potential observable actions and internal emotions, thoughts, and bodily reactions that are either maladaptive or adaptive)

- **C**onsequences (i.e., subsequent events or changes in the external environment or the client's internal experience that increase or decrease the likelihood of the behaviors stopping, continuing, or starting)

The term "functional" is used because the focus is on the function that antecedents and consequences (which may include the thoughts, beliefs, emotions, and bodily processes that constitute the person's internal environment as well as stimuli in the external environment) play in both problematic/symptomatic and healthy/adaptive behavior. Following from the behavior analysis paradigm of operant and instrumental conditioning, the antecedents set the stage for the behavior, and the consequences are the outcomes that either increase or reduce the likelihood of the behavior going forward. Therefore, to change behavior, it is necessary (although not always sufficient) to change its internal and external antecedents and the consequences.

In a crisis, the behaviors of primary concern are the external or internal (e.g., maladaptive cognitions) actions (or inaction) that express or contribute to emotional dysregulation and the adaptive forms of emotion regulation and associated feelings, thoughts, bodily states, and actions that could help resolve the crisis. The goal is to enable clients to change the antecedents that lead to, and the consequences that reinforce, emotional dysregulation as well as to enable clients to find, create, or increase their access to antecedents and consequences that lead to and reinforce adaptive self-regulation. This is also called *behavioral chain analysis* because the psychotherapist helps the client develop many links between antecedents, behavior, and consequences (ABC) in a chain leading to self-regulation.

ABC chains can be identified both within and outside the therapy setting and relationship (Follette et al., 2009). In client–therapist interactions in the psychotherapy session, a maladaptive ABC chain can be identified in many types of crises. For example:

- A: The client angrily accuses the therapist of a betrayal and incompetence.

- B_T: The therapist reacts defensively by interpreting the client's anger as displaced from the client's troubled relationship with an emotionally invalidating parent.

- B_C: The client interprets this as criticism and rejection, feels abandoned and betrayed (again), and is both enraged and ashamed, and threatens to quit therapy and commit suicide.

- C_T: The therapist feels frightened and helpless to prevent the client from self-harm, and calls an ambulance to come for the client.

- C_C: The client is involuntarily hospitalized and receives an increased dose of medication.

A more helpful chain could be developed if the therapist creates a different antecedent (A) by responding (B_T) nondefensively and inviting the client nonjudgmentally to talk about what has happened in the therapy, and in the client's life, that was upsetting for the client. The therapist might know that the anger is likely to be at least, in part, a transference reaction from the client's troubled relationship with a parent. The therapist probably also knows, from history and by basic deduction, that other difficult emotions are likely to accompany that anger, including fear, hurt, shame, guilt, and grief. Furthermore, the therapist probably knows that positive emotions related both to the client's primary relationship(s) and their therapeutic relationship might be complicating the client's emotional turmoil, including an idealized admiration of the therapist and an ambivalent and vulnerable wish to be loved. While all of those psychodynamics could not possibly be explored in the brief time frame of the immediate crisis, nonjudgmentally and empathically helping the client to consider and reflect on even one of them is a therapist behavior (B) that might lead to a very different client behavior (B_C) and to a more therapeutic outcome for the client ($_C$) and the therapist (C_T). The therapist also could consider how the consequences (C_C) that are occurring currently or have occurred in the past following episodes of emotional dysregulation (B_C) might perpetuate or exacerbate the client's current emotional dysregulation in order to not interact with the client in a manner that inadvertently replicates those maladaptive consequences (B_T).

Clients' lives are complicated, and so the behavior chains that occur in their lives are correspondingly long and complex (i.e., ABC–ABC–ABC . . .). However, when broken down into small ABC "links," even the most complex chain can be carefully examined and incrementally modified to change from a cascade of escalating avoidance and dysregulation to the development and implementation of ABC chains that provide the client with a new set of consequences that reinforce self-regulation. A key point is that emotional dysregulation can serve as the antecedent for therapeutic responses by the therapist (e.g., nonjudgmental empathic validation), which can be an antecedent for new adaptive behavior by the client (e.g., attachment security and self-regulation) with a key consequence: the averting or resolving of therapy crises.

Metacognitive Psychotherapy

What clients want from life and how they believe they need to (and are able to) go about achieving core goals is the focus of metacognitive psychotherapy. One metacognitive model—motivational interviewing (MI; Arkowitz, 2008; W. R. Miller & Rollnick, 2002) and motivational enhancement therapy (MET; W. R. Miller & National Institute on Alcohol Abuse and Alcoholism, 1995), or MI/MET—offers systematic principles and techniques to guide therapists in aligning with and enabling clients to draw on their motivation to achieve the personal goals that they (the clients) view as their top priorities. MI/MET begins with the premise that goals are embedded in every problem but that goals often are overlooked or discounted when problems seem unsolvable or involve emotional turmoil and dysregulation.

To help a client in crisis to recognize the goals that best represent a positive outcome (both objectively and from the client's point of view), motivational enhancement begins by the therapist's continuing to directly and indirectly express a client-centered affirmation of the client's worth and autonomy (e.g., asking open-ended questions; deferring to the client's decisions; seeking to understand and nonjudgmentally accept the client's emotions, beliefs, and preferences). Further elaboration of this attitude of respect, collaboration, and positive regard for the client is provided by active reflective listening (i.e., taking the client's viewpoint, paraphrasing the core messages the client is conveying, checking with the client on the accuracy of the paraphrasing) and rolling with the resistance (i.e., accepting disagreement or challenges from the client nonjudgmentally without attempting to change the client's mind with logical persuasion, objective analyses, or citations of "facts"; discrediting the client's views or authoritative edicts; W. R. Miller & Rollnick, 2002).

MI/MET builds on this foundation by engaging with the client in an exploration of goals that could serve as a basis for solving problems (i.e., "change talk") and supporting the client in making decisions consistent with core personal goals (i.e., "sustain talk"; W. R. Miller & Rollnick, 2002). Engaging in change talk is done by posing questions to help the client to define and commit to achieving their core goals. This includes five steps that are summarized by the acronym, DARN-C (W. R. Miller & Rollnick, 2002):

- **D**: "What are the goals that are based on most my most fundamental hopes and **d**esires?"

- **A**: "What are my **a**bilities and strengths that can enable me to achieve these goals?"

- **R**: "What are **r**easons why achieving personal goals can make a difference in my life?"

- **N**: "How much do I **n**eed to achieve these goals and how much of a difference will this make?"

- **C**: "How strong is my **c**ommitment to do whatever it takes to achieve these goals?"

MI/MET also offers a basic set of principles to guide therapists, summarized by the acronym, RULE: **R**esist the urge to fix, correct, or demand compliance from the client; **u**nderstand the client's motivation; **l**isten and support change talk and sustain talk; and **e**mpower the client to set and achieve their own personal goals (W. R. Miller & Rollnick, 2002).

When goals are being explored and set in MI/MET, it is crucial to shift from a focus on the "problem" to one on the positive outcome that the client seeks to achieve and what the client is willing and able to do to achieve that outcome (i.e., potential solutions). Solution-focused therapy (SFT) involves principles and techniques that guide therapists in assisting clients to creatively identify potential solutions that build on the clients' abilities and past successes (Berg, 1994; de Shazer, 1988; O'Connell, 2012). In SFT, solutions are developed by helping the client explore how life will be different if problems are solved and goals are achieved: What will the client be feeling and doing? How will relationships and other life pursuits change? and What is standing in the way of that brave new world that is within the client's power to alter or overcome? In SFT, solutions also are generated by exploring exceptions, that is, instances in the client's life in which the desired outcomes actually have occurred, even if only temporarily or partially. SFT thus focuses the therapist's and client's attention on what has worked in the past that the client can draw on currently as well as what the client actually hopes to achieve (to strengthen the connection between proposed solutions and the client's core goals).

A third metacognitive model, acceptance and commitment therapy (ACT), emphasizes mindfulness (S. C. Hayes et al., 2006; Lee et al., 2015; Lindsay & Creswell, 2017). The mindfulness perspective extends MI/MET and SFT by teaching two interconnected strategies for thinking about goals and solutions. The first strategy is radical acceptance (i.e., taking circumstances as they are, not attempting to rewrite history or to change what is not within the person's power to change). The second strategy is to make a commitment to taking actions that are within the person's power. Similar to meditation practice and models of complementary medicine (S. Smith & Ford, 2020), acceptance and commitment therapy emphasizes a universal goal and solution that underlies all unique individual goals and solutions: achieving peace of mind (A-Tjak et al., 2015).

The metacognitive perspective thus offers another way to formulate the dynamics of clients' problems and to tap into and strengthen their personality integration. Taken together, MI/MET and SFT, and ACT provide a framework for helping clients to change not only the ABC leading to emotional dysregulation but also how they think about (i.e., metacognize) the dynamics of emotional dysregulation and their ability to self-regulate. Metacognitive psychotherapy also offers therapists an important way to engage with clients that can enable clients to develop an increased sense of attachment security by experiencing the therapist as fully accepting of them and dedicated to helping them to set and achieve the goals that are of most importance to them with solutions that come from (and are respectful of) their own personal experiences, preferences, and abilities.

Psychodynamic Psychotherapy

An integrative psychodynamic perspective with great applicability to crisis resolution has been developed using the concept of CCRTs (Kächele et al., 2002). CCRTs are formulated based on a three fundamental intrapsychic aspects of relationship episodes: wishes (i.e., what the person wants from the other person or people and how the person wants to participate in their interaction), response from other (i.e., how other people react to the person, actually, potentially, or in the person's imagination), and response of self (i.e., how the person reacts to other people's interactions, behaviorally and emotionally, and how the person feels emotionally and views herself or himself as a result; Loughead et al., 2010; Luborsky & Crits-Christoph, 1989).

Examples of wishes are to be loved, appreciated, and understood; to be emotionally close or distant; to be unnoticed or the center of attention;

to be assertive and self-expressive or to be passive and hidden; or to achieve recognition or to be left alone. Examples of responses from others include real, anticipated, or imagined rejection; liking; appreciation; coercion; anger; deference; distress; fear; or indifference. Examples of responses of the self include helping and feeling helpful; being isolated and feeling helpless and alone; achieving success and feeling respected and accepted; being avoidant and feeling anxious and self-doubting; arguing, fighting, and being cruel; or feeling ashamed and detached. A reformulation of CCRTs (Kächele et al., 2002) grouped the themes into two overarching domains, harmonious and disharmonious relationships, each of which has several useful themes for psychotherapy. Harmonious relationship themes include the following:

- engaging (exploring, admiring, accepting, understanding)

- supporting (explaining, confirming, helping, giving independence)

- loving and ensuring well-being (being close, confident, satisfied, loving, interested, healthy)

- having self-determination (being trustworthy, thankful, tolerant, calm, considerate, constructive, enduring, patient, proud, autonomous, a role model; developing, improving; being thoughtful, in control, courageous, responsible, self-critical)

Disharmonious relationship themes include the following:

- being depressed and resigned, being dissatisfied (guilty, ashamed, frustrated)

- being anxious (confused, nervous, tense, hysterical, unrestrained, shocked, outraged)

- being controlled by others (dependent, alone, lonely, clinging, passive, doubting, stagnating, weak, helpless, exposed, unprotected, inferior, injured, a disappointment, failing, unimportant, ugly)

- being angry and unlikable (feeling disgust, contempt, jealousy, offended, hate, resentment, impatience, ungenerous, uninteresting, unfriendly, unfaithful, impolite)

- being unreliable (neglectful, selfish, insensitive, destructive, foolish, abandoning, superficial, irresponsible, heartless, lazy, unfair, egotistical, greedy, dishonest)

- being rejecting or subjugating (exploiting, cheating, betraying, denying, ingratiating, deceiving, dominating, demanding, controlling)

- being annoying or attacking (hurting, embarrassing, humiliating, being malicious, being cynical, harassing, distracting, threatening, provoking, tormenting, being hostile, punishing, exacting revenge, being violent, abusing)

- withdrawing (distancing, being distrustful, avoiding, complying, being submissive, being reserved, being compulsive, acquiescing, being inhibited, being exhausted, being ill, dying, killing oneself)

A four-step approach based on the CCRTs framework has been proposed to enable the therapeutic interaction "to rise above relational enactments in a supportive way and how it can provide a corrective emotional experience to enhance the emotional bond between the patient and the therapist" (Leibovich et al., 2018, p. 231). Leibovich et al. (2018) proposed an ICEF approach: Identification, Countertransference, Empathy, and Freedom. In the first step, identification, they distinguish between clients' wishes in regard to core relationships that are progressive (e.g., to be seen and respected as a full and worthy person) and regressive (e.g., to avoid or substitute superficial pleasure or relief for intimacy). Underneath every regressive wish, the authors posited, lies abandoned, lost, or shattered progressive wishes. When psychotherapy helps the client to find a progressive wish, that can change the client's fundamental view not only of relationships but also of self—and this can be comforting, a source of relational security, and remoralizing (Frank, 1971).

To help the client to achieve this shift from seeing only the regressive wish to recognizing their progressive wishes, psychotherapists must be able to perceive the client's inner life without blinders based on the client's transference or their own countertransference (as I discuss in detail in Chapter 6). "Understanding the countertransference can open space in therapy to deepen the therapist's understanding of the patient" (Leibovich et al., 2018, p. 235), and this, in turn, can enable the therapist to communicate more accurate and therapeutically helpful empathy for the client's inner experience from the client's point of view. In this manner, psychotherapy can be the experience of a relationship in which the other (the psychotherapist) shows authentic interest in and respect for their personal perspective without the kinds of emotional reactions that have caused them to feel hurt, doubt, and even hopelessness in previous (or current) formative relationships, and, moreover, also sees their core healthy hopes and wishes for themselves and their relationships despite their more obvious conflicts and compromises. This fundamental relational shift is posited to provide a basis for enabling the client to achieve a corrective emotional experience

(Alexander & French, 1946) that provides a new freedom from enactment of the regressive relational wishes—that is, to enable the client to choose to engage in relationships (including psychotherapy) on the basis of progressive rather than regressive wishes.

Rather than viewing a client's difficulties in engaging in meaningful self-reflection and dialogue merely as "resistance" to be overcome, it is more productive (and respectful) to view these difficulties as opportunities for the therapist to protect and guide the client in regaining self-regulation by finding new solutions for the client's core conflictual relationship issues. It is not "resistance" that the client is struggling to express but persistence in seeking solutions (despite often being communicated in surface terms as an unwillingness to seek or even hope for a solution).

From this perspective, which is consistent with the psychodynamic paradigm shift of self-psychology and its empathic valuing of the client's point of view over the therapist's or any other external perspective (Kohut & Wolf, 1978), crises in the therapy session are a twofold challenge: first, to restore the therapeutic alliance, and second, to demonstrate a genuine commitment to collaboratively assisting the client in clarifying the problem by finding solutions. When the therapist is able to identify CCRTs that reflect the client's fundamental personal goals and the problems the client is (or has historically) faced in achieving those goals, this can provide a focal point for engaging the client in productive self-reflection and thereby help the client to begin to escape the self-perpetuating trap of escalating rumination and emotional dysregulation as well as to engage in adaptive self-regulation.

From a psychodynamic perspective, this can be understood as the therapist's helping the client to engage and strengthen the client's observing ego. When people engage in self-reflection on their own emotions, beliefs (about self, relationships, the world, and the past and future), goals, conflicts, thought processes, and ways of coping and pursuing personal goals, this is the observing ego (Glickauf-Hughes et al., 1996; A. A. Miller et al., 1965; Winnicott, 1955). In a crisis or at a stuck point in psychotherapy, the core process in psychotherapy—self-reflection—has been largely displaced by emotional dysregulation. Thus, intervening to help the client to resume self-reflection can provide a fundamental shift in the client's emotional state by reframing the problem (i.e., emotional distress, despite being a legitimate concern, is interfering with the client's ability to achieve important goals), goals (i.e., to fulfill core personal wishes and hopes), and solutions (i.e., to stop and think clearly so as to access the personal knowledge and abilities needed to achieve those wishes and hopes). "An important function of the observing ego is the ability to monitor and reflect upon one's feelings, impulses, and thoughts rather than impulsively acting them out" (Glickauf-Hughes et al., 1996, p. 431). By observing inwardly rather than reacting outwardly, the client can shift from emotional reactivity to adaptive self-/emotion regulation (i.e., by attending to emotions and using them as information to guide decisions rather than reacting impulsively to them and failing to give them sufficient attention so that, like a fractious child who is not given attention and meaningful reassurance, they become unmanageable and escalate problematically).

The therapist's ability to "not behave in a reactive manner when clients express strong affects or are in crisis" (Glickauf-Hughes et al., 1996, p. 434) demonstrates to the client that the therapist can be trusted as a helpful ally and emulated as a role model when the client is feeling and expressing a sense of anger, grievance, disappointment, abandonment, hopelessness, or even betrayal, exploitation, or violation in relation to the therapist or therapy. This includes "not too quickly resort[ing] to problem solving," modeling "the observing ego function of understanding and thinking through one's strong feelings prior to taking action," and "continual self-monitoring [by the therapist] of his/her non-verbal expressions of affect . . . and speaking slowly in a calm tone of voice [to communicate] a sense of confidence about managing a problem" (Glickauf-Hughes et al., 1996, p. 434). Keys to the therapist's ability to access their own observing ego and serve as a role model for adaptive emotion regulation are recognizing and managing their own emotional reactions, including countertransference reactions, rather than enacting those reactions with the client (see Chapter 6, this volume).

Four specific techniques for engaging and strengthening the client's observing ego have been identified by Glickauf-Hughes et al. (1996). The first is to help the client clarify the nature and meaning of emotions after a cathartic (i.e., intense) expression or enactment of emotional distress. This can be done during as well as following a crisis, and is just as important when a client withdraws and mutes their expression of emotions as in cathartic discharges. It can begin with a paraphrasing of the client's expressed emotions (e.g., "I hear that you're feeling very angry right now"), but to fully engage the client in self-reflection, it is also is crucial to include the client-centered and motivational enhancement component of affirmation or validation (e.g., "It makes sense that you're feeling this way. Can you tell me more about what you're feeling and thinking about this?") and to invite the client to join in a collaborative effort to understand the problem and unfulfilled goals that are creating a core relational conflict for the client (e.g., "I'm listening carefully and take your concerns very seriously, so let's figure out what I need to understand so that I can best support you and help solve this problem"). The clarification process provides openings for the therapist to tentatively reflect to the client other emotions (e.g., "This kind of betrayal can be very hurtful and sad as well as angry-making") and meanings about self and relationships (e.g., "It sounds like you're being as critical of yourself as you are of me for letting you down, even though you've been very dedicated to our work together and you're the one who's being responsible and courageous in bringing this up"). Ultimately, clarification of emotions and their meaning and relationship to the client's core goals can reduce emotional dysregulation by reducing the anxiety that clients often feel about both having and expressing distressing feelings (e.g., "It's not easy and can feel risky to give voice to emotions, but by doing so, you're making it possible for me to better understand and help you, and you're making a very important statement that you, and what you feel, always counts").

Two related approaches to engaging and strengthening a client's observing ego are to serve as the client's auxiliary ego and to increase the client's reality testing (Glickauf-Hughes et al., 1996). These interventions involve the therapist's temporarily and tentatively (so as not to usurp or undermine the client's authority and autonomy) speaking for the client to help the client to recognize, organize, and trust what they are feeling, and how those emotions and related thoughts and impulses make sense in relation to current antecedents and consequences that are occurring in the client's life (and in the psychotherapy) as well as in relation to formative life experiences and relationships. Often best expressed in terms of "I wonder if . . .," therapists can jump-start and free up their clients' ability to stop, think, and self-reflect by extending the assistance they provide through coregulation (i.e., focusing on and expressing calm confidence and genuine interest and caring in the client and their ability to work together, and enable the client to achieve core personal goals) by coreflecting (i.e., modeling self-reflection and hypothesizing potential insights that the client might explore in reflecting on themselves).

A fourth approach to engaging and strengthening a client's observing ego points the client's attention away from self-reflection to paradoxically enable the client to increase their capacity for and motivation to engage in self-reflection. These "distancing" techniques (Glickauf-Hughes et al., 1996, pp. 437–438) seem like distractions or tangential diversions away from self-reflection, but they actually enable the client to step back mentally and emotionally from overwhelmingly intense or distressing thoughts and feelings to regain a sense of calm confidence while simultaneously gaining a fresh perspective that opens up new options for solutions that can enable the client to achieve blocked goals (i.e., reframing). Distancing can be accomplished by shifting the focus of therapeutic discussion from the client's being on the spot and having to deal with a problem immediately to being the observer. This can be done by asking the client to reflect on the problem as if it were happening to someone else (e.g., "What would you think, and what would you advise your best friend, if she was dealing with this?"), by using the Gestalt therapy empty chair technique (i.e., inviting the client to separate their conflicted feelings or thoughts about problem and have a vicarious conversation of both—or several—sides of the issues with an empty chair representing one or more of the conflictual perspectives), or by journal writing outside the session and, in subsequent psychotherapy sessions, sharing and figuring out the meaning and value of insights that arise from the writing. Distancing also can be accomplished by the hypnotherapy technique of telling a story that metaphorically encapsulates or symbolizes the client's dilemma, enabling the client to simultaneously vicariously experience and escape the problem so as to reflect on it while also being temporarily freed from the pain, pressures, and confusion actually involved (Erickson & Rossi, 1976).

In the midst of a crisis, these methods of therapeutic distancing often are not sufficiently immediate to provide the client with a sense that the therapist is affirming the seriousness of the client's concerns and willing to take action in collaboration with the client to work toward solutions. However, distancing also can be accomplished while simultaneously demonstrating to the client that the therapist is joining with and actively supporting them in resolving the problem. The therapist can do this by focusing on a careful examination with the client of the specific current circumstances that are the antecedents and consequences directly associated with emotional distress or dysregulation for the client in their life and in the psychotherapy.

Modify Modes of Relating, Communicating, and Coping

The therapist's jurisdiction is process, *not content, the process of how each [client] can achieve the hopes which the problem-solving process represents [and] to add to that process so that [clients] can resolve their own problems without further assistance. Then, each new conflict is an opportunity for every [client] to get what he wants.*

–Richard Bandler, John Grinder, and Virginia Satir (1976, pp. 155-156)

Another key principle of psychotherapy is that it should be a dialogue and not an interview or interrogation (Ford, 1984; Markowitz et al., 2020; Vohs et al., 2018). "Perhaps the most effective way in which a therapist can foster spontaneous production of material is by interviewing without asking questions . . . [and] without lengthy commentaries and elaborate reconstructions of the therapist's impressions" (Weiner, 1975, pp. 101–102). Psychotherapy fundamentally is a process of self-reflection by the client, not a test or quiz in which the client must answer questions that are determined primarily by the therapist's interests, priorities, or desire to develop a clinical formulation of the case and the client. The questions posed by the therapist should be the questions that clients are asking themselves. They may be based on the client's direct statements but also require that the therapist read between the lines and observe the implied, denied, omitted, or hidden messages that the client is nonverbally communicating or that are logical based on the client's personality and personal history as well as current circumstances. In so doing, the therapist deliberately and consistently speaks with (and not at) the client, offering (but not imposing as a challenge or test) questions that they can explore together without putting the client on the spot to answer "correctly."

To put this principle into practice, "the therapist should listen closely for words that have individual meaning and should encourage the patient to elaborate on them" (Weiner, 1975, p. 109). For example, the linguistic approach to psychotherapy emphasizes clarifying missing information but in a form that asks the client for their perspective on the matter at hand (e.g., "What does _____ mean to you?"). The behavior analytic approach to therapy uses a more fact-based format for questions (Follette et al., 2009) but emphasizes the client's perspective to help both client and therapist develop an understanding of key events and how complex situations have unfolded over time—and therefore may be modifiable when potential solutions are under consideration (e.g., "How did that actually happen? What happened next?").

In addition to listening carefully to and seeking to empathically (i.e., from the client's point of view; Wolf, 1993) understand the client's specific words and phrases, it also is essential to listen for and "call . . . attention to what is not stated" (Weiner, 1975, p. 110). This can take the form of information that logically fits with what the client is describing but had omitted (i.e., what linguistic-based therapists refer to as deletions and missing referential indices; see the later section, Linguistically Focused Systemic Psychotherapy). As emphasized by experiential/emotion-focused approaches to therapy (Fisher, 2020; Fosha et al., 2009), this also can take the form of emotions, attitudes, and thoughts that are expressed via body language or vocally but nonverbally (e.g., tone of voice, inflection, emphasis, pacing of speech). And, from the perspective of somatosensory psychotherapies (Fisher, 2020; Ogden, 2020), physical movements (both macro- and micro-) and symptoms, such as pain, exhaustion, tension, unintended movements, or lack of mobility, and difficulties with basic bodily functions, such as sight, hearing, eating, or sleep, can speak volumes without words. Everything the client communicates directly, indirectly, and by omission is potentially important for the therapist to understand and to help the client to understand.

Systemic Psychotherapy

Crises in psychotherapy occur in the context of relationships—both the client's relationships outside of therapy and the client–therapist relationship. The family is a prototypical network of relationships that are interconnected in ways that parallel the workings of living and mechanical systems. Systemic psychotherapies (Ford, 2020b; Goldenberg et al., 2017) capitalize on these parallels to help therapists and clients to understand and change relationships that have an impact on the client (and in which the client impacts others). In crises and at stuck points, relationships often are dysregulated, both reflecting and contributing to the emotional dysregulation that the client is experiencing. Informing the client about the systemic processes that occur in key relationships and assisting the client in navigating and initiating or responding to changes in their relationships can be vital in a crisis. Five systemic processes are of particular relevance: coalitions, boundaries, triangles, rules, and secrets (Giacomo & Weissmark, 1987; Goldenberg et al., 2017; Kantor & Neal, 1985).

Relational Coalitions. Families and other groups (e.g., friends, coworkers, teammates, community or faith-based organization members) often spontaneously divide into subgroups. When subgroups form as a means of including some people and excluding others, whether purposively or inadvertently, this can lead to ingroup/outgroup or us-versus-them conflict and discrimination or stigmatization of people who are either in or out of a subgroup. The people in each subgroup tend to band together initially based on some shared goals or interests but, over time, become increasingly in an adversarial relationship to nonmembers or to other subgroups. These subgroups thus are coalitions of people bound together by a common purpose or identity and competing with and intent on maintaining separation from other groups or individual nonmembers (Goldenberg et al., 2017; Minuchin, 1999). Being included in a relational coalition can lead to problems, emotional dysregulation, and crises or stuck points in psychotherapy, as can being excluded from a coalition.

For example, a client's family relationships might be such that she and her father are extremely emotionally close, but both feel estranged from the client's mother and brother (who, in turn, have a close emotional bond with each other). This family has subdivided into two dyadic coalitions, which also have the added complication of being intergenerational (i.e., father–daughter and mother–son). The coalitions were not formed intentionally and are not explicitly acknowledged among the family members but are informally accepted by the client as "just the way things worked out with the differences in our personalities." This client might experience a number of stressors as a result of these unspoken structural ties and divisions in her primary family relationships, for example, emotional over-involvement, a sense of dependency, and anxiety about any potential conflict with or separation from her father; self-doubts about her self-concept, identity, and roles as a woman because of feeling emotionally disconnected from or in conflict with her mother; difficulty in developing or trusting close relationships with peers as a result of having a primary relational focus on being a "child" in relation to an adult (her father) and having an unfamiliar feeling with or estrangement from the one member of her peer group in her family (her brother). If stressors occur in this client's life that activate and intensify those relational stressors (e.g., having a falling out with her father, her mother and father divorcing, becoming involved in a romantic relationship with a person who reminds her of her father but who also can be emotionally distant like her brother), this could precipitate or play an important role in a crisis or in the client's feeling stuck and withdrawing from the therapy. The coalitions also could be a source of strong transference reactions to her therapist (e.g., if she idealizes the therapist in ways similar to her feelings toward her father while also being critical based on similarities she perceives between the therapist and her mother), which might lead to or exacerbate a crisis or stuck point, especially if the therapist disappoints her or seems to her to be abandoning her (e.g., announcing a change in their scheduled appointments or an increase in the fee).

Relational Boundaries. The psychological and physical boundaries separating people are important to preserve the autonomy and unique identity of each individual as well as each person's privacy and safety. Boundaries, however, can lead to isolation when they close off desired contact and can lead to conflict if they are defended aggressively (Minuchin, 1982). When boundaries are so open that a person can be psychologically or physically intruded on or imposed on with little or no recourse, this can result in relationships that are coercive or enmeshed and, as a result, undermine the individual's sense of self, safety, and control as well as subject the individual to intimidation, devaluation, exploitation, neglect, betrayal, violation, and exhaustion. In crises in psychotherapy, an absence or loss of relational boundary integrity both outside of therapy and in the client–therapist relationship (either directly, if a therapist does not maintain professionally appropriate and therapeutically attuned boundaries, or indirectly, if a client has transference reactions based on boundary problems in external relationships) often play a role and are an important potential focus for resolving the crisis.

For example, the client described in the previous section is likely to have some degree of enmeshment in her relationship with her father, which could take the form of subtle emotional pressures to live up to his standards or meet some of the emotional needs he doesn't feel his wife is meeting, or could be as severe as paternal emotional, physical, or sexual abuse. The client's boundaries with her mother and brother, on the other hand, are likely to be overly rigid and impermeable, such that she might have difficulty accepting, or even recognizing, genuine love, affection, or respect and appreciation from either of them, while also reducing the likelihood that they would be able to develop or maintain, let alone communicate, those feelings to her because she has persistently denied having any positive feelings in her interactions with both of them. This combination of enmeshment and detachment in formative family relationships can play out across the full spectrum of other relationships, leaving the client vulnerable to many relational complications (e.g., difficulty in tolerating either emotional closeness or separation, fears of both being vulnerable and exposed to hurt or being isolated and shut out emotionally). A host of CCRTs can develop as a result of compromised or problematic relational boundaries, which, in turn, can contribute to or exacerbate crises and stuck points in therapy.

Triangulation. Many relationships involve more than two people, as do all relational networks, such as families, work or faith-based groups, teams, friendship circles, and entire communities. Relationships are essentially dyadic on a psychological level because it is not possible psychobiologically for humans to multitask. (We can shift attention rapidly between multiple foci, which simulates but does not actually achieve true simultaneous multitasking.) However, every dyadic relationship also exists in a larger context of a network of interconnected relationships. Although all complex relational networks can be complicated, the three-person network has proven to be particularly problematic. Visually, it can be depicted as a triangle with each individual having a connection to the other two people. Relational triangles can have a synergistic effect and heighten the benefits that accrue in each of the three dyadic pairs if none of the dyads devolves into a coalition and the boundaries within and between each dyad provide a balance of closeness and separateness. However, if coalitions form or the boundaries are excessively open or closed, dyadic relationships can devolve into triangulation.

Triangulation is a condition in which two people use a third person as their go-between (Davis, 1961; Pam & Pearson, 1994). That third person is caught in the middle. This can take the form of two people each going to a third person to complain about or play out conflict with each other (i.e., the middle person is caught in two adversarial coalitions). Or, two people can gang up on a third, displacing conflict between them (or between them and other people) onto the third person. Or, the triangle may be based on the three people adopting interconnected roles that perpetuate psychological and relational problems, such as the drama triangle involving a victim, a persecutor, and a rescuer (who also may be an enabler; Nichols & Davis, 2020). As the emotional strain of being caught in an interpersonal triangle grows over time, crises or stuck points in therapy can emerge.

For example, several triangles may have developed in the family in which there are two coalitions (father–daughter/client; mother–son) and multiple boundary issues. The client and her father might play out conflicts between themselves, which they want to minimize so as to preserve their sense of closeness with each other by each engaging in arguments with either the mother or brother instead. If the client or her brother experiences problems in their respective dyadic coalitions (e.g., brother feels frustrated with their mother), they might put aside their past estrangement and take their complaints or hurts to their sibling for support or collusion. If the client or her brother develops substance abuse problems, the parent with whom they are enmeshed could take on the role of the rescuer while the other parent might be critical of both the adult child and of their spouse (i.e., the role of the persecutor). If these triangulated relationships are contributing to or being played out in a crisis or a stuck point in therapy, the therapist is best able to intervene constructively if aware of the impact that triangulation is having on the client and able to recognize and therapeutically work through any transferences of the triangulation into the client–therapist relationship. For example, the client might shut down or withdraw from therapy if she perceives the therapist as a persecutor or as not nurturing and triangulates by complaining to her father about the therapist instead of bringing up those concerns directly with the therapist.

Relational Rules. Expectations develop, grow, change, and also die over time as a relationship evolves, and most of these expectations are implicit and unstated—but emotionally powerful. The unstated but consistently enacted expectations in a relationship have been described as the rules of the relational system (Lederer & Jackson, 1968). Relational rules can be beneficial when they promote harmonious core relationship themes (e.g., mutual respect, valuing of individual differences, honesty, kindness). However, as relationships are adapted when people experience stressors and difficulties in their lives, relational rules can become a source of conflict, hurt, disappointment, and ultimately of emotional dysregulation and crises. Implicit relational rules often spill over into the therapist–client relationship because they are so second nature that they are readily transferable. Crises and stuck points in psychotherapy thus often hinge on or at least involve some degree of influence by unspoken rules that the client brings from other relationships into the therapist–client interaction. Key options for crisis management are explicitly stating the rule and helping the client to recognize it to determine whether and how the rule is applicable to the current problem or crisis—in the therapy as well as in the client's outside life—and to decide whether to modify or adapt the rule, or how best to prevent the rule from leading to problems in those relationships and to emotional distress.

For example, the client described in this section might be bringing several unstated rules from her formative experiences in family relationships into her current life and relationships, including with her therapist. She might believe, without consciously articulating those beliefs, the following:

- Feelings cannot be expressed; this only leads to rejection of falling apart emotionally.

- It's the two of us against the world; the only person who really loves me and whom I can trust is my father.

- Some people are important and others are worthless, and I'm afraid I'm worthless.

- Women should sublimate their desires and aspirations to not show up men in their life.

- If you just don't like someone, it's not worth it to try to have a relationship with them.

- Happy families are all alike; every unhappy family is unhappy in its own way.

Relational Secrets and Myths. A final linchpin for the systemic approach to therapy is the concept that all relationships have secrets and myths that limit the options and can adversely affect the ability of their members to find fulfillment in the relationship and in their lives (Giacomo & Weissmark, 1987; Kantor & Neal, 1985). These can be deeply hidden secrets, but often they are either supposedly hidden but are actually in plain sight or they are known by the client and are a source of emotional distress because of the burden of holding the secret or of being a truth-teller who reveals it and faces condemnation for that act. The myths in relationships tend to be either repetitively told and retold stories about actual (or semimythical) family experiences and family members who exemplify the family's rules while also keeping embarrassing or morally conflictual truths about the family past and present hidden. When clients describe family relationships and formative experiences, they often inadvertently (and sometimes intentionally, as a form of testimony or confession) reveal secrets and myths that are sources of distress and, like relational rules, tend to be viewed as "just the way things are" and not subject to change in the client's current life and across all of their relationships. As such, secrets and myths can come to define, dominate, and constrain people's sense of self, how relationships work (or fail), and what the future holds within and outside of the family.

Identifying the influence of a relational secret or myth when a crisis or stuck point occurs in therapy—as a potential contributing factor but not as the main or only problem—can enable the client to recognize both the influence that the secret or myth has had in their life and that it might be possible to not be burdened by continuing to hold the secret or to perpetuate the myth. This can help to transform crises and stuck points into an opportunity to make changes—albeit with caution and careful planning and support—that increase personal freedom and open up new possibilities in relationships and for the future that had been closed off by the secret or myth.

Linguistically Focused Systemic Psychotherapy

Systemic psychotherapists joined with a linguist to extend the insights of systemic psychotherapy by focusing on the intricacies of moment-to-moment communication between people. They identified several specific ways in which communication can appear meaningful on the surface but actually have gaps and inaccuracies in its deeper structure (i.e., the meaning or meanings sent and received)—"distortions" (Bandler et al., 1976). In crises and stuck points in psychotherapy, these communication distortions often contribute to confusion and trigger emotional dysregulation.

> The therapist's task is *not* to say who is right or who is wrong; it is not his domain to arrange a compromise. The resolution of the problem is not the main

task of the therapist. Even if this problem is resolved, the . . . communication which caused this problem will just produce another one. The task of the therapist, then, is to break the . . . communication loops and to provide an environment for learnings about what choices and resources the [clients] have which they can use to solve *any* specific problems. (Bandler et al., 1976, p. 156)

When communication distortions are identified and clarified in the therapeutic dialogue, this can enable the client to regain trust and security in the therapist and the therapeutic alliance, clarity in defining the problem and their goals and potential solutions both in therapy and in their broader life and relationships, and confidence and hope in themselves and their future.

Integrative Psychotherapy

Briere (2019) drew on a wide array of "well-established treatment approaches, ranging from psychodynamic psychotherapy and interpersonal therapy to dialectical behavior therapy, mindfulness training, and exposure therapy" and "philosophies that focus on increasing self-determination, empowerment, skills development, and psychological growth, and that deemphasize pathology-based perspectives" (p. 3). The focus in this integrative approach is on preventing and resolving crises in psychotherapy by enhancing emotion regulation, increasing attachment security and hope, maintaining the therapeutic relationship, communicating nonjudgmental acceptance, and avoid controlling or confrontational therapist behavior (Briere, 2019; Lyon et al., 2014; Weisz et al., 2012). Examples of specific tactics include the following:

- trigger reduction (Briere, 2019, p. 72) involving assisting the client in planning and implementing practical changes that reduce exposure to situations that trigger emotional dysregulation

- proactive resilience (Briere, 2019, p. 73) involving engaging the client in developing a physically health-promoting lifestyle (e.g., diet, exercise, sleep) and getting needed health care

- relaxation and breathing techniques

- grounding (i.e., mindful present-focused awareness of self and environment)

- self-soothing and strategic distraction activities

- positive self-talk

- mindful self-awareness, metacognitive awareness (i.e., that symptoms are transient and changeable experiences, and recognizing but not acting on impulsive urges; Briere, 2019, pp. 86–87)

Briere (2019, p. 99) also provided a sequential guide for managing and preventing distress reduction behaviors that parallels the FREEDOM (focusing, recognizing triggers, emotion awareness, evaluating thoughts, defining goals and options, making a contribution; see the Introduction) sequence for self-regulation that I describe in Chapter 5. The acronym, ReGAIN, involves the following five steps that clients as well as therapists can use:

1. **Re**cognize that you are triggered.
2. **G**round yourself.
3. **A**llow yourself to experience whatever is coming up with self-compassion.
4. **I**nvestigate how you are triggered and why the triggers are so upsetting.
5. **N**onidentify by recalling that triggered thoughts, emotions, or memories are just experiences.

In the case vignettes and psychotherapy session transcripts in Chapters 7 through 12, these integrative techniques often are used and are seamlessly interwoven into the therapeutic dialogue as aids for the client in managing and reducing the distress and emotional dysregulation that underlies each crisis or stuck point. These techniques also assist the therapist in maintaining or regaining self-regulation when experiencing their own emotional dysregulation and countertransference.

CONCLUSION

Psychotherapy offers many valuable tools for crisis prevention and resolution. Before we turn to case vignettes illustrating the application of those tools in psychotherapy sessions, in Chapter 5, I propose a concise seven-step approach to handling crisis in the psychotherapy session based on the essential principles and practices of both crisis intervention and psychotherapy. Then, in Chapter 6, I turn our attention to the user of the tools—the therapist—and specifically to a crucial double-edged sword—the therapist's countertransference reactions.

5

AN INTEGRATIVE APPROACH TO RESOLVING CRISES IN THE PSYCHOTHERAPY SESSION

In crises, clearly no one size will fit all clients when it comes to how the therapist can best assist the client in regaining or attaining self-regulation and a sense of hope and motivation to continue in psychotherapy (or to live, in the case of acutely suicidal clients). However, therapists do need a practical structure to guide them in systematically applying the principles of crisis intervention (Chapter 3) and psychotherapy (Chapter 4) while flexibly responding to assist each unique client in crisis. Therefore, in this chapter, I describe a step-by-step template designed to provide structure while also enabling the therapist to take an individualized approach to helping clients in crisis to restore self-regulation (Ford, 2020c).

That template, described by the acronym FREEDOM (focusing, recognizing triggers, emotion awareness, evaluating thoughts, defining goals and options, making a contribution; see the more complete description in the Introduction to this volume), is the organizing framework and skill set for an empirically supported psychotherapy designed to treat complex traumatic stress disorders: Trauma Affect Regulation: Guide for Education and Therapy

https://doi.org/10.1037/0000225-006
Crises in the Psychotherapy Session: Transforming Critical Moments Into Turning Points, by J. D. Ford

(TARGET; Ford, 2020c; see also Ford et al., 2011, 2012, 2013; Ford, Grasso, Greene, et al., 2018; Ford, Grasso, Levine, & Tennen, 2018; Ford & Hawke, 2012; Marrow et al., 2012). The TARGET model of therapeutic intervention includes psychoeducation about how the brain and body adapt to stress, and how those adaptations can result in symptoms of anxiety, depression, posttraumatic stress disorder, and other emotional and behavioral disorders. In the TARGET model, therapists help the client to understand how they can apply this knowledge using the step-by-step FREEDOM process to shift out of the state of emotional dysregulation and achieve a state of adaptive emotion regulation. The FREEDOM framework has proven applicable for clients and psychotherapists who are dealing with a wide variety of complex psychiatric and psychosocial problems, including acute crises (Ford, 2020c).

In addition, the FREEDOM framework was developed to map onto the core principles of both crisis intervention and psychotherapy that have been discussed in the previous two chapters. The FREEDOM steps follow the crisis intervention process by helping clients to progress from regaining safety and stability to becoming aware of emotional dysregulation, and then helping them to regain adaptive emotion regulation to ultimately be able to engage in productive problem-solving and accessing of resources. In line with the first core principle of psychotherapy, the FREEDOM steps provide the therapist with an approach to engaging empathically with the client in a collaborative relationship that highlights and draws on the client's personal strengths and competencies. Consistent with the second core principle of psychotherapy, the FREEDOM framework enables the therapist to nonjudgmentally help clients to recognize the specific ways in which chronic and acute stress reactivity have led to the affective and cognitive disruptions that create emotional dysregulation, and to recover emotions and beliefs that are based on their core values and provide a foundation for regaining adaptive emotion regulation. In line with the third core principle—the systemic principle that psychotherapy is a dialogue that facilitates self-reflection and adaptive engagement in relationships (Ford, 2020b)—the FREEDOM steps engage clients in a deliberate process of open-minded and rigorous self-reflection and reevaluation of how they can make a positive contribution to key relationships by becoming genuinely emotionally regulated. Thus, the FREEDOM framework represents an effort to consolidate the core principles of both crisis intervention and psychotherapy into a single, practical template to guide therapeutic engagement with clients throughout the course of therapy, but, of particular relevance here, when crises occur.

OVERVIEW OF FREEDOM

The psychoeducation that serves as the foundation for FREEDOM is based on research on three areas in the brain that coordinate stress reactions (Wheelock et al., 2018):

- an alarm signaling the presence of a situation requiring attention and corrective action (represented by the amygdala)

- a contextual memory filing (i.e., encoding and retrieval) center (represented by the hippocampus)

- an executive thinking (i.e., knowledge generation and organization, decision making and planning) center (represented by the prefrontal cortex)

The introductory psychoeducation in the TARGET shows how, optimally, these brain centers seamlessly interconnect and form a self-correcting system (see Figure 5.1). The brain's alarm activates the body's autonomic nervous system and the stress hormones that create the stress response. The brain's memory filing center retrieves information from memories to provide a map for reacting to the stressor based on lessons learned from life experiences and transmits this information to the executive thinking center for analysis. Then the brain's executive thinking center translates the memories or information into conscious knowledge and formulates decisions and action plans. The executive center completes the circuit by resetting the alarm to signal that the stressor has been handled. The alarm then signals the body to reset.

Although self-regulation is more complex than stress management alone and involves other areas throughout the brain, a coordinated stress response among these three brain centers is the foundation for self-regulation:

- physiologically: by adjusting the body's levels of activation to mobilize when necessary and relax, reset, and rejuvenate as a counterbalance

- emotionally: by recognizing and finding meaning in emotions when the executive center translates salience input from the alarm and contextual input from the memory filing center into conscious and verbally mediated awareness of emotion states

- cognitively: by formulating meaning, goals, decisions, and action plans in the executive center based on the input from the alarm and memory filing centers

FIGURE 5.1. Normal Stress: The Brain and Body Working Together

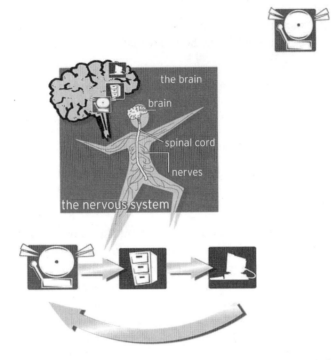

Note. From *Trauma Affect Regulation: Guide for Education and Therapy (TARGET) Manual–Adult/Adolescent Individual* (p. 5), by J. D. Ford, 2001. Copyright 2001 by the University of Connecticut. Reprinted with permission.

- relationally: by translating physiological, affective, and cognitive input from the body, alarm, and memory filing center into executive-center-mediated motivations, goals, plans, and actions that are communicated in relationships

- identity: by translating physiological, affective, and cognitive input from the body, alarm, and memory filing center into executive-center-mediated self-concepts

On the other hand, when the cycle linking these three brain centers is not completed and stressors continue to trigger the brain's alarm without this crucial resetting, the brain's alarm can essentially hijack the memory and executive systems (and the body) in what is experienced as an unresolved stress reactivity, which can lead to emotional dysregulation and ultimately escalate into a crisis in life or in psychotherapy (Ford & Wortmann, 2013; see Figure 5.2).

FIGURE 5.2. Extreme Stress/Trauma: The Alarm Takes Control

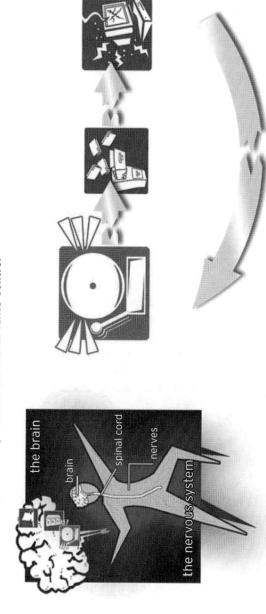

Note. From *Trauma Affect Regulation: Guide for Education and Therapy (TARGET) Manual–Adult/Adolescent Individual* (p. 5), by J. D. Ford, 2001. Copyright 2001 by the University of Connecticut. Reprinted with permission.

The FREEDOM template provides a step-by-step process to activate the brain's thinking and memory filing centers and reset a hyperaroused alarm. The sequence is based on empirical research demonstrating that self-regulation requires (a) awareness of bodily states, maintenance of bodily arousal within a window of tolerance (i.e., neither too intense nor numbed or dissociated); (b) recognition and inhibition of impulsive emotional reactions and triggers; (c) awareness of one's own emotion states and tolerance of distress; (d) translation of feelings into thoughts to make meaning; (e) translation of emotions and thoughts into self-enhancing prosocial goals; (f) formulation and enactment of behavioral choices consistent with the prosocial goals; and (g) positive self-perceptions based on a sense of personal control and efficacy (Ford, 2020c).

Correspondingly, the FREEDOM framework involves seven steps: (a) choosing a core personal value or commitment that serves as an initial focal point (called an orienting thought); (b) recognizing triggers that set off the alarm (i.e., both external stimuli and contexts as well as internal physiological states); followed by reappraisal in four domains, including (c) emotion awareness; (d) evaluation of thoughts and beliefs; (e) defining goals and motivations; and (f) option identification (i.e., plans and behaviors); and a final integrative step; (g) making a contribution. This final step involves heightening awareness of how being self-regulated not only can lead to personal gains but also makes the world a better place for everyone whose lives one's own touches.

Rather than attempting to eliminate or replace reactive physiological responses, emotions, thoughts, goals, and behaviors, the FREEDOM framework validates the importance of these "alarm" reactions and engages the person in reflection on the adaptive aspects of each reaction (i.e., drawing on the brain's memory filing and thinking centers). Let's see how this framework is put into practice as a guide to real-time crisis intervention in the psychotherapy session.

STEP 1: PROTECTING SAFETY AND SHIFTING TO PRESENT-CENTERED FOCUSING

The first priority in a crisis is client safety, with the safety of the therapist a close second. Taking steps to guard against any immediate in-session physical danger or imminent extra-session threat to a client's life or health is the most immediate concern. The therapist's physical safety both in and outside the session also is paramount. The psychological safety of both clients and the therapist is the next priority, requiring a careful but rapid assessment of the immediate situation and interaction to identify actual or potential sources of covert as well as overt emotional abuse, verbal aggression devaluation, exploitation, or identity-based microaggressions that need to be called out and stopped—including those that the therapist is knowingly or unwittingly engaging in by acts of omission as well as commission. Establishing or regaining a context of safety begins the process of shifting to a present-centered focus by temporarily setting aside all but the most immediate concerns and experiences occurring in the therapy in order to be fully in the moment. The larger context of the past and future remains a crucial backdrop at this initial stage of dealing with a crisis, but the immediate interaction as well as the client's and therapist's immediate experience both internally (e.g., immediate bodily reactions, emotions, thoughts, goals, actions) and in their interaction are the starting point for resolving the nascent crisis.

Protecting Safety

The critical first concern in any crisis is focusing rapidly on ensuring the physical and emotional safety of the client and others. In the context of psychotherapy sessions, this includes ensuring the safety of the therapist, the client and significant others in the client's life, or other people who may be affected by the client's actions (i.e., including office staff or colleagues). Protecting safety obviously begins with safety in the moment, which warrants a clear, immediate statement from the therapist; for example:

> We've both/all agreed to first focus on making sure that we are all safe here together. Is anything happening here, or has anything happened in this therapy, that is making you/anyone feel unsafe right now? If there is, we need to deal with it immediately so that you feel safe to continue.

Safety in the moment may also require an immediate intervention by the therapist to de-escalate clients' actions that pose an immediate or imminent threat to self or others (i.e., with a client who has brought a weapon into the session and is threatening to use it or one who is threatening to assault the therapist or others or who is holding others hostage). Intervention may include verbal statements or nonverbal actions to reaffirm limits on behavior that is potentially acutely dangerous, such as aggressive actions toward others or self; immediate negotiation regarding turning over a weapon or agreeing to not engage in physical violence; or immediate negotiation for the release of any hostages. Maintaining a stance of calm and reason as well as remaining in visual and vocal or auditory contact with the client while sustaining a comfortable degree of physical proximity and distance communicates to a severely dysregulated client relational availability and respect for the client's need for space, and, in the process, maintains a nonintrusive and nonadversarial psychological connection to the client. Physical confrontation and restraint are a choice of absolutely last resort only when there is no other way to offset harm; however, it is a strategy that risks inadvertently increasing harm to the client and therapist. Moreover, with previously traumatized clients, it can create an unintended reenactment of clients' memories of traumatic physical or sexual assault, entrapment, domination, or violation, and thus further dysregulate them.

Intense escalation of anger or implosion of despair often are drivers of potential or actual aggression or other unsafe behaviors. When anger reaches or approaches the point of a dangerous explosion or despair reaches or nears a shutdown by the client, it is likely that the client is experiencing intense dissociation as well as distress. This can involve feeling as though they cannot think clearly enough to have control over their actions—as if possessed by out-of-control emotions and impulses, that is, a state of depersonalization or derealization, or the emergence of acute identity fragmentation ("It's as if someone else inside me takes control"). Intervening to preserve safety and prevent harm thus often begins with assisting the client in reorienting to the present in remembering their values, including valuing their own and other people's safety. Rather than attempting to directly suppress the client's distress or impulsive behavior, the therapist's focus is instead on helping the client to restore security and safety in the moment by reorienting their attention to their bodily state and to a single guiding thought that they find reassuring (e.g., "I'm with a therapist whom I trust, and together we are safe").

Being able to maintain safety may also depend on the client's external situation. When external conditions threaten a client's safety or the safety of someone else and it is within the client's ability to either prevent or mitigate that harm, a key first priority in session is for the therapist to affirm both that core goal and—with the support of the therapist as an active partner—the client's ability to achieve it. For example, the therapist might say,

> You're courageously facing and dealing with a relationship that has become dangerously violent and that can feel overwhelming. We need to put everything else aside and together make a safety plan that starts right now and that includes how I and others can assist you so that you're not alone with this.

Exactly what that safety plan will be is unique to each individual, although it always involves universal precautions, including specific plans to prevent revictimization; engage appropriate private and public resources; and preserve or restore the client's control of their own body, relationships, decisions, and life choices. The safety plan is not put aside at this point but instead is carefully considered and (when relevant) referred to explicitly and woven into each of the remaining steps in crisis intervention to ensure that there is no imminent danger or that the best possible protections are in place if imminent danger is unavoidable.

Although physical assaults or other seriously destructive behavior is rare in most psychotherapy settings, it is important for therapists to know that they can and do occur up to and including the murder of the therapist, or an estranged spouse/partner, or both, in a couple session. Numerous protocols have been developed for systematic prevention or management of violence (Price & Baker, 2012), although the evidence is limited that training in these techniques actually lead to not only knowledge and confidence but also to effective acute violence prevention (Price et al., 2015). In addition, evidence of their effectiveness with nonpsychotic (Spencer et al., 2018) and psychotic (Du et al., 2017) aggression also is limited. With every client, it is important for the therapist to be prepared with proactive safety precautions if there is any history of violence or risk by the client either within or outside of therapeutic contexts. If such history is the case, a clear (and nonjudgmental) statement is important by the therapist to affirm—and to get a confirmation of full agreement from the client—that physical violence is out of bounds in the therapy setting to ensure the safety of all parties. It is helpful for therapists to have developed a professional safety plan (e.g., a panic button or other signaling system to alert colleagues or security personnel of the need for immediate assistance as part of their office practices), yet many do not have such a plan. In the event a plan is in place, the therapist who assesses that physical violence is an imminent possibility should operationalize it by taking measured steps to protect the safety of everyone involved while also attempting to de-escalate the potentially violent client.

Shifting to Present-Centered Focusing

A defining feature of crises is the loss of homeostasis, including a loss of orientation to time, place, and current circumstances. Ruminative perseveration on past frustrations, disappointments, and injuries is typical as are preoccupation with anxiety and a sense of hopelessness about the future. Therefore, helping the client to shift as soon as possible from this state of distress and confusion to a achieve a clear and mindful focus on the present moment is of critical importance. Joining with the client sets the stage for this shift because through the act of validating the client's goals and affirming the intention to actively assist them in achieving those goals, the therapist has already shifted the focus of the therapeutic interaction to the immediate present. The message that is metacommunicated is: "I am here with you, and together we can find a way to take steps to make things better, starting now."

Encouraging and modeling a present-centered focus builds on and extends the process of joining with the client—in "coming back into the room" even while still experiencing distress or hopelessness. The act of intentionally refocusing in the present moment on bodily state, emotions, and thoughts as well as of the other person or people and the nature of the relationship shared with them can begin to restore the physiological and psychological balance that has become disrupted. Mindful, present-focused awareness may be facilitated by grounding techniques that assist the client in recognizing and nonjudgmentally interpreting stress reactions in their body and emotions as useful information or as guides toward solutions (or steps to solutions) to the otherwise apparently unsolvable problems at the core of the crisis. These techniques include helping the client to use physical awareness and the presence of the therapist to bring their arousal level within a window of tolerability. They also include helping the client to shift from feeling confused and flooded with or devoid of sensations, emotions, and thoughts to a position of being in the role of an actively reflective observer and problem solver.

In addition to encouraging the client to engage in and facilitate present-centered focusing, having a present-centered focus also is an immediate priority for the therapist. Psychotherapy involves constant attention by the therapist to simultaneous dual process their own internal state of body and mind along with that of the client—and of the client's degree of self-awareness or lack thereof. The therapist must consciously maintain present-centered self-awareness and unobtrusively self-regulate their own bodily state, emotions, and internal cognitive narrative in a manner that directly parallels the client's present-centered mindfulness. By virtue of their training and role, therapists are in a position to maintain—or relatively rapidly regain—self-awareness, self-regulation, and an inner sense of calm. Although therapists can't simply snap their fingers and achieve optimal self-awareness and self-regulation, they can purposefully focus their attention on their own inner state while also monitoring their client.

As such, the most immediate and powerful way the therapist can assist a client in crisis in (re)gaining a present awareness is by serving as a role model for self-awareness and self-regulation, and intentionally monitoring and modulating their own internal physiological and emotional balance and sense of calm. Of course, particularly when interacting with a client who is in crisis, this does not mean that the therapist can, or should, maintain a constant state of calm imperturbability. Instead, the therapist's willingness and ability to reset physiologically and psychologically when thrown off balance in crisis interactions (as in all other psychotherapy encounters) provides the client with immediate tangible evidence that mindful, present-centered self-awareness are desirable and achievable goals (and by extension, awareness that the therapist and the psychotherapy session can provide genuine safety and support).

The focusing step in TARGET's FREEDOM—specifically the SOS template, described as follows—provides a concise practical approach for therapists to intervene to protect safety and establish (or restore) present-centered reflective awareness by themselves as well as on the part of the client in crisis. SOS stands for the following:

- **S**lowing down and sweeping the mind clear: These intentional acts may seem paradoxical in a crisis; yet this is exactly what first responders often report intuitively doing when in an emergency. Slowing down does not mean acting slowly; rather, it refers to slowing the flood of information that must be processed and sifting through it to sweep away all but the most crucial data. It also means intentionally paying attention to the external environment and to one's internal (bodily) status and reactions. As a result, it is possible for the therapist to be acutely aware of the most crucial focal points in the external environment that will determine the safety (or lack thereof) of the client and the therapist. Simultaneously, the therapist is tuned into signals from their own body as it "keeps the score" (van der Kolk, 2014, p. 1) so they can use stress reactions either warning signs or resources for responding in a timely and emotionally regulated manner to the client's distress.

- **O**rienting to a thought involving safety: In an acute crisis, safety is the most important thought to which a therapist must be paying full attention. Using safety as an orienting thought increases the therapist's ability to maintain a steady focus on this goal while reducing the distraction that could be caused if other thoughts, emotions, or goals are allowed to supersede safety. Focusing on safety as the orienting thought also can increase the therapist's ability to stay on message in communicating with the client; nothing is more important at that moment than ensuring that everyone, especially (but not only) the client, is safe. Doing so can prevent extraneous reactions or messages from confusing or overloading the client with information that inadvertently escalates their sense of being unsafe or otherwise unable to trust that the therapist has their best interests at heart.

- **S**elf-checking one's stress level and level of personal control: Performing this self-check can facilitate crucial internal calibration by the therapist ("Does my stress level indicate that this is more or less imminently dangerous or out of control than I've been thinking?" "Independent of how stressful this is for me, am I thinking clearly?"). It also can remind the therapist to communicate to the client a nonjudgmental validation of the stress the client is experiencing and expressing, and is a nonjudgmental reminder and support for the client in maintaining or regaining personal control despite the stress.

STEP 2: JOINING AND PARTNERING COLLABORATIVELY

Joining and collaborative partnering may seem incompatible with a therapist's responsibility to take charge on behalf of the client's and their own safety in a crisis. However, restoring the dysregulated client's ability to self-regulate and think clearly depends on restoring that client's sense of security in a true partnership with the therapist. That security depends on knowing that the therapist recognizes and takes seriously the severity of the dilemma(s) that the client is experiencing, which begins by the therapist's clearly and authentically acknowledging the triggers that are creating the sense of desperation for their client and the intense emotions that the client is experiencing as a result. Recognizing triggers and acknowledging emotions therefore are the second and third steps in the FREEDOM template. There also is a cognitive dimension to joining and partnering, which is reflected in the FREEDOM template's second "E" step, evaluating thoughts: As triggers are identified and emotions are expressed, thoughts about the meaning of those triggers and emotions naturally arise and provide an additional basis for joining with the client. Those three steps in FREEDOM thus provide a basis for the therapist to join and begin (or resume) collaboratively partnering with the client who is in crisis. Ultimately, as you will see, fully restoring the collaborative partnership also requires an active affirmation of support for the client's core goals, which involves applying the FREEDOM "D" step of defining goals.

Joining

The most prevalent threat to safety in the psychotherapy context is the potential emotional threat of a rupture in the therapeutic relationship (Eubanks, Burckell, & Goldfried, 2018). Establishing a strong and secure therapeutic alliance is the single best way to prevent ruptures from developing into (or fueling and exacerbating) emotional or relational crises in the therapy. The therapeutic alliance also is based on identifying transference themes and reactions based on a client's unique history, personality, and circumstances—and developing and communicating an empathic and nonjudgmental understanding of these issues and their often subtle or unrecognized early warning signs with regard to their emergence as a crisis. With this foundation, which is ever a work in progress, by reaffirming the intention to support the client, the therapist can join and reengage psychologically in the psychotherapy session with a distressed or dissociated client who is at an early, middle, or an emergency or breakdown stage of crisis.

Calmly and firmly reaffirming the partnership and steadfast intention to provide support of the client is of particular importance with those who are experiencing (or have previously experienced) significant betrayal and abandonment by significant others (Freyd, 1994) or psychologically primitive or regressive self-states and transference reactions (Kohut & Wolf, 1978). Even the highest functioning client may experience episodes of critical distress and disorientation as well as a crisis of confidence in relation to the therapist (Levy et al., 2018; Slade & Holmes, 2019). Crises in psychotherapy tend to involve an intense disorganization of the client's attachment working models that can escalate into dissociation (Lahav & Elklit, 2016) or impulsive acts of aggression (toward self as well as toward the therapist or others; Critchfield et al., 2008; Fossati et al., 2009). By taking a stance of active and empathic joining, and active nonjudgmental reassurance, the therapist can reassure the client that together, they can resolve the crisis.

Joining with a client in crisis begins with clearly acknowledging the seriousness of the triggers that the client is facing and attuning to and affirming the client's emotions (Fosha et al., 2009; Greenberg & Pascual-Leone, 2006; Paivio, 2013). In a crisis, the emotions that the client is most aware of are negative or numbed emotions, which in the TARGET framework are considered to be reactive emotions linked to the inner alarm. Of course, those emotions are the product of complex interactions between multiple systems within the brain and body as well as external interpersonal interactions between the client and many other people (past and present), including the therapist. However, viewing emotional distress as a message from the inner alarm in the brain and body that is intended to be protective of one's own and others' safety and well-being provides a nonjudgmental perspective for acceptance of distressing emotions (Follette et al., 2009). Viewing emotional distress as a protective mechanism also communicates nonjudgmental acceptance by the therapist of the client and a willingness by the therapist to understand and assist the client in finding ways to understand the message that the distressing emotions are expressing about problems, hurt, or danger that the client wants to solve, heal from, or prevent.

Joining with a client in crisis also involves affirming the client's sustaining "positive" emotions, which may seem absent or very difficult to access in a crisis. The emotion recognition "E" step in the FREEDOM template includes helping the client to recognize or recall emotions that relate to their core values (e.g., determination, courage), primary relationships (e.g., love, reassurance), and sense of self (e.g., confidence, pride). In TARGET, these are described as "main" emotions because they are not always experienced as euthymic, but they provide a base for trust, hope, and the ability to seek solutions rather than a reliance on reflexive reactions when under stress. When a therapist is able to point to ways in which these main emotions are reflected in the adaptive features in the client's current goals and actions—therefore acknowledging the validity of the client's more evident reactive emotions—this provides the client with a view of themselves as a person who has the presence of mind to join with the therapist in resolving the crisis.

Emotions are an essential focus for the therapist in empathically attuning to and joining with the client who is experiencing emotional dysregulation; however, empathic attunement and joining therapeutically also involves a cognitive dimension. Clients often experience emotional dysregulation as a diffuse sense of distress that is organized around specific thoughts or beliefs (e.g., "Everyone I count on lets me down," "I'm unlovable and a failure," "My therapist thinks I'm unimportant and only wants my money," "I have no choice but to end it all"). Identifying the thoughts that are at the heart of the distress and helping the client to consciously recognize them are central features of virtually every approach to psychotherapy. In a crisis, empathic attunement requires that the therapist affirm (rather than attempt to dispute or devalue) those thoughts to provide the client with a sense of being heard and taken seriously with nonjudgmental acceptance. However, it is equally important to not inadvertently seem to endorse the extreme implications of these thoughts, especially in a crisis. Rather, the therapist must help the client to contextualize those negative and dysregulated thoughts by highlighting the adaptive metacognitions that are embedded within the extreme and negative surface version of each such thought.

In the TARGET model, the second "E" in the FREEDOM framework (evaluating thoughts) represents this two-step process of validating the seriousness and importance of the reactive (dysregulated) thoughts while also affirming the adaptive underlying thoughts embedded within them. Thus, a client's main thoughts embedded in the reactive or crisis thoughts described earlier might be:

- "I'm determined to find people whom I can trust to stand by me and not let me down."
- "I am lovable and valued by people who really know me and who share my values."
- "I succeed when I am given a genuine opportunity to do what I'm capable of."
- "I need to understand why my therapist seems distracted, frustrated, and impatient."
- "I deserve a therapist who values me and not just my money."
- "I need to find the peace of mind that makes life seem worth living."
- "I need my therapist to see that I can't keep going along like this. Something has to change."

When the client's reactive crisis thoughts are treated as important and the underlying thoughts that express the client's core goals, hopes, and sense of self are clarified, then the client does not have to resort to desperate measures (i.e., crisis behavior) to get the therapist's attention. Helping to articulate the dialectic that the client is living with—the evident crisis emotions and thoughts but also the less evident but self-affirming, core, main emotions, and thoughts—is a crucial first step in empathically attuning and joining with the client in crisis.

Partnering Collaboratively

As clients experience the therapist as joining with them, they become correspondingly more able to also experience the therapist as a calming and reassuring source of safety, support, protection, and hope—as a source of coregulation and as a genuine partner. Partnering with a client in crisis takes place on at least two levels. The explicit aspect of therapeutic partnering is based on the therapist's communicating to the client, in action as well as through words, that they are working together. The practical and tangible aspect of the therapeutic partnership is based on respect for the client as the expert on their life, goals, and the problematic situation. The therapist's role in the partnership is as a guide with expertise on finding the information and defining the problem(s) in a manner that opens new options (or revises and updates old options to fit new or changed situations) that the client can decide to use (or not). Partnering to enable the client to define and achieve goals that are of importance can serve as a direct counterbalance to an essential dialectic that drives every crisis: the sense of desperate unwillingness to give up despite feeling hopeless and demoralized by a sense of personal failure and a conviction that the goals are unattainable.

In the FREEDOM framework, the "D" step (defining goals) is the practical application of this concept of partnering. Partnering involves clearly communicating nonjudgmental validation of the importance of the reactive goals that are expressions of the client's distress and emotional dysregulation. Attempting to steer or direct the client away from their crisis-driven reactive goals and toward a priori "adaptive" goals usually is experienced as critical invalidation rather than as helpful guidance. The client's emergency goals can instead be explicitly taken seriously as expressions of the client's sense of urgency without endorsing the aspects of the goals that are likely to exacerbate the crisis or to otherwise be self-defeating or harmful to the client or others. The client's emergency (reactive) goals are a statement that there are problems that seem insurmountable but yet somehow must be overcome or resolved. This apparently internally inconsistent and contradictory statement can be understood as a valid combination of the client's striving for goals that are based on emotional dysregulation (i.e., the view that the crisis problems are unsolvable yet must be resolved) and at the same time is striving for more fundamental underlying goals that the client can actually attain (i.e., the client's main goals).

Simultaneously to intervening on an explicit verbal level by affirming both the client's reactive and main goals, partnering occurs on a level that is largely implicit and nonverbal. This aspect of partnering involves the provision of affective coregulation by the therapist. It would be awkward and could be perceived by the client in crisis as ingenuine and unhelpful if a therapist simply says, "Let's partner together." It's the therapist's actions that offer an authentic and meaningful invitation to the client to partner, and in a crisis, the actions that count involve coregulation.

Coregulation is an extension of the therapist's self-regulation. As the therapist focuses consciously and unobtrusively on maintaining awareness and regulating their own bodily state, emotions, and cognitions, this provides the client with a lifeline and a copilot as they struggle to cope with intense confusion, distress, and disorganization. Even when a crisis involves hostile or fearful transference reactions that include the client's perception that the therapist is part of (or the principal source of) the problem or is an adversary or source of threat, the therapist strives to remain a potential ally. Similarly, when crises involve transference reactions characterized by devaluation (e.g., perceiving the therapist as weak, defective, impotent, a failure, worthless), the therapist strives to remain steady and to not retaliate or withdraw. Thus, the therapist is a lightning rod not only for crisis-escalating transference reactions but also for the client's faint but persistent hope that the crisis can be overcome and an inner sense of peace can be restored. That hope often is opaque to the client's conscious awareness, but it is a link to the therapist that can enable the therapist's active efforts to self-regulate to activate and engage their corresponding capacities for self-regulation. Coregulation takes place largely on a preconscious physiological and affective basis, but it need not be left to chance because the therapist can consciously facilitate it by intentionally engaging in mindful self-regulation.

On a practical basis, the coregulation aspect of partnering with a client in crisis can be accomplished when the therapist applies the "D" step of the FREEDOM framework to themself. Specifically, the therapist can intentionally pay attention to their own goals in relation to the client while simultaneously affirming and helping the client to be aware of their reactive and main goals. For therapists, as I discuss in more detail in the next chapter, there are many potential reactive goals when a client is in crisis in a psychotherapy session. These are the goals that therapists usually try not to think about, such as "I want to make this client calm down so I don't have to take drastic measures like an emergency hospitalization"; "I wish this client would just end the therapy so I don't have to deal with this anymore"; "I'm tired of dealing with this client's constant devaluation of me, so I'll show him how stupid he's being and how smart I am"; or "I'm frightened of this client and just want to make her stop harassing me."

Simply being aware of those reactive goals (and emotions and thoughts) is an important first step to not inadvertently acting on them but is not sufficient enough to enable the therapist to regain self-regulation. It is essential to explicitly counterbalance these reactive goals with the core goals that are the basis for not only working with this specific client but also for making psychotherapy a career. Each reactive goal has one or more main goals embedded within it for the therapist—no less than for the client. The main goals that can provide a therapist with a sense of confidence when dealing with a crisis and the reactive goals thus elicited might include the following:

- "I am helping this client calm down by providing empathy, acceptance, and genuine hope."

- "I am dedicated to seeing this through with this client because that's my duty as a professional and as a caring human being."

- "If I am not the right therapist or this is not the right therapy for this client, I will help the client find a therapist or therapy that is a better fit for them."

- "I know this client is showing me how they feel they have been devalued, and I can help them to recognize that neither they nor I have to be flawless to be of worth."

- "I am going to show this client that I care and that I'm smart by helping them recognize how they are a caring and very intelligent person."

- "I am going to talk with my trusted colleagues to get advice about how to deal with the threats and harassment this client is directing toward me."

This crucial inner work by the therapist not only provides a model for self-regulation but also communicates nonverbally and in words to the client that the therapist is a true partner who is willing to walk the walk as well as talk the talk. It also sets an important example to the client of how it is possible to start with reactive goals in a crisis but use them as a starting point for finding and focusing on the more fundamental main goals that can be attained and, moreover, that make life worth living. This is a point of emphasis in the next chapter.

STEP 3: AFFIRMING CORE VALUES, OPTIONS, AND RESILIENCE

When crises occur, it is easy not only for clients but also for therapists to lose track of the larger context of clients' lives when under pressure to deal with the immediate problems and escalating distress. Although making the shift to focusing on the immediate present and reaffirming the therapeutic relationship can help clients (and the therapist) to begin to modulate intense stress reactions and reduce the dysregulation they are experiencing, these "grounding" approaches to crisis intervention may not be sufficient to enable the client (or the therapist) to fully restore self-regulation. What may be missing is a reaffirmation of the client's core values and the restoration of the client's sense of personal control and efficacy, and their capacities for resilience (e.g., personal strengths, supportive relationships). Therefore, in the midst of a crisis, it is not only possible essential to help clients restore self-regulation by renewing their awareness of their core values and the options that they have available based on those values and their capacity for resilience.

Affirming Core Values

By affirming the therapeutic partnership and the client's resilience, the therapist thus has begun to help the client to make a crucial shift in focus from desperation and hopelessness to a sense of having a worthwhile purpose and valuable capabilities. This affirmation opens the door psychologically for the client to make a complementary shift in perspective from focusing on what has gone wrong and needs to be "fixed" to what they are attempting to achieve in a positive sense based on their core values, beliefs, and priorities. This shift can be a powerful antidote for the rumination and perseveration on problems and failures that drive and escalate crises. The therapist can best catalyze and support this shift in focus by reflecting back to the client what they have communicated, often indirectly, about their core values, beliefs, and priorities. This should *not* ever be an attempt on the part of the therapist to instill or endorse new or "better" values, beliefs, or goals than those the client endorses. That would be an imposition and intrusion, and would communicate precisely the opposite of the empathic understanding and respect of the client. The therapist's listens for the subtle as well as the obvious signs of the values and goals that are of greatest importance to the client.

Psychotherapists (Banks, 1965; Frank, 1971; Horowitz, 2014; Mickleburgh, 1992; Rogers, 1964; Schmideberg, 1958) and psychological theorists and researchers (Chadwick et al., 2006; Crone et al., 2018; Graham et al., 2011; Korner, 1963; Ng et al., 2017; Pittel & Mendelsohn, 1966; M. B. Smith, 2000) have articulated a number of core values that can guide the therapist's attempts to identify or infer those that are expressed indirectly as well as directly by the client's words and actions. Several taxonomies of core human values and aspirations have been formulated that identify the following cross-cutting themes:

- care/nurturance, kindness, compassion, friendliness, charitableness, generosity
- justice, loyalty, freedom/liberty, equality/equity, cooperativeness
- modesty, honesty, trustworthiness, integrity, authenticity/genuineness, humility
- courage, determination/dedication
- creativity, efficacy/productivity, achievement, individuality
- knowledge, wisdom, expertise
- purity, selflessness, transcendence, poise/gracefulness, temperance/restraint

In the midst of moments of crisis in psychotherapy, it may seem counterintuitive for the therapist to focus on the client's core values and life goals. However, doing so signals that the therapist has not lost track of the fundamental hopes and moral standards that are the bedrock for their hopes and aspirations. It also reminds clients that no matter how discouraged and stressed they feel when in crisis, they have vital personal reasons to persevere. Thus, while in no way diminishing the difficulty and distress that the client in crisis is experiencing, helping the client to not just reactively cope but also to actively remember and rededicate themself to the pursuit of core values and goals can spark a revival of hope, purpose, and determination.

Identifying Meaningful Options

Resolving crises requires practical actions yielding outcomes that match the client's main goals (i.e., goals based on their core personal priorities and values). Effective action begins with stepping back from approaches that aren't working and developing new ways (or creative variations of familiar but unsuccessful ways) to break through or go around the brick wall, the dead end, or the revolving door of escalating frustration, disappointment, and discouragement at the heart of the current crisis. With core values and priorities as a North Star, and some renewed confidence in one's own resilience and in the partnering, role modeling, and coregulation provided by the therapist, the client can begin to consider practical steps (i.e., options) to achieve meaningful progress toward solutions.

Options have two essential features: First is the desired outcome. Deciding what needs to be—and can be—different to make improvements is the perquisite to making any apparently unsolvable problem potentially solvable. This is essentially setting a target toward which action will be directed and that will provide evidence of success. In crises, large goals are at stake, but it is essential to break those larger goals down into smaller parts, or else the larger goal will always seem (and typically will actually be) out of reach. "Small wins" (Weick, 1984, p. 40) is an approach to solving large-scale social problems that is based on individual-level psychological research and has direct applicability to resolving individual-level crises. The essential concept is to create "a strategy of small wins wherein a series of concrete, complete outcomes of moderate importance build a pattern that attracts allies and deters opponents" (Weick, 1984, p. 40). The slogan "one day at a time" attributed to Alcoholics Anonymous (Canada, 2017) epitomizes this approach.

In the context of a crisis in psychotherapy, small, meaningful wins from the point of view of a client might include being heard and validated by another person (including the therapist and significant others), working out a plan to achieve a compromise that includes some of the larger goal, or repairing a rupture in a conflicted or separated relationship. They might also involve being able to reduce the immediate pressure, conflict, or lack of privacy or autonomy that a client is experiencing, or receiving meaningful reassurance that a dreaded or distressing event is not going to occur or will occur in a way that is tolerable. A common denominator across all types of small wins is that these are outcomes that affirm, in a small but meaningful manner, the client's capacities. Thus, the values clarification that began in the prior step is carried forward in down-to-earth practical terms when the therapist helps the client to identify small wins that make a difference from the perspective of the client.

The second feature of options are action steps that the client can take that, similar to the small wins, are small enough to be practical, manageable, and yield relatively immediate positive outcomes with acceptable costs. Once outcomes are defined, the brainstorming process that is central to effective problem-solving can be put into play to formulate varied approaches to immediate action that might make a positive difference. In crises, even if all of the aforementioned steps have been taken to help clients to self-regulate sufficiently to be able to brainstorm, the emotional intensity experienced by the client typically is sufficiently strong and persistent to limit their immediate ability to put aside judgments and freely consider all possible courses of action. Therefore, the therapist should expect to help develop a menu of potential action steps that the client can choose from and modify.

A useful tactic in stimulating and supporting brainstorming of target outcomes and action steps is for the therapist to base any suggestions on what has worked in the past for the client. Recognizing small wins that the client has made in their life in similar or relevant contexts can provide a catalog of possible options for the current dilemma(s) that build on the client's core values and priorities, and are familiar to the client. This of course does not mean suggesting actions that the client has taken repeatedly with some degree of benefit (perceived or actual) but that have had serious short-term or long-term costs. It could, though, include variations on those past actions that are modified to achieve the desired outcome without the unacceptable adverse outcomes. In that light, another potential source of options involves the actions that the client currently is taking that are not succeeding in achieving the desired goals or that have serious costs to the client. However, those actions could potentially be of benefit if the intended outcome is revised (e.g., scaling back from a large victory to a small win), or the action is modified to directly achieve an intended outcome (e.g., expressing a grievance in the form of a respectful request based on a statement of core values).

Affirming Resilience

A true collaborative partnership involves active participants who each make contributions of comparable value to the relationship and the achievement of goals. Psychotherapy clients are in a one-down position in their partnership with the therapist—not because they do not actually bring equal (or greater) value to the relationship in comparison with the psychotherapist but because of cultural beliefs and societal norms that elevate the status of the professional as the authority and diminish the status of the client as the supplicant seeking help as a result of their ostensible inability to manage psychological problems. Those tropes vastly understate the status of the client as a person and as a partner in therapy. Crises in psychotherapy often are fueled or exacerbated by the client's struggling with (and against) a sense of being (or being treated as) "less than" (i.e., of little value) in relationship to the high-status therapist and in their lives as a result of difficult and apparently intractable psychological and other life difficulties. We see this in bold relief in the awakening of awareness that Black lives matter and in the terrible damage that authority based on intimidation, devaluation, and an unjust sense of privilege has caused for Black and Indigenous People of Color. With all clients, and especially those who come from marginalized races, communities, and cultures, it is essential that therapists not inadvertently provoke or fail to resolve crises by adopting an elitist attitude that discounts the worth and competencies of clients who are experiencing dysregulation and crises. Instead, crises are a critical opportunity to be antiracist and truly therapeutic by genuinely affirming clients' resilience.

The crucial next step in resolving crises in psychotherapy therefore is for the therapist to explicitly demonstrate respect and recognition for the client's resilience. Clients in crisis might seem to a naive observer to be showing few signs of resilience and many signs of not being able to deal effectively with the stress and distress they are experiencing. Often, that also is the way that the client in crisis perceives themself (i.e., as helpless, incompetent, needy, explosive, or an empty shell) even if they deny it outwardly intensely or aggressively. What is crucially missing from these superficial assessments is recognition and valuation of the admirable and often remarkable resilience that clients in crisis possess and demonstrate even in the midst of crises.

Aspects of resilience that warrant close attention include the courage and determination required to persevere in the face of apparent failure, the persistence and dedication to achieve goals despite their apparent unattainability, the creativity with which adaptations have been made, the compassion and love they feel for others, and the integrity to hold true to core values at great personal cost. Also missing is the recognition of the talents, qualities of character, and interests and passions that these individuals bring to their relationships, work and studies, community involvements, and psychotherapy. These are the strengths that any person in crisis needs to draw on to regain the presence of mind and self-regulation to resolve a crisis and to develop ways to achieve the goals—or meaningful revisions of those goals.

Affirming the client's resilience involves shifting the focus of the inter-action in the midst of the crisis from rumination about irresolvable problems to identification of areas of strength, abilities, and personal and relational resilience and resources that provide a sense of reassurance, connection, and self-affirmation. This is not an artificial exercise in boosting the client's self-esteem with inauthentic or empty praise, nor is it a celebratory congrat-ulation intended to uplift the client's spirit with genuine praise. Instead, affirming resilience requires the therapist to recognize the core values, qualities, and choices that the client is making in attempting to deal with the crisis and to accomplish the as yet unattained goals. In that sense, this is an empathic statement confirming that the therapist respects and takes seriously the client's character, courage, capability, and persistence in struggling to overcome barriers. This is a fundamental shift in perspective for most indi-viduals who are in crisis, opening up the possibility of viewing themselves as not just failures or victims but as courageous and capable.

Affirming core values and resilience requires more than generic praise intended to boost a client's self-esteem. Specific examples of behavior—past as well as present—that demonstrate the client's core values and resilience must instead be identified and affirmed. This can be difficult when behavior that appears dysfunctional is what is most evident to the client and to the therapist. In the TARGET model, the "O" step in the FREEDOM framework is designed to enable the therapist to help the client reflect on the difference between what they are doing that is survival or alarm driven versus what they could alternatively choose to do or are already doing based on their core values. These are identified as reactive and main options to be a down-to-earth practical comparison that the client can make to nonjudgmentally determine the choices and actions that they believe best reflects who they are as a person. This is not a call to the client to be a "better" person but an invitation to the client to remember and base decisions on their strengths, capabilities, and core values. It also is purposefully a way for the therapist to affirm their commitment to empowering rather than controlling or devaluing the client by nonjudgmentally highlighting the contrast between the reactive actions that the client is taking as a result of emotional dysregulation versus options that reflect the client's resilient capabilities.

STEP 4: DEVELOPING A COLLABORATIVE ACTION PLAN

In life, and especially in crises, talk is cheap, and action is the ultimate coin of the realm. The goal of crisis resolution is not simply to calm a person who is highly distressed or to prevent that person from acting in a way that is harmful to self or others. The immediate culmination of crisis intervention, in general and specifically when crises occur in psychotherapy, is an action plan (along with a safety plan as needed) with specific steps that the client and the therapist will take immediately and over the intervening period until they meet again (whether that is an hour, a day, a week, or longer). The importance of therapists' having responsibility for developing plans and assisting the client in putting a plan into action by taking defined action steps cannot be overstated. If the therapist "assigns" (or more tactfully, "suggests" or "encourages") action steps for the client but none for themselves, the meta-message is that the responsibility is entirely on the client, and the client is alone in handling the crisis (even if the therapist is in the background— in the audience, so to speak—cheering the client on with well-intended but ultimately distancing and even invalidating attempts at encouragement).

On the other hand, if the therapist takes responsibility for action steps that are within their purview (while carefully not preempting the client in steps that are the client's purview), the metamessage is that "this is your life, and I am here to guide and assist you, but you're not alone because we're in this together." Fully collaborative action planning thus is an extension of the earlier stages of joining and partnering, and represents a practical way to walk the walk in genuinely affirming the client's resilience and core values.

The form of the collaborative plan that the client chooses and that the client and therapist take together (each with their own defined areas of responsibility) can be an experiment designed to test and revise (as necessary) different possible approaches. The goal is not to get it exactly right on the first attempt (although small or partial successes warrant recognition and celebration). Instead, the goal is to learn on a trial by trial basis, refining the action steps and the intended outcomes to make progress toward the immediate and the larger goals. The action steps and small win outcomes are hypotheses that are based on the best educated guess by the client and therapist about what will result in meaningful change. Each action step is a test of the hypothesis, and the actual outcome yields information to guide the next iteration of the experiment. This process is itself a part of the resolution of the crisis because it is an approach to setting and achieving goals that maximizes the likelihood that goals (albeit often with many revisions) can be attained, and crises averted.

In the FREEDOM framework, the action plan is a combination of main goals and options that enable the client to not only handle a specific crisis but, moreover, to express their core values and make a positive difference in their relationships and community. This is the final FREEDOM step: "M" for making a contribution. The formulation of the action plan and steps for its implementation is a practical matter that involves the client's defining of goals and committing to options (actions) to achieve goals based on their core values as described in Step 3. However, the therapist can help the client to fully commit to the action plan by invoking a context for collaborative planning that is based on highlighting how the client's goals and actions not only benefit them but also make the world a better place.

It is important that this discussion of making a contribution does not inadvertently reenact past experiences in which the client sacrificed or devalued themself or was exploited to take care of or meet others' expectations or demands. Making a contribution is an expression of the belief that actions must be fair and beneficial to everyone involved—including the client as well as their significant others and community. Often, psychotherapy clients have felt, or been told, that they only take from other people and don't have anything of value to give. When a client develops a way to genuinely resolve a crisis, this involves actions and effort that have direct and indirect benefits for other people as well. Highlighting that possibility can make crises seem more amenable to resolution because it emphasizes the value the client and their actions can have as well as the challenges that the client is dealing with.

STEP 5: ACCESSING RESOURCES AND ENSURING CONTINUITY

The resolution of crises depends on the client's having access to resources and the security of knowing that their relationship with the therapist will be one of those resources that can be counted on going forward. Feeling a sense of relief, reduced distress, affirmation, and hope is important in resolving crises, but without ongoing resources and a continuity of treatment, those immediate gains are not likely to be sustained, and new crises may develop.

Accessing Resources

No action plan is complete without marshaling the resources necessary to put it into action and complete it successfully. In the intense and typically focused and reflective dyadic or systemic interactions that occur in psychotherapy, it is easy for the client—and the therapist—to lose track of the resources that are potentially accessible to the client within and outside of the psychotherapy relationship. On the one hand, the client or therapist may rush to identify the resources outside psychotherapy that can help the client to navigate a crisis—family, friends, work, school, activities, material or financial tools and supplies, other helping people or organizations—while overlooking the help that the therapist can provide not just in the moment of crisis but on an ongoing basis. Just knowing that the therapy will continue and the therapist is not critically judging, is not disappointed or angry with, or is not rejecting or abandoning the client in reaction to the crisis is an essential resource. Affirmation by the therapist of a genuine willingness to continue to help the client to understand and master problems that have culminated in a crisis is crucially reassuring to a client in crisis. Knowing that this resource will continue to be accessible may seem obvious, but for many clients in crisis, their fear of rejection or abandonment calls the therapist's continued support into question—especially when the client already is feeling desperate, alone, and overwhelmed while in crisis.

On the other hand, it's also easy for the client, and also the therapist, to become so focused on their immediate relationship that they lose track of viable external resources in the client's life. In a crisis, that focus under-standably can narrow to just the immediate present such that the client's and the therapist's attention is completely absorbed in the working through of the client's immediate sense of overwhelming distress "in the room." Although external resources often cannot be drawn on instantly to help resolve a crisis, statements by the therapist that remind the client of important external resources can serve as an important reassurance (primarily for the client but also not insignificantly for the therapist—who may also be feeling alone in dealing with the client's crisis). It also may be possible to make contact with external resources or to make a plan for how the client, the therapist, or both can recruit those resources, for example, with a phone call to a source of help while still talking together in the therapy session.

Identifying and helping the client to access crucial resources is crucial to enable the client to have the fullest possible range of helpful resources outside the therapy setting and to ensure that neither client nor therapist views therapy as the sole solution to the crisis. This should take the form of an action plan—and not just a general statement of intent—that should include specific steps to assist the client in connecting with resources and relationships outside of therapy that may be sources of positive support. In addition, because "resources" are not always helpful and can increase rather than ameliorate the client's distress and difficulty in achieving key goals, it also is important to address external resources by developing a plan for how the client can set limits with or disconnect from resources and relationships that exacerbate or drive any problem(s) that contribute to (or originated) the crisis.

Ensuring Continuity

Ultimately, crises are resolved when the person in crisis becomes hopeful that they have the ability to resolve the stressor at least partially and that they do not have to face the current—or future—challenges to their goals alone. It is not possible to promise any client that they will always be able to overcome any future obstacle and avoid any form of failure. The approach of framing collaborative action planning as an experiment makes it clear that there will be both trials and errors, and some goals may simply be unattainable—but those goals can be modified, and action steps can be creatively developed and tested such that the ultimate result may not be ideal, but it also will not be the total failure that sparks a crisis.

Of greatest importance to the sustained resolution—rather than merely a transient deferral—of a crisis in therapy is the client's knowledge that the relationship with the therapist can be counted on to continue without an arbitrary ending. This does not mean that the therapist should, or could, promise to always be available in precisely the same way in perpetuity or will never leave in recognition that the therapist cannot control what is out of personal control. The therapeutic bond will continue while the real relationship between the therapist and client (e.g., visit schedules, session timing and length, intersession contacts) will shift over time as the client progresses. It is the knowledge that there is a bond that is not, and will not, be broken on an emotional level with the therapist that—as in all types of attachment working models—is of the essence. Therefore, in the wake of a crisis, when the client's sense of secure attachment is likely to be frayed even if the crisis has apparently been resolved, it is crucial that the therapist take steps to metacommunicate that their bond is intact and will continue into the foreseeable future.

This final step in resolving a crisis (and preventing or mitigating the severity of future crises) in the psychotherapy session is primarily the responsibility of the therapist as a provider of professional services to the client. As such, by doing more than simply engaging in a helpful conversation with the client in the session but actually connecting their clients in crisis to crucial resources and being an ongoing resource that the client can count on, therapists are making a contribution (the FREEDOM framework's final

"M" step). Therapists don't have to have all of the resources or contacts for them immediately available, but as the transcripts beginning in Chapter 7 illustrate, offering to work with the client to find or access those resources is key. That communicates the message that the therapist is genuinely committed to the client's well-being and safety, and that the therapist is offering to be a collaborative partner on an ongoing basis (i.e., to provide continuity). One of the greatest fears that can drive a crisis is that of feeling abandoned and having to face stressors and distress alone. Even when the therapist doesn't have all the answers or all the resources, working toward helping the client find those answers and access key resources is a crucial contribution to the client's sense of trust in the therapist.

CONCLUSION

In this chapter, the focus has been on what the therapist can do in a practical step-by-step manner to handle and resolve crises in the psychotherapy session. The role of therapist self-regulation has come up explicitly or implicitly at every step. It takes considerable poise and personal control for therapists to be with and guide clients through a crisis—let alone to transform the crisis into a positive turning point in psychotherapy and in the client's life. Before we turn to transcripts of crises in psychotherapy sessions, it's important to consider carefully what the therapist can, and must, do to provide that therapeutic presence and guidance when confronted by a client in the emergency or breakdown stages of a crisis.

6 CRISES AS A CHALLENGE TO THERAPIST SELF-REGULATION

When clients are in crisis and experiencing emotional dysregulation, they rely on their therapist not only for support and guidance but also to communicate a sense of calm confidence that is crucial in helping the client to regain emotional regulation by experiencing a sense of secure attachment (Bowlby, 1969) and hope (Frank, 1961). Handling crises in psychotherapy sessions therefore requires technical knowledge and skill on the part of the therapist as well as the ability to maintain (or regain) emotional regulation "in the heat of the moment" (Abblett, 2013, p. 1). Therapists are only human, and none of us actually is "free from neurotic difficulties" (Weiner, 1975, p. 30) or immune to personal reactions, such as frustration, fear, confusion, doubt, or compassion when sitting with a client who is in crisis. A central principle across all theoretical approaches to psychotherapy is: Therapist know thyself. Self-awareness enables therapists to "differentiate clearly between patient behavior and [their own] reaction to that behavior." For that reason, the "therapist must be keenly aware of his own personality dynamics—in particular, what tends to make him angry or anxious, how he feels about the important figures in his life, and why he behaves as he does" (Weiner, 1975, p. 31).

https://doi.org/10.1037/0000225-007
Crises in the Psychotherapy Session: Transforming Critical Moments Into Turning Points,
by J. D. Ford

When therapists are unaware of or try to ignore or minimize their personal reactions to a client, they can commit a fundamental error that undermines the therapeutic process and erodes or directly damages the therapeutic relationship. This is the therapist's error of letting personal reactions to the emotional issues and distress that clients play out in their interaction with the therapist be deflected back onto the client in the form of emotional demands, frustration, avoidance, devaluation, criticisms, or attempts to rescue the client or gain the client's approval. This countertherapeutic phenomenon has been described as *countertransference*: a reciprocal transfer by the therapist back onto the client of the distress the client is transferring into the therapeutic relationship (Weiner, 1975). Psychotherapists are affected, often deeply, by the intense emotional dilemmas expressed by clients. When these sympathetic responses trigger personal issues that are painful and largely unresolved for the psychotherapist, rather than experiencing compassion, the psychotherapist may develop emotion-laden beliefs regarding the client as a defense against experiencing the elicited distress. For example, the psychotherapist might feel frustration or even contempt while viewing the client as lacking motivation or intelligence, as needy and dependent, or as purposefully sabotaging the psychotherapy. This emotional intensity and the associated beliefs can profoundly compromise even the best intentioned and most experienced psychotherapist's crucial ability to maintain a position of nonjudgmental interest in the client's well-being and unconditional positive regard toward the client. In many such cases, the psychotherapist is reacting not just to any random behavior on the client's part but to interactions in which the client is displacing or projecting emotional conflicts onto the psychotherapist—that is, to transfer enactments by the client. For this reason, these reactions by the psychotherapist are countertransference.

Crises in the psychotherapy session can be precipitated or significantly exacerbated by therapist countertransference, but when therapists are self-reflective and self-aware of their understandable human reactions to their clients and the distress their clients are experiencing, countertransference can be a valuable source of therapeutic information that can be used to prevent or safely resolve crises. Therapists therefore need to intentionally apply to themselves the same skills for self-awareness and emotion regulation that they teach to and support in their clients. The FREEDOM framework (discussed in the Introduction to this volume; the letters refer to focusing, recognizing triggers, emotion awareness, evaluating thoughts, defining goals and options, making a contribution) can provide an efficient practical means to do exactly that. The FREEDOM steps for self-regulation are not just for clients; they are also for therapists. By following the FREEDOM steps in processing their own personal reactions in the therapy session, therapists can develop the self-awareness and emotion regulation that enables them to be highly focused; to provide empathic, nonjudgmental, and genuine acceptance and guidance; and to serve as a source of collaborative guidance and security for the client while maintaining the boundaries necessary to protect the client's emotional safety, strengthen the client's autonomy, and support the client's coherent sense of self.

In this chapter, I examine how countertransference plays out in-session in client–therapist interactions and how it can lead to, exacerbate, or impede the resolution of crises in psychotherapy sessions. I also consider how counter-transference can be managed and potentially used therapeutically, and how it can prevent or facilitate the resolution of crises in psychotherapy sessions. Although the emphasis is on the client's safety and the benefit accrued by the client from preventing or resolving crises, a focus on countertransference provides an opportunity to also consider how psychotherapists are affected personally by crises and how managing countertransference benefits not only the client in crisis but also the therapist.

COUNTERTRANSFERENCE AS THE HUMAN CONDITION– AMPLIFIED IN PSYCHOTHERAPY

Psychotherapists are only human. Like anyone else, we are affected emotion-ally in our life experiences—particularly so when the experiences involve emotionally charged relationships. Psychotherapy is an inherently emotionally charged relationship with another human who is experiencing distress and seeking help. To provide meaningful help, psychotherapists must achieve an exquisite balance between encouraging the client and providing for the client an unprecedented degree of psychological openness while simulta-neously maintaining relational and psychological boundaries that preserve the client's individual integrity and safety. This balance involves rigorous attention to, and reflection on the meaning of, the client's emotional and relational experience in the moment and historically as well as simultane-ously paying attention to one's own experience.

In this context, countertransference is inevitable. Countertransference is a bidirectional interpersonal—or, more specifically, "intersubjective" (Atwood & Stolorow, 1984, p. 119)—experience that occurs when psychotherapists are affected personally by the intense emotions expressed by their clients. The client and psychotherapist experience emotions, impulses, and thoughts that are in reaction to their immediate interaction together (what Weiner, 1975, described as the "real relationship" [p. 217]) and to memories, both conscious and unconscious, from their life histories. "The transference," wrote Atwood and Stolorow (1984), "is actually a microcosm of the patient's total psychological life. . . . Countertransference, in turn, refers to how the structures of the analyst's subjectivity shape his experience of the analytic relationship and, in particular, of the patient's transference" (p. 47).

The emotion-laden reactions involved in the transference–counter-transference dance are elicited and experienced by both the client and psychotherapist, hence the term "intersubjective." Countertransference is not "caused" by the client nor by the psychotherapist any more than transference is "caused" by—or is solely the responsibility of—either the client or the psychotherapist. Both individuals' life experiences accompany them in every interaction in the psychotherapy, predisposing each to experience personally relevant emotions, impulses, and beliefs that can be elicited or intensified—but not caused—by behavior by the other that is associated with their own past formative life experiences and relationships. As the psychotherapist and client interact overtly in their behavior with each other, their subjective inner worlds of emotions and thoughts also are interacting, influencing not only one another's behavior but also each other's ways of feeling (on bodily and affective levels) and of interpreting the meaning of their experience (i.e., perceptions and beliefs about self, others, relationships, the world, and the past and future).

How this intersubjective dialogue and dance of mutual engagement and influence play out depends partly on the personalities and life experiences of the client and the psychotherapist, as it does in all relationships. However, what is unique about psychotherapy is the shared commitment to not just interacting but, moreover, to observing and reflecting on their interaction to enable the client to find ways of understanding the client's perceptions, emotions, motivations, actions, and relationships that can free them from incapacitating emotional dysregulation and provide a path toward fulfill-ment in relationships, primary life pursuits, and day-to-day living. In this therapeutic process of finding and making meaning, countertransference can cut either way. It can potentially enable the psychotherapist to draw from their own personal experience to see meaning in the client's behavior and life experiences that is illuminating and helpful to the client. Counter-transference, though, also has the potential to lead the psychotherapist to misunderstand or unhelpfully formulate and communicate the meaning of the client's behavior and life experiences such that the client is burdened, trapped, or even injured by the psychotherapist's words and actions (Westra et al., 2012).

Not only can countertransference prevent psychotherapy from being a "success," but it can—when not filtered through and processed by rigorous self-awareness by the psychotherapist—dominate or dictate the psychotherapist's emotions, attitudes, and behavior toward the client. The client may seem to be only an object on to which to project personal attributes that the psychotherapist cannot accept in themself or from which the psychotherapist seeks to gain gratification for personal needs. Left unrecognized and unchecked, psychotherapy can then become an intersubjective enslavement rather than a dyadic—let alone, therapeutic—relationship. This inevitably undercuts the client's sense of trust and security in the therapeutic relationship and saps the client's sense self-confidence, self-regard, and hope sufficiently to make them vulnerable to precisely the kind of escalating emotional dysregulation that erupts in crisis.

Fortunately, although countertransference is inevitable, it does not inevitably lead to enactments by the psychotherapist that can trigger or exacerbate crises in the psychotherapy. Atwood and Stolorow (1984) described the antidote for contratherapeutic countertransference as "reflective self-awareness and [the] capacity to decenter" (p. 47). To understand how reflective self-awareness can turn countertransference into a therapeutic asset and what is involved when a psychotherapist decenters while engaging in the client–therapist interaction, it's first necessary to take a closer look at the phenomenon of countertransference.

COUNTERTRANSFERENCE AS THE PSYCHOTHERAPIST'S UNRESOLVED PERSONAL ISSUES

The earliest formal description of countertransference was provided by Freud in his 1910 speech to the Nuremburg Psychoanalytic Congress in which he stated, "We have become aware of the 'countertransference' which arises as a result of the patient's influence on [the analyst's] unconscious feelings" (Freud, 1910/1957, p. 144). Countertransference originally was viewed as an impediment to psychotherapy that arose from the psychoanalyst's unconscious conflicts (Gabbard, 1999). For example, the problem of negative countertransference was described as creating

> in the therapist an unconscious need to reject, dominate, or over-protect the patient, or to be punitive, demanding, prohibitive, moralistic, restrictive or impatient towards him. It is clear that such unconscious attitudes within the therapist will make a cure impossible. (Hora, 1951, p. 560)

Psychoanalysts therefore were urged to strive to overcome this personal vulnerability by engaging in a thorough self-analysis (Gabbard, 1999).

Freud (1910/1957) strongly recommended that the psychoanalyst "shall begin his activity with a self-analysis and continually carry it deeper while he is making his observations on his patients" (p. 145). A lengthy course of successful (i.e., resulting in insight into one's own unconscious conflicts, needs, and defenses) personal analysis with a training psychoanalyst was thought to be a prerequisite for conducting psychoanalysis (and still is among traditional psychoanalysts). Hora (1951) followed that line in recommending that "personal psychoanalysis should make the therapist aware of his own 'blind spots' and the predilections to the extent that he is able to resolve his own resistances" (p. 560).

Gabbard (1999, pp. 5–6) gave a down-to earth example of how countertransference can emerge when a client's actions take a psychotherapist by surprise and tap into unresolved issues in the psychotherapist's personal life and inner world. This client accuses her therapist of hating her, and the therapist reacts with surprise and questions the client's reasons for making that accusation. Asking "why" questions (e.g., "Why do you say/think/feel that?") is a way of putting the other person on the defensive, and when a psychotherapist does so, it often is a sign that the psychotherapist is experiencing a countertransference reaction to something the client is doing (or not doing). In the vignette, the client becomes increasingly upset in reaction to being questioned by the psychotherapist and even more upset when the therapist denies feeling hate toward the client or knowing why the client would have this belief. The client then escalates the tension and intensity of the interaction by accusing the therapist of lying and pretending to be unaware of the problem. Subsequently, the therapist becomes indignant and protests being labeled as a liar, which leads the client to conclude that her accusation has been proven true by the therapist's angry demeanor. Gabbard (1999) concluded that

> the client, having project[ed] a hating internal object into the therapist . . . then behaves in such an infuriating manner that she coerces the therapist to take on the characteristics of the 'bad object' . . . with his obvious anger. (p. 6)

This vignette presents a stereotypical "hateful patient" (Groves, 1978, p. 883) and a therapist who seems clumsy and inarticulate. However, the dilemma it illustrates could apply to clients who are not "hateful" but instead are anxious about their therapist's emotional trustworthiness and opinion of them, or who are interpreting (accurately or not) their therapist's behavior as showing an attitude of criticism, impatience, or indifference and labeling that behavior as an expression of "hate." The example also could apply to situations in which therapists are poised and adept but cover up their internal reactions by interacting in a manner that conveys (albeit only superficially) a high degree of therapeutic and interpersonal savvy despite being caught off guard by a client's intense exclamations and persistent interrogation. Even if a psychotherapist is able to disguise (i.e., sublimate, deny, or minimize) or apparently rise above (e.g., via displacement, projection, reaction formation) countertransference reactions by maintaining a superficially professional demeanor, those defenses are no more likely to prevent even the most well-defended psychotherapist's needs and conflicted reactions from leaking into the client–therapist interaction than they are for a well-defended client. The result is that even the most savvy psychotherapist's felt reactions of shock and defensiveness—if not recognized and understood before action is taken—can be expressed nonverbally or in words communicating opprobrium that is thinly masked by a pedagogical attitude ("This is for your own good"; A. Miller, 1981) and wrapped in a mantle of professional decorum (e.g., as an interpretation or as cognitive restructuring).

It also is important to note that, although psychotherapists rarely are the primary "cause" of crises, this can happen when a psychotherapist violates boundaries of professional ethics and treats a client in a manner that is emotionally, economically, or sexually dishonest, cruel, exploitive, or otherwise harmful. Seducing or coercing a client into a personal, financial, or sexual relationship, or colluding with a client by passively allowing such actions to occur at what appears to be the client's behest always leads to a crisis for the client and to the end of the psychotherapy regardless of whether the client and psychotherapist continue to maintain a semblance of ongoing treatment. Countertransference takes many forms, most of which are not as obvious as egregious boundary violations. However, professional boundary violations are a vital reminder of the seriousness and potential harm that can occur when psychotherapists transfer their personal lives into what should be an exclusively professional helping relationship. By viewing, and interacting with, the client mainly on the basis of personal needs or biases, the psychotherapist is abdicating their professional responsibility to serve the client (Courtois, 2020). For the client, a psychotherapist's abdication of professional responsibility can lead to crisis because this is a fundamental betrayal of trust and a breach of the therapeutic contract. Even if the client receives some personal gratification of conscious or unconscious wishes or desires (e.g., feeling that the psychotherapist is treating them as a very special person and providing the love or affirmation that has been lacking in other key relationships), that gratification comes at the cost of becoming a servant for the psychotherapist (i.e., existing primarily to serve the psychotherapist's personal needs) rather than a partner in a relationship dedicated primarily to serve and protect the client's personal well-being.

With due regard for the fundamental principle of primum non nocere (first, do no harm), it also is vitally important to recognize and prevent or mitigate the adverse consequences of less obvious forms of countertransference by the psychotherapist. Subtler manifestations of the transference of personal biases, reactions, and needs on the part of the psychotherapist into the client–therapist interaction are far more common; less easily recognizable; and, over time, potentially just as much of a concern as precipitants or intensifiers of crises in psychotherapy as obvious ethical breaches. Like the drip . . . drip . . . drip . . . of a leaky faucet that corrodes the pipes and can lead to a flood, the persistent, repeated subtle countertransference enactments over time can result in an emergency or breakdown that constitutes a crisis.

Of course, the perfectly analyzed psychoanalyst or therapized psychotherapist is a rarer than a unicorn, existing only in myth and fantasy. No psychotherapist can flawlessly recognize with 100% success the intrusion of unresolved personal issues and the accompanying countertransference reactions. Therefore, unintended countertransference enactments (e.g., empathic failures, moments of transparent frustration or impatience, hesitance or avoidance based on self-doubt or fear of a client's emotional reactions) are inevitable. However, the ability to decenter from one's own psychological perspective and focus empathically on learning, understanding, and affirming the validity of (and also the possibility of change in) the client's psychological perspective depends upon first knowing oneself. The self-analysis that Freud (1910/1957) recommended can occur in many contexts and many ways, but the most difficult challenge is the same one that each client faces: coming to recognize, acknowledge, and understand the needs, impulses, conflicts, aspirations, and motivations that are hidden in plain sight, are masked by psychic defenses, and thus are almost always disillusioning or downright painful to acknowledge.

COUNTERTRANSFERENCE AS OBJECTIVE REACTIONS TO CLIENTS' UNCONSCIOUS ISSUES

A paradigm shift was underway more than 70 years ago, as exemplified by Winnicott's (1949) observation that there may be an "objective" basis for countertransference in the form of reactions by the psychoanalyst to the client's unconscious conflicts and defenses that are independent of the psychoanalyst's own unconscious conflicts and needs. Racker (1957/2007) noted that countertransference may be concordant (i.e., an empathic response by the psychoanalyst to the client's inner experience and self-representation) or complementary (i.e., the activation of unconscious conflicts within the psychoanalyst by the client's projections of unacceptable characteristics onto the psychoanalyst). Thus, countertransference is not necessarily a reflection of unanalyzed (i.e., unresolved) personal conflicts or issues by the psychotherapist, although this is a possibility that requires careful attention so the psychotherapist is not led to defensively act out conflicts toward a client. At that same time, Heimann (1960) provided a major redefinition of countertransference as a window into the client's unconscious rather than a problem of insufficiently analyzed unconscious needs or conflicts on the part of the psychoanalyst. Countertransference reactions thus may reveal psychological or interpersonal issues for a client that are being played out in the client's interaction with the psychotherapist.

Psychotherapists' personal reactions to their clients—especially the transference of emotional and interpersonal dilemmas by clients into the client–therapist interaction and projection of attributes that they have found unacceptable in themselves or hurtful in others onto the therapist—can guide the psychotherapist in gaining a clearer and more empathically accurate understanding of how those dilemmas play out in their clients' inner lives and their external relationships and activities. Just as understanding transference reactions and enactments can enable clients to better understand themselves, so, too, recognizing countertransference reactions can provide psychotherapists with a mirror into their own personal issues and a window through which they better understand their client's inner and interpersonal experiences and dilemmas.

TRANSFERENCE-COUNTERTRANSFERENCE ENACTMENTS

When transference sparks an emotional reaction from the psychotherapist, some form of enactment is almost inevitable. Indeed, it is primarily, and perhaps only, through the enactment that a psychotherapist can be consciously aware of countertransference (Hunter, 1998). The key seems to be to attain insight into the countertransference reaction without impeding the client's progress in the psychotherapy or compromising the client's safety and well-being by violating professional or ethical boundaries with actions driven by countertransference reactions.

As difficult as it is to manage the more obvious manifestations of counter-transference, perhaps the greatest challenge facing psychotherapists is recognizing and managing the subtle and typically covert enactments of countertransference—what Jacobs (1986) described as the "covert, scarcely visible, yet persistent reactions that pervade [the psychotherapist's] listening and responding" (p. 292). This can lead to the kinds of problematic metacommunications that Bandler and Grinder (1975) described as a key mechanism underlying psychopathology and a critical focus for change in psychotherapy. For example, in Freud's (1905/1953) famous analysis of his patient Dora, he covertly adopted a complex and contradictory attitude and demeanor that was romanticized yet detached, sexualized yet puritanical, paternalistic yet childlike, hierarchical yet dependent, avoidant yet intrusive, and collaborative yet misogynistic. His actions were overtly appropriate as a doctor providing the indicated treatment according to his culture's and his own standards of care, yet his emotional history, conflicts, and blinders led him to treat Dora like a servant rather than a patient and also alternately as a mature adult or a wayward child rather than as an adolescent (Glenn, 1986; Mahony, 1996).

Countertransference enactments are actions through which the psychotherapist seeks to meet a personal need that either has not been met or has been responded to with punishment or rejection. In the case of seeking to meet a personal need, countertransference may lead the psychotherapist to accept a client's positive transference reactions (e.g., idealizing the psychotherapist) without helping the client to recognize and acknowledge both the psychotherapist's imperfections and the same or similar qualities in themselves. If the psychotherapist is kept up on a pedestal, that may gratify their need for approval, recognition, admiration, and love but reifies rather than helps the client to resolve their sense of unworthiness, dependency, and inferiority. It also makes affirmation of the psychotherapist the priority over affirmation of the client, which is exactly the opposite of a decentered and client-centered approach to psychotherapy.

In cases in which the psychotherapist accepts the client's idealization of them, countertransference is driven by unresolved feelings and unhealed emotional wounds: losses and grief, unachieved strivings and frustration, unrealized expectations and disappointment, threats to safety and terror, threats to security and anxiety, isolation or separation and loneliness, sexual or physical abuse and dissociation, emotional abuse or neglect and detachment. In these enactments, the psychotherapist is playing out personal dramas and tragedies by either joining with the client in perpetuating a belief that there is no way to come to terms with the feelings nor to heal the emotional wounds or by projecting the feelings and wounds onto the client when they are not actually the client's true experience or dilemma.

Alternatively, countertransference may be based on a need or desire that has put the psychotherapist personally in conflict with other people, with social norms or cultural mores, or with the psychotherapist's own moral or ethical standards or idealized view of themselves. This includes viewing the client as having feelings, needs, or motivations that are unacceptable for the psychotherapist to acknowledge in themselves (e.g., narcissism, anger, voyeurism, doubt, contempt, guilt, shame, hopelessness). In this context, the psychotherapist may find themselves engaged in a "formidable, if unconscious, battle" (Jacobs, 1986, pp. 299–300).

Countertransference enactments can be acts in which the psychotherapist joins with or actively opposes the client as well as those in which the psychotherapist actively confronts the client based on projection or displacement of the therapist's own emotional conflicts or otherwise imposes their unresolved issues on the client. When a client's transference projects a certain attitude (e.g., "You hate me") or role ("You're lying to me") on the psychotherapist, it is a natural human reaction to either object ("That's not true. You're seeing me in a distorted way") or take on the projection ("I think we've come as far as we can in this therapy"). Unless the client's transference reactions, and the psychotherapist's counter-reactions "are grasped by the [psychotherapist], he may find himself simply accepting the role imposed on him by the patient and joining him in a piece of mutual acting out" (Jacobs, 1986, p. 293).

Jacobs (1999) described how even the silence by a psychotherapist that is ostensibly in the pursuit of empathic understanding can conceal countertransference. Silence can serve as a way for the psychotherapist to avoid facing personally conflicted emotions (e.g., envy, anger, shame) when they are stimulated by a client who is experiencing an internal and relational dilemma with which the psychotherapist can identify as well as empathize based on their personal experiences. Similarly, efforts to maintain and convey an attitude of nonjudgmental neutrality can lead to avoidance of helping the client to recognize and work through internal or relational conflicts and binds that are familiar to the psychotherapist from their personal life. Silence also can become an expression of aggression. In such cases, psychotherapists may refrain from communicating with a client as an unconscious means of withholding contact or affirmation because of frustration when the client's dysregulation or transference reminds the psychotherapist of similar encounters that were unresolved in their own formative personal experiences.

COUNTERTRANSFERENCE PRECIPITATING OR EXACERBATING CRISES

Although countertransference can be a valuable source of knowledge about the client (as well as about the psychotherapist themself), Freud's (1910/1957) original cautionary note about countertransference remains a cogent warning. Countertransference reactions not only can impede psychotherapy but also can lead a psychotherapist to place demands on a client or to react explicitly or covertly in an impatient, harsh, dismissive, detached, or critical manner. Klein (1955) in "On Identification" cautioned psychoanalysts to recognize the powerful impact that clients' transferential projective identifications can have in stimulating their inner conflicts and emotions so as not to hold the client to blame (Gabbard, 1999). When psychotherapists react to their clients without awareness and empathic understanding because of countertransference, this constitutes an empathic failure (Kohut & Wolf, 1978). Empathic failures can trigger or exacerbate states of extreme emotional dysregulation by a client (e.g., experiencing a sense of betrayal, abandonment, shaming, or rejection). In other words, countertransference reactions, if expressed by the psychotherapist without self-reflection and empathic understanding and validation of the client's adaptive strivings, can precipitate crises in psychotherapy and serve as a major impediment to their resolution. Several examples follow.

THE PSYCHOTHERAPIST'S AGENDA TAKING PRECEDENCE OVER THE CLIENT'S ESSENTIAL SELF

One form that subtle countertransference enactments can take is *hierarchical elitism*, described by Schwaber (1992) as when "the analyst . . . retreat[s] from the patient's vantage point" (p. 349). Schwaber recounted a case that illustrated how even psychotherapists who are dedicated to taking a client-centered nonhierarchical position can unintentionally impose their own "agenda" on their clients based on "what I felt was good for you" (see also A. Miller, 1983, for how this can replicate what primary caregivers do when dictating their children's feelings, choices, and sense of self "for your own good"). She courageously and insightfully described how an unrecognized desire on her part as a psychotherapist that her client move forward with applying to graduate school had contributed to the client's "feeling like a zero . . . a feeling of being so alone" (p. 352) that he had reverted to engaging in risky behavior and was noncommunicative in the psychotherapy—that is, verging on, if not actually in, crisis in the therapy.

THE DISINTERESTED AND UNRESPONSIVE PSYCHOTHERAPIST IN THE GUISE OF NEUTRALITY

Another form of subtle countertransference enactments is detachment and abdication. The profound developmental and relational impairment that can occur when primary caregivers are emotionally disengaged and unresponsive to their children in the earliest years of life is well documented (Bowlby, 1969; Tronick et al., 1978). Enid Balint (1963) described how children who are met with an unresponsive primary caregiver when seeking emotional security and affirmation of their emotions and strivings can learn to stave off fear, grief, anger, shame, and aloneness by profoundly isolating themselves—by "being empty of oneself" (p. 470). In so doing, they create an inner life but often at the price of living in a terrifying inner fantasy world that can escalate into a breakdown (e.g., severe depression, paralyzing anxiety, unresolved bereavement, dissociative detachment and fragmentation) as they transition into adulthood. The crises that brought that Balint's client into psychotherapy and that emerged as the client relinquished her protective isolation and began to experience her body, self, and relationships as real were not the result of countertransference enactments by her psychoanalyst— nor were the crises that occurred when that client retreated back to a position of detachment and a state of internal and relational emptiness. But had the client's psychoanalyst reacted to her emotional emptiness based on countertransference, for example, with either persistent silence or intrusive attempts to get her to reveal and relinquish her fantasy life (e.g., to "correct" or "console" or "rescue" the client), those countertransference enactments could have iatrogenically replicated either the nonresponsivity that led initially to the client's psychological struggles or the terrifying intrusiveness of her fantasy world. In either case, at best, the analysis would have become stuck, and at worst, crises could have eventuated.

Thus, crises are precisely what can occur in even more extreme and potentially countertherapeutic, debilitating, and even dangerous ways (e.g., dissociative fragmentation and disengagement, aggression toward self or others, suicidal threats or acts) as a result of countertransference enactments in which the psychotherapist communicates disinterest or is otherwise disengaged and nonresponsive. Detachment is not the same as maintaining a therapeutic position of professional neutrality because neutrality involves genuine interest in and positive regard for the client in combination with being nonjudgmental and nonintrusive to be respectful of the client's point of view, privacy and integrity, and self-determination. Detachment as a result of countertransference is implicitly judgmental and invalidating (i.e., communicating that the client is not of sufficient worth or interest to warrant understanding their experience and perspective) as well as exploitive and intrusive (i.e., placing the burden on the client to "perform" so as to live up to the psychotherapist's expectations or standards)—far from "neutral" and completely at odds with maintaining a collaborative therapeutic alliance.

Here, too, countertransference enactments more often emerge subtly despite a conscious dedication by the psychotherapist to find value and meaning even when a client presents with flat and constricted affect or focuses only on what seem, at first glance, to be only mundane minutia, trivial complaints, or superficial concerns. The difficulty that a psychotherapist has in engaging with interest and without judgment in such cases may be further magnified if the client tends to seek advice and then respond with "yes, buts" when the psychotherapist offers a way that they can together come to an understanding of the issue that can enable the client to make informed and self-determined choices with the therapist's support and guidance. The "boring" or "frustrating" (or help-seeking and help-rejecting) client is less obvious a challenge than the extremely narcissistic (Modell, 1976) or "hateful patient" (Groves, 1978, p. 883) but no less likely to elicit countertransference that can trigger or fuel crises in therapy. Such clients often have experienced profound detachment and nonresponsivity in key relationships with caregivers at formative periods of their life, and can become profoundly psychologically "empty" or desperately dissociative, self-harming, or suicidal (in crisis) when a psychotherapist's countertransference replicates that detachment and nonresponsivity.

POSITIVE COUNTERTRANSFERENCE REACTIONS FROM THE PSYCHOTHERAPIST

Positive emotional reactions to clients (e.g., liking, admiration, inspiration, twinship) are a crucial therapeutic condition as demonstrated by clinical observations and research on the crucial role of unconditional positive regard in psychotherapy (Farber et al., 2018). The "too much of a good thing" phenomenon can occur, however, when positive regard becomes entangled with admiration and idealization of a client based on personal experiences. Jacobs (1986) described how countertransference can occur when a therapist replays a core personal experience in a manner that seems benign or even therapeutic but actually reduces the therapist's ability to provide empathic attention to the client:

My listening had taken on a special quality . . . something akin to awe, and I realized that although I had missed nothing, neither had I offered much in the way of interpretation. I became aware [that] I had been listening to [the patient] as, for years, I had listened to my father holding forth at the dinner table, expounding his personal view of world history. . . . Only later did I realize that the particular way in which I listened was serving an old and familiar purpose—to keep from my awareness the negative and competitive feelings I was experiencing toward [my father]. (pp. 295–296)

FEELINGS OF SYMPATHY FROM THE PSYCHOTHERAPIST AND A DESIRE TO RESCUE OR PROTECT

The duty to protect the safety of the client is a fundamental priority for psychotherapists. Unrecognized countertransference, however, can distort this aspiration, leading the therapist to perceive or exaggerate threats to a client. As well, the client's strengths, competence, and ability to effectively handle stressors or conflicts may be overlooked or undervalued, thus diminishing the client (and their self-valuation) in the process of attempting to sympathize and protect.

Atwood and Stolorow (1984) provided a telling example of a psychotherapist's reaction to a client whom she felt (based on countertransference) she needed reassurance of love. The client's

difficulties centered around a profound ambivalence . . . in close relationships . . . around her deep conviction that her hostile feelings constituted a deadly threat to those she loved. . . . She experienced the people on whom she relied for support and security as fragile and vulnerable . . . while her aggression seemed savagely destructive. . . . The therapist, too, had experienced difficulties with the expression of anger during her developmental years and had acquired a conviction that if she became hostile toward those she loved they would reject her and hate her. The therapist assured [the patient] that the expression of anger was permissible and even desirable in the analytic relationship . . . [seeking] to give reassurance. . . . The patient rejected these reassurances and her anxiety intensified, for she was experiencing this encouragement as an invitation to disaster. (pp. 50–51)

In this case, the psychotherapist was trying too hard to protect the client because of her own fear of the destructive power of anger. Doing so did not help the client to understand how she could express and experience anger in safe ways but instead left the client feeling rather more than less fearful of experiencing anger. The psychotherapy was able to progress when the therapist was able to recognize her own countertransference issues related to anger so that instead of simply attempting to reassure her client, she could engage the client in a genuinely therapeutic reexamination of how and why the client viewed important people in her life as fragile and vulnerable and her anger as destructive (Atwood & Stolorow, 1984, p. 51).

COUNTERTRANSFERENCE ENACTMENTS CROSSING MULTIPLE DOMAINS: TWO EXAMPLES

I recall two psychotherapy clients from many years ago with whom I experienced a complex mix of countertransference reactions and enactments. The first case illustrates how countertransference can amplify and exacerbate a slow-moving crisis that occurred over the course of psychotherapy. In the second case, my countertransference contributed to escalating distress by the client that resulted in an intense crisis involving the threat of suicide.

Each client was very intelligent, articulate, and charismatic interpersonally. One was a young adult; the other, in midlife. The client in Case 1 was focused on being popular socially and being seen with the "in-crowd"; she had no clear career or educational aspirations or interest in a committed primary relationship. The client in Case 2 was a career woman who wanted to have children but had delayed it for the sake of career advancement. She feared she would never find her true mate and had waited too long to ever have the family she dreamed of. Neither client felt able to live up to what she, and one or both of her parents, felt was her "potential." Both clients described their primary reason for seeking psychotherapy as overcoming chronic intense feelings of anxiety, including panic attacks and episodes of depression in which they felt unable to leave home to socialize or work. Neither had any history of suicidality or current thoughts of suicide, although both described struggling with increasingly strong feelings of hopelessness when depressed. These were two clients with serious legitimate reasons for being in psychotherapy and psychological issues worth attention. Furthermore, this was the first attempt at psychotherapy for each of these women.

I rarely have difficulty in taking a genuine interest in the lives, concerns, and questions raised by the clients with whom I work. Psychotherapy sessions, in my experience, usually begin with the client recounting recent experiences in waking life or dreams that might seem ordinary on the surface but that represent meaningful personal, relational, moral or ethical, and spiritual questions and dilemmas. Helping clients hear, and find meaning in, these essential concerns and aspirations as well as to see their core self that emerged in formative life experiences and relationships (including those that were affirming but also disappointments, unmet needs, and emotional wounds) are consistently emotionally moving and intellectually engaging challenges that hold my interest so completely that my attention to the client is entirely authentic. But not so in these cases: Try as I might, I could not find a way to move out of a position of being simultaneously frustrated, anxious, bored, and withdrawn or intrusive with these clients.

Case 1: Countertransference's Contributions to a Breakdown in the Psychotherapy

With the younger woman, I found myself falling into a virtual stupor while trying to listen to what seemed to be a nonstop narrative of people, places, and activities that was like a never-ending soap opera. When I attempted to offer a summary comment, she would not pause for a beat before continuing with her narration as if I'd not spoken. I realized that her pressured manner (which apparently also characterized her day-to-day life) and preoccupation with being popular with and seen by the world as a vital member of the in-crowd represented defenses against a pervasive sense of inadequacy and self-doubt, and anger, hurt, and loneliness in relationship to an emotionally absent father and an intrusively competitive and critical mother.

I felt stymied in seeking a way to help her recognize how, by avoiding facing those primal emotional dilemmas, she was perpetually repeating them in her adult life and as a result was failing to recognize and actualize her essential competence and worth. At some point, I realized that I had given up on helping this client to gain understanding and to come to know her true self, and had withdrawn into the stance of a passive audience member who listened but did not really hear this client. I told myself that she needed that audience to offset the ongoing criticism she described receiving from her mother and the indifference she perceived from her father. I was able to be neither critical nor indifferent on the surface, but I could not prevent myself from feeling both disappointed (with the squandered potential I saw in her) and bored with the soap opera.

Although not long by psychoanalytic or psychodynamic therapy standards, this therapy continued essentially on automatic pilot and life support for 2 years with no progress that I could discern. The client did not seem concerned about progress, never seeming to have any difficulty filling 50 minutes once or twice weekly with her narrative. I felt guilty that I looked forward to any break in the therapy when the client occasionally canceled when traveling. I questioned whether I should be taking her time and (her family's) money while I did nothing of value for her, and considered suggesting that we terminate therapy but then berated myself for being so insensitive as to replicate the rejection and abandonment that this client was attempting to cope with in her family. I also obsessed about whether this case was some form of poetic justice and evidence of my own narcissistic grandiosity and overvaluing of my knowledge, skill, and ability to be helpful as a psychotherapist. When the client announced that she was ending the therapy because she decided to move to "a bigger pond" in a city on the other coast, I felt both unburdened and relieved that she, rather than I, had been the one to decide to terminate therapy.

In retrospect, I'm not sure what difference it would have made if I had recognized several countertransference issues at the time, but I suspect that I could have at least left this client with the seeds of self-awareness had I not adopted the stance of a sympathetic, passive, and minimally attentive audience. The countertransference barriers that arose for me mirror those just discussed.

First, my agenda took precedence over the client's: My personal experience with a father who always seemed to know more than anyone else and to have all the answers (literally as a former debate champion and as a chief executive officer) but who was easily wounded by any criticism or challenge to his knowledge and authority played out in several ways with this client. I felt angry that she would not confirm my knowledge and authority by showing deference to my attempts to enlighten her. I viewed her as an immovable object who would never be overcome by the irresistible force of my psychotherapeutic skill.

Second, I felt disinterested in her narrative, her life, and her inner self: I had observed my father seemingly constantly communicating profound boredom with and disinterest in my mother's life, opinions, and feelings, and I found myself trivializing rather than finding personally valuable and illuminating meaning in my client's personal narrative. I had attributed my father's apparent indifference both to his lack of empathy and emotional depth, and also to a superficiality in my mother's intellectual and emotional life. In parallel, I faulted myself for being judgmental and unempathic with this client while also viewing her as an emotionally and intellectually an empty vessel that could not be filled.

Third, I admired this client for her spunk and chutzpah, and her ability to dominate relationships with her often incisive observations (about everyone else but herself) and storytelling. In that respect, I felt somewhat intimidated by her, as if I could never reach the celebrity status she described achieving (albeit largely by simply positioning herself in the right places at the right time as a celebrity groupie)—just as I had felt admiration for my father and was intimidated by him and the powerful people who associated with and respected him. In that position, I joined with my mother as an admiring outsider who never would be in that in-crowd or deserve that respect. As a result I succumbed to doubts as to whether, as a therapist, I could have anything of value to offer a client from that lofty circle.

And fourth, at the same time that I admired the client's spunk, I also viewed the client as extremely emotionally fragile and in need of protection: I saw the client as a person who was falsely pretending to be knowledgeable, confident, and strong but who, in reality, was easily emotionally wounded and potentially on the verge of collapsing like the Wizard of Oz, as I viewed my father—and, simultaneously, as legitimately emotionally vulnerable and in need of compassion and affirmation, as I viewed my mother. As a result, when I felt rebuffed in my attempts to help the client to see behind the screen of her defenses and to stop her frenzied attempts to keep running (emotionally, verbally, and interpersonally) fast enough to not be caught and overrun by her fears and doubts, I decided it was hopeless and potentially even cruel to help her with active therapeutic interventions that could emotionally immobilize her.

Case 2: Countertransference's Contributions to a Psychotherapy Crisis

With the midlife client, there was no lack of back-and-forth in the psychotherapy interaction. This client also had an intense narrative to recount in each session, but she did so with a range of emotions that revealed vulnerability (unlike the Case 1 client's angry or detached emotional constriction). Furthermore, she frequently interspersed questions about herself for which she expressed a genuine desire in help with her search of answers (unlike the Case 1 client's apparent disinterest in raising any questions or seeking any help involving self-exploration).

At times, this client would push the boundaries of the therapeutic contract. She periodically expressed frustration at having to end sessions when she felt she had so much left to say and so many questions unanswered. She also would request a telephone consultation when feeling distressed in between sessions and began several sessions by disclaiming that she knew that other therapists would take the time to talk with their clients when an immediate need arose and would not make them wait until the next in-person session. Over time, she increasingly voiced frustration that nothing was changing in her life despite all the effort she was making by doing the hard work of dealing with painful feelings in psychotherapy. It seemed to me that nothing was changing in her outer life—which largely involved work in an administrative job that she found frustrating and unfulfilling, and short-term involvements with men that always ended in disappointment—because nothing was changing in her inner life. Her expressed feelings seemed more like complaints and solicitations of sympathy than authentic emotions, and her reflections seemed more like rationalizations and demands than genuinely introspective contemplation and questions in search of meaning.

In this context, it perhaps is not surprising that a crisis might be expectable, although in retrospect, I believe that had I been more aware of my countertransference, there could have been a better resolution of the therapeutic dilemmas without a crisis. What did happen was that the client arrived at a scheduled session atypically late and in an atypical state of evident emotional disarray that included disheveled clothing (in contrast to her usual presentation with a demeanor of emotional poise and extremely neat and stylish accoutrement). She had been crying in her car and could not stop until she had sat in the parking lot for a very long time, she said. I expressed surprise and genuine concern for the emotional pain she was experiencing. She said,

> Thank you, but your sympathy is really not doing me any good right now. I know you're trying, but you just don't seem to understand my life, what I'm going through, and no one else cares enough about me to even try to help, let alone to really help me change this miserable life that I'm existing—not living—in.

After a moment, while she appeared immersed in inner thoughts, I replied,

> It seems like things have really come to a head in a way that's deeply painful and discouraging for you, and I take that very seriously. Can you help me understand what's happened, or what's happening, so that we can see if there is a way that we together can help you with the misery and aloneness that you're feeling?

She looked up, appearing quite taken aback and angry, and said,

> I'm not here to help you! If you can't understand what I need or help me change my miserable and pointless life, then I think I've done all that I can, and it's time for me to get off this merry-go-round and do what I should have done years ago: just end it all.

We had talked about times in the past when this client had contemplated suicide, but she had said that she never actually intended to follow through even with a suicidal gesture because she didn't want to give up on herself and she didn't want to hurt family members (primarily nieces and nephews with whom she had developed a close quasimaternal relationship) whom she felt would feel betrayed and guilty if she ever tried to end her life. She had expressed a sense of doubt that she could ever free herself from the

anxieties and disappointments with which she had struggled since childhood—but never outright hopelessness. My immediate reaction was that
this was a crisis of imminent suicidality, and I responded by telling her that
we needed to make sure that she was safe. She took this as a challenge and
a coercive demand or threat on my part:

> You're not going to help me. You just want me to calm down and not do
> anything to disturb this neat little world you therapists all have. My life is too
> messy, so I'll do you a favor and end it.

At that point, I was reeling internally. Clearly, what I was saying and
doing was making things worse, not better. I felt as though I was trying to
stop a hurricane that I was powerless to stop as it tore through the psychotherapy and was heading on a path of destruction. In retrospect, I realized
that I had come full circle through several phases of countertransference
with this client. Initially, my reaction was to sympathize with her sense of
bravely enduring a life in which she was unappreciated, alone, and burdened
by the expectations and needs of other people who viewed themselves and
were viewed by society as more important than her. In this respect, there were
numerous parallels to how I'd viewed my mother as a dedicated caregiver
to my father and our entire family who stoically endured his neglect while
putting his and others' needs ahead of her own. I feared that, without help
in extricating herself from the isolation and exploitive relationships in which
she constantly described herself as being trapped, my client would reach
her limit and fall apart—as I had seen my mother do periodically, when
she would retreat to her bed for days at a time with what were described as
attacks of neuralgia (and that, as a child, I feared might cause her to die).
I admired the client for her courageous willingness to stand up for herself
and protest the emotional pain she was suffering as well as to call out the
people in her life whom she felt were letting her down and falsely pretending
to be more important than her, and stronger and intellectually, vocationally,
and interpersonally superior to her—acts of truth telling and pursuit of
justice that I'd wished my mother had been willing or able to do.

As a result, I tried to overlook or rationalize the client's contributions to
her emotional dilemmas. For example, I viewed her as valiantly struggling
to assert herself but overlooked how she was thinly concealing unrealistic
expectations and harsh criticisms that she imposed on others by faulting
them for doing the same to her. In that process, I also discounted her true
strengths and capabilities. For example, I viewed her as an alienated victim
in need of rescuing and then as frustratingly help-seeking and help-rejecting
rather than affirming her determination to find genuine caring, respect,
and mutuality in relationships. I'd become frustrated with her for filling

the hours with what seemed like a broken record of complaints, external-ized blame, and "yes, buts" to my efforts to help her shift from focusing on unsolvable problems to building meaningful solutions. I became convinced that she was too stubbornly invested in secondary gain to even consider, let alone put into action, real solutions. She came to seem more like my father—critical, never satisfied, entitled, and belittling of others, including me—than my mother, and my mother's patient perseverance and uncondi-tional acceptance seemed a better path for the client to follow. As I kicked the client off the pedestal on which I had put her, not surprisingly, she felt abandoned, unappreciated, and misused by me, and needed to both knock me off my pedestal and show me the intolerable suffering and burden that people like me had forced her to endure.

All of this came to a head in the crisis session. Only after I finally had the presence of mind to stop trying to force her to renounce her determination to end it all did I learn that she had had two major emotional injuries that very day. Instead of pressuring her to make a safety plan (which, later in the session, we were able to do collaboratively), I acknowledged that I was not listening to the message that she wanted me to understand and that I was pressing my own agenda rather than supporting her in expressing what was important to her and helping her to recover from what must be deeply distressing experiences. I said that her anger at me made sense as an honest and insightful statement to step up to my responsibility to under-stand what she was telling me in a way that would be helpful on her own terms and not based on my prejudgments. I wondered if she would be willing to tell me what had been on her mind right from the start of the session that I had been missing in my rush to pursue my own professional agenda.

After some challenges to test my authenticity (e.g., "You'll probably think this is too trivial, that I'm just falling apart for no reason"; "You probably can't do anything to help me with this; nothing ever seems to get better"), the client disclosed two disappointments that had just occurred that day and were emotionally wounding for her. She described how she had been criticized publicly at work by her usually affirming and appreciative super-visor, and then told by a male coworker, whom she thought was working up the courage to ask her out on a date, that she was making too much of the situation and that she shouldn't let her supervisor's having a bad day make it seem like the end of the world. We discussed her fear that this meant that she had irrevocably lost two important allies at her workplace who also were among the few people whom she felt respected and supported her as a person rather than just for her work skills. The plan that we developed was not a superficial no-self-harm safety contract but a series of steps she felt she could take—and wanted to take—to reconnect with her supervisor (and let her know how much she appreciated her supervisor's respect and support) and to talk with her coworker to let him know that she appreciated his intent to reassure her and to check out whether he really was the kind of person whom she wanted as a friend (withholding judgment on any potential further involvement until she felt she knew whether he could be a true friend).

This session illustrates a crisis that might have happened even if I had been aware of my countertransference reactions but that was intensified by the countertherapeutic attitude and enactments that I brought into the therapeutic interaction because of my unrecognized countertransference. Had I paid more attention to my own personal reactions and how they were based not only on the client's behavior and transferences to me but also on my personal history, I would have had a greater understanding of this client's chronic struggle with a sense of being unappreciated and burdened rather than cared for and supported in her relationships. I also would have recognized that, when she brought emotional and interpersonal conflicts into her perception of the therapeutic relationship and of me as a person, this transference represented attempts by her to find new ways to understand and resolve those long-standing dilemmas. Rather than falling into the countertransference traps of idealizing, devaluing, or infantilizing her, I could have taken transference enactments as an opportunity to better understand the meaning for her, based on her personal history of formative relationships and experiences, of crucial experiences in her current life and to help her develop ways to respond to those experiences that reflected her core values, aspirations, needs, and personal talents and interests. That is what we began to do when I was able, albeit belatedly, to decenter and focus on validating her perceptions and pay attention to what she was trying to get me to understand—both about our interaction in the psychotherapy and about her life outside of therapy. Although the client chose to stop therapy while still grappling with her internal and interpersonal dilemmas, there were no further crises of suicidality or other extreme expressions of desperation and hopelessness in the psychotherapy.

COUNTERTRANSFERENCE AS AN OPPORTUNITY TO PREVENT OR RESOLVE CRISES

As the examples from my own and other psychotherapists' experiences illustrate, the recognition and management of countertransference potentially represents a key to preventing and resolving crises in psychotherapy.

Countertransference represents not only a window into clients' inner life and their effects on others in relationships but also an opportunity to help clients to understand emotional and interpersonal difficulties without shame or blame. Bion (1963) likened psychoanalysts to containers who could transform and detoxify their clients' unconscious conflicts and projections so that the clients ultimately could reinternalize a more adaptive view of themselves and their relationships (beginning with the therapeutic relationship).

Along similar lines, Winnicott (1963) described the therapeutic relationship as a "holding environment" in which

> the analyst is holding the patient, and this often takes the form of conveying in words at the appropriate moment something that shows that the analyst knows and understands the deepest anxiety that is being experienced, or that is waiting to be experienced. (p. 240)

To safely and therapeutically provide psychic containment and understanding of the client's "deepest anxiety" and unconscious conflicts, the psychotherapist must in parallel manner recognize, contain, and understand their own inner needs, conflicts, and emotions.

Thus, knowing (i.e., recognizing, nonjudgmentally accepting, and finding meaning and value in) one's own countertransference reactions can enable a psychotherapist to understand and provide their clients with a therapeutic process for knowing and resolving the inner and interpersonal dilemmas that have led to, and continue to perpetuate, emotional dysregulation. When psychotherapists recognize and take responsibility for the personal emotional reactions that are elicited by clients and their interaction in therapy sessions, this also strengthens essential professional boundaries by reducing the likelihood that the psychotherapist's countertransference reactions will become enactments. It is no less true for psychotherapists than for their clients that awareness and conscious reflection are the best way to prevent impulses from becoming enacted.

When the psychotherapist recognizes their own distinct emotional reactions to a client, those reactions can be a valuable clue to a better understanding of the client's emotional reactions and the relational experiences that historically have contributed to those reactions by the client. When the reactions have a negative valence, as tends to be the case when clients are grappling with problems with emotional dysregulation, the psychotherapist can draw on their own experiences to formulate nonjudgmental and affirming ways of understanding the legitimacy, meaningfulness, and value of the client's emotional reactions and conflicts. Thus, by containing countertransference reactions (i.e., recognizing and accepting personal feelings and thoughts that are elicited by the client and their interaction) and reflectively developing a nonjudgmental understanding of the origins and potential meaning of those reactions in their own life, the psychotherapist can formulate and communicate to the client new and affirming ways of understanding the client's inner distress and interpersonal or other life difficulties.

Managing and using countertransference by intentionally focusing on recognizing, owning, and finding meaning and value in emotional reactions experienced when interacting with clients also is crucial to enabling the psychotherapist to be simultaneously empathically attuned and responsive to the client while maintaining a degree of separateness that supports the client's autonomy and their ability to be simultaneously self-sufficient and meaningfully engaged in the psychotherapy and in the client–therapist relationship (Modell, 1976). When the psychotherapist acknowledges their emotional reactions as their own responsibility, this provides the client with a role model for mature individuation and respectful participation in a primary dyadic relationship. Lapsing into the negative relational stances that can occur when countertransference is unacknowledged and unmanaged (e.g., rejection, blame, impatience, infantilization of the client; Hora, 1951) is a recipe for alienating clients and provoking (or escalating) crises in psychotherapy. Managing countertransference reactions with awareness and self-reflection, and using those reactions to nonjudgmentally understand the meaning and value of both one's own and ultimately the client's inner and interpersonal experience, is a recipe for preventing or resolving crises in psychotherapy.

COUNTERTRANSFERENCE: RECOGNIZING AND PREVENTING ENACTMENTS

Through clinical observation, J. A. Hayes et al. (2018) identified five factors as essential to the management of countertransference. They identified research that supports the value of each of these characteristics of therapists and noted that they "do not reflect what a therapist actually does to manage CT [countertransference], but . . . are . . . characteristics that are positively associated with CT management" (p. 498):

> [T]herapist *self-insight* refers to the extent to which the therapist is aware of his or her own feelings, including CT feelings, and understands their basis. Therapist *self-integration* refers to the therapist's possession of an intact, basically healthy character structure . . . [which manifests] . . . in the therapy interaction . . . as a recognition of interpersonal boundaries and an ability to differentiate self from other. *Anxiety management* refers to therapists allowing

themselves to experience anxiety and also possessing the internal skill to control and understand anxiety so that it does not bleed over into their responses to patients. *Empathy*, or the ability to partially identify with and put one's self in the other's shoes, permits the therapist to focus on the patient's needs despite difficulties he or she may be experiencing with the work and the pulls to attend to his or her own needs . . . which in turn ought to prevent acting out of CT. . . . Finally, *conceptualizing ability* reflects the therapist's ability to draw on theory in the work and grasp the patient's dynamics in terms of the therapeutic relationship. (p. 498)

Although several studies have shown association between negative countertransference attitudes and actions by psychotherapists and poorer psychotherapy outcomes (Table 1 in J. A. Hayes et al., 2018), there is limited empirical evidence demonstrating precisely how the five factors translate into effective management of countertransference (Table 2 in J. A. Hayes et al., 2018). Psychotherapist self-awareness has been found to be inversely related (i.e., potentially protective against) negative countertransference enactments, but the other four factors have not been tested in relationship to countertransference attitudes or enactments. With the exception of a self-report Countertransference Management Scale (Pérez-Rojas et al., 2017), precisely what constitutes effective countertransference management has not been systematically operationally defined. The items in that scale essentially replicate the five domains of psychotherapist attributes that have been hypothesized to mitigate the adverse effects of countertransference. By definition, the five factors describe a psychotherapist who can modulate anxiety sufficiently in session to be aware of their own reactions and the sources or those reactions in their personal history, and to be able to distinguish those from the client's personal reactions and history while focusing on valuing and understanding the client's inner and interpersonal life based on the client's viewpoint and personal history. With that foundation, the psychotherapist is in a good position to be able to formulate a conceptualization of the client's psychosocial difficulties and personal strengths and weaknesses, and to use that formulation to understand and assist the client by developing a therapeutic alliance and interventions promoting new or enhanced personal insight and skills.

Thus, the effective management of countertransference essentially parallels the process of effective psychotherapy but with a crucial addition. The psychotherapist's frame of reference must encompass not only an understanding of the client as a person but also themselves as a person and how their personal reactions to and with the client (and their origins in their personal history) affect their perceptions and conceptualizations of the client in ways that can interfere with (or even cause harm; i.e., be iatrogenic) or enhance the psychotherapy. Awareness of and managing countertransference reactions and enactments provide a practical framework for psychotherapists to use themselves as a therapeutic tool rather than adopt the counterfactual position of a being purely objective professional deliverer of therapeutic services.

The result of a psychotherapist's intentional deployment of these five factors is elegantly illustrated in a case example (Mr. B) described by Schwaber (1992, pp. 356–357). In response to Mr. B's hesitant expression of sexual feelings toward the psychotherapist and his description of feeling anxious that she was "repelled" by him, the psychotherapist suggested that he might have felt "scared" if she hadn't stepped back from him in a recent situation in which he had approached her in the waiting room. Mr. B had agreed with that interpretation at the time but then "no longer felt that there was anything in particular on which he wanted to work, and he sounded somewhat flat." Mr. B later told the psychotherapist,

> It was like you were saying I couldn't handle your sexuality . . . [that] you're not man enough, . . . just like my mother, always emasculating me. . . . I felt put down by you. . . .

At that point, the psychotherapist expanded her conceptual focus from sexual anxiety to an empathic understanding of a deeper sense of "humiliation and belittlements" that could be traced back to "old hurts" in the formative relationship Mr. B had with his mother. The psychotherapist subsequently engaged in rigorous self-reflection, seeking self-insight.

Schwaber (1992) did not explicitly refer to the role of anxiety management in her approach to managing countertransference enactments, but it is evident that by being open to "resist . . . my inclination to teach, and [seek] instead to learn what I did not yet understand, about [my client], and perhaps about me too" (p. 357), she is describing a willingness to confront the anxiety of not "knowing—even about ourselves—what is the correct reality" (p. 359). She also illustrated, with humility, the importance of having sufficient self-integration to be able to acknowledge that "repeatedly I stumble, seeing through my own pre-fixed lens" (p. 358).

Schwaber (1992) concluded with a summary of both the problem of countertransference and a very practical (albeit extremely challenging to actually put into action) way to manage it:

> Countertransference interferes when, knowingly or not, I won't let go of the supposed greater wisdom of my own vantage point. . . . If there is a discrepancy between my view and the patient's, I must ask the question, do I not use this difference to guide the patient, however subtly . . . in my direction, or even to arrive at some compromise between us; or is it evidence of something I have yet to learn, which I don't now understand? (p. 359)

In most, if not all cases, the answer to this essential question is: both. The answer that there is more to the client's experience than even the most sensitive expert psychotherapist can fully understand unless they listen carefully and is guided by the client is an essential frame for preventing and therapeutically resolving crises in the psychotherapy session.

THE FREEDOM FRAMEWORK: APPLICATION TO COUNTERTRANSFERENCE MANAGEMENT IN CRISES

Thinking back to our discussion in Chapter 5 of the FREEDOM framework as a template for therapists in assisting clients in crisis, let's now look at how the FREEDOM steps can serve in addition as a template for countertransference management in crises in the psychotherapy session. When therapists are faced with an emotionally dysregulated client, the first FREEDOM step, the SOS approach for focusing, provides therapists a way to rapidly enhance self-insight (J. A. Hayes et al., 2018). The first SOS substep is to clear one's mind and concentrate on noticing but letting go of immediate thoughts and nonjudgmental awareness of bodily signs of stress (the slow down and sweep your mind clear starting point). The first substep in the SOS is essentially a shortcut to mindful acceptance and awareness of stress-related thoughts and bodily state and reactions (Niles et al., 2020).

The second SOS substep is identifying an orienting thought. Orienting involves circumscribing one's awareness by focusing on just one thought or image that represents whatever is most important to the therapist at that moment. Orienting is of particular importance in the midst of a crisis because it serves as an integrative counterpoint to the flood of reactive thoughts that are inevitable as the therapist experiences the freeze (and subsequently the fight–flight) phase of the stress response in reaction to the client's emotional dysregulation. Consciously (but silently) putting into words or imagery what's most important from the therapist's perspective is a way to engage self-integration (Dales & Jerry, 2008): focusing on core values, goals, and sources of security that strengthen the therapist's sense of having a coherent stabilizing identity in the face of the crisis. In a crisis, a therapist's orienting thoughts might include ones such as "I need to listen carefully and empathically" or "My client's safety is my priority" or "I've got this. I'll figure out how we can get through this" or "I know this client trusts me, but he's having a hard time remembering that while he's feeling so desperate."

The third substep in the SOS, the self-check, provides therapists with a quick way to monitor their own stress level using the Personal Stress Rating

Scale (1 = *no stress* to 10 = *worst stress ever experienced*). The self-check also includes a separate rating of one's *degree of personal control*, which is defined as the ability to think clearly under stress (Ford, 2020c). Recognizing and quantifying one's level of stress and personal control are a means of both self-monitoring (Maas et al., 2013) and engaging executive function (i.e., intentional self-reflection or mentalizing; Fonagy & Campbell, 2017). In this way, the therapist can transform a diffuse freeze, fight, or flight stress reaction into a meaningful self-appraisal that acknowledges the stress reactions while also affirming the therapist's ability to be emotionally regulated. Once focusing has been initiated, the SOS can be repeated as needed for the therapist to remain emotionally regulated despite experiencing additional stress reactions in response to the client's emotional dysregulation and transference enactments.

The recognizing triggers step in FREEDOM involves identifying the specific behavior and communications by the client as well as aspects of the immediate context that are eliciting stress reactions for the therapist and those that may be eliciting client stress reactions. This can include obvious actions by the client that are expressions of emotional dysregulation (e.g., angry accusations or threats, self-harm or suicidality, dissociative fugue states) but also subtler triggers (e.g., the perseverative monologue described by Jacobs, 1986, and in my case example). Contextual triggers might include the emergence of practical issues (e.g., payment of fees); separations (e.g., the therapist's recent absence because of a vacation or illness); major changes in the client's life or well-being that evoke hope or demoralization, or evidence of progress (or lack thereof); or regression or the emergence of new symptoms by the client.

Recognizing triggers is a crucial part of anxiety management (J. A. Hayes et al., 2018). When the therapist consciously identifies the most likely or impactful triggers for their personal stress reactions in the midst of a crisis, this shifts the therapist's focus from their client's distress to managing their own stress reactions. This might seem to be a distraction from devoting full attention to the client, but it actually can increase the therapist's ability to attend to the client: When triggers for personal reactions are identified, they are less likely to elicit the kinds of countertransference enactments than triggers that go unrecognized (Gabbard, 1999; Jacobs, 1986). Recognizing personal triggers also can enhance the therapist's acuity in recognizing the triggers that are eliciting stress reactions for the client by facilitating the detection of similar patterns of triggered stress reactions that are affecting the client. Thus, by taking a few seconds to focus on and identify triggers, the therapist can create a grounded foundation for responding to a client's crisis in an emotionally regulated manner. The remaining FREEDOM steps build on that foundation.

Once focused and consciously aware of potential stress triggers, the next four steps in the FREEDOM framework are a guide for the therapist in doing a rapid silent inventory of the stress reactive emotions, thoughts, goals, and behavioral options that those triggers are eliciting. These are the reactive emotions (e.g., frustration, worry, guilt), thoughts (e.g., "I have to rescue this client"; "This client only listens to themselves"), goals (e.g., to endure the boredom, to convince the client that their anger is healthy, to show the client that they are not repellent), and behavioral options (e.g., pretend to pay attention, give advice, avoid upsetting topics) that are often the product of countertransference. At the very least, they are inconsistent with best practices in psychotherapy (see Chapter 4), but they are understandable human reactions. By making these aspects of one's own stress reactions in a crisis transparent to oneself, the essential antidote for countertransference enactments can be achieved: The "EEDO" steps provide a rapid conscious inventory of countertransference reactions so that these reactions are reflectively acknowledged by the therapist rather than reflexively enacted in interacting with the client. The examples described earlier in this chapter show how this self-reflective process often does not occur until after a session has ended—sometimes too late to prevent or contain a crisis. Instead, using the "EEDO" steps as a practical guide, therapists can intentionally engage in self-reflection to clarify their personal reactions in crises in real time rather than only after the fact.

The EEDO steps also provide a structure for therapists to move from a state of reactivity to emotion regulation. Using the principle of orienting to core values and goals from the SOS, the EEDO steps can be used to do a rapid inventory of sustaining emotions (e.g., interest, caring), core beliefs (e.g., optimism, compassion, confidence in self, client, and the therapeutic relationship), core goals (e.g., supporting client resilience and self-esteem, strengthening a collaborative partnership with the client), and therapeutic behavioral options that are consistent with those emotions, beliefs, and goals (e.g., acknowledging the client's distress, validating the client's core goals, affirming the commitment to partner with the client). This provides a basis for calmly and confidently engaging collaboratively and empathically with the client, as illustrated, for example, by Schwaber's (1992) willingness to "resist . . . my inclination to teach, and [seek] instead to learn what I did not yet understand, about [my client], and perhaps about me too" (p. 357). Such acts of therapeutic integrity are the key to transforming crises into turning points in the psychotherapy and in clients' lives—and, as such, they are the completion of the FREEDOM steps with the therapist's willingness to be responsible for their own emotion regulation: **m**aking a contribution as a role model and guide for the client in crisis.

CONCLUSION

The act of engaging in truly client-centered listening and of incrementally acquiring and therapeutically communicating to the client an empathic understanding of the client's inner and interpersonal history and life are keys to both preventing and resolving (i.e., therapeutically transforming) crises in psychotherapy. Countertransference—when recognized and managed—paradoxically can inform and guide the therapist in the process of resolving crises. At the very least, recognizing countertransference through an active process of self-reflection will contribute to the therapist's emotion regulation in the midst of a crisis. With that foundation of emotion regulation, the therapist is in a position to intervene mindfully and effectively with the crisis intervention and psychotherapeutic strategies discussed in Chapters 4 through 6. Let's turn next to a series of case examples that bring to life how crises emerge and are resolved by real therapists who are faced with life-and-death dilemmas in their psychotherapy sessions.

PART **II** CASE SESSION
TRANSCRIPTS OF
IN-SESSION CRITICAL
MOMENTS

7

SUPPORTING A RECENTLY TRAUMATIZED YOUTH IN A CRISIS OF DISSOCIATION AND SELF-HARM

CASE BACKGROUND[1]

Samantha, a 15-year-old African American young woman, was referred for psychotherapy by the hospital where she was taken after she was gang raped while passed out at a party after drinking more than she ever had. This is Samantha's first ever outpatient psychotherapy session, and she finds herself experiencing disorienting and, at times, overwhelming waves of depression and hopelessness as well as dissociative fugue states. Trying to calm herself, Samantha also finds herself involuntarily scratching at her arm and sucking her thumb, both of which give her a comforting sense of emotional and physical numbness.

---

[1]To view the webinar associated with this case, including a video of the psychotherapy session, go online (https://learn.nctsn.org/course/view.php?id=478). Alternatively, you can go to the main website (https://learn.nctsn.org), click "Clinical Training" in the menu bar at the top of the page, click "Identifying Critical Moments and Healing Complex Trauma," and then click the webinar associated with this case: "Supporting a Recently Traumatized Youth in a Crisis of Dissociation and Self-Harm." Although you will need to create an account ID and password, there is no fee to access the webinar.

https://doi.org/10.1037/0000225-008
Crises in the Psychotherapy Session: Transforming Critical Moments Into Turning Points, by J. D. Ford

Samantha's friends describe her as beautiful, a kind and honest person with a great sense of humor, an A student, and a star athlete. Samantha attends an exclusive private high school on scholarship; there, she is one of very few students of color. Her dream is to get a scholarship to an Ivy League university. When not studying or on the lacrosse field, she volunteers to help children and families in need in the community and for human rights causes. Older boys have frequently asked Samantha out, but she has never agreed because her parents are strict about dating and don't want her to get entangled in a romantic relationship and lose her focus on college.

Samantha's family lives in urban public housing, where drug abuse and community violence are common occurrences. When she was 10 years old, Samantha witnessed her older brother, Andre, get shot and killed. He was walking her home from school, and they were caught in the cross fire of a gang fight. At the time, she didn't understand what had happened when he suddenly fell down and blood was all over the sidewalk around him. She tried to get him to wake up and get up, but he wouldn't open his eyes, move, or speak. She remembers neighbors taking her home and her mother screaming and sobbing when told that Andre had been shot. Samantha recalls that her mother "never was the same" after that: She wouldn't go out except to go to work and return home. Samantha frequently found her mother seemingly in another world, sobbing and saying, "My boy, my boy!" After the shooting, Samantha's father also started drinking alcohol to the point of intoxication several times a week. Samantha has learned to stay away from him when he is drinking because he changes from being a loving and kind man to an angry and violent person she doesn't recognize.

Samantha's parents kept their jobs; they work long hours and encourage her to get scholarships and do well in school and sports. Samantha feels very grateful but also guilty that her parents are stressed and working hard while she seems to be enjoying school and sports in a sheltered school setting. Girls in her neighborhood, though, call her an "Oreo" (because she is Black but they see her as trying to act like a White girl) and have stopped being friends with Samantha. At school, girls pick on the way she speaks, saying she sounds like a "ghetto girl" and that she only got into the school because of charity or government handouts. She has a solid group of male friends but sometimes feels like she doesn't really fit in with the other girls at school. Girls are also jealous of her because of the attention she gets from boys, which has made making girlfriends even more difficult. She has one close female friend, Lily, who is also on the lacrosse team.

At the end of Samantha's junior year, after she had aced a very difficult AP (Advanced Placement) chemistry exam, Lily convinced her to go to a senior summer kickoff party. A graduating senior, Jack, who had been asking Samantha out since she was a freshman, was hosting the party and wanted both girls to come. After prodding from Lily, Samantha decided to "let loose" for one night and attend the party. Samantha told her parents that she was sleeping over at Lily's. Jack made a big deal of Samantha's being at the party and offered to "grab drinks." Although he was enthusiastic, Jack had always been friendly and had never been aggressive in his pursuit of Samantha. Samantha had only experimented with alcohol, but she wanted the full party experience, so she decided to "go for it."

Samantha began by slowly sipping on a drink, but then got pulled into a drinking game with Jack and his guy friends. She quickly became intoxicated. Jack asked her if she wanted to go somewhere quiet to talk, and Samantha agreed. Jack helped her walk precariously to his bedroom, and the moment she sat on his bed, Samantha passed out. Realizing that she needed to be taken care of, Jack went to find Lily. This took quite a while with the raucous party spilling over into all parts of the house. When Jack and Lily returned, they saw four very intoxicated guys nervously coming up the hallway from the direction of Jack's room. When Jack and Lily entered the room and turned on the lights, they saw Samantha sprawled out and mostly undressed on Jack's bed, still unconscious. Lily called an ambulance and Samantha's parents.

Samantha woke up in a hospital room with Lily, Jack, her parents, and a nurse. "What happened?" she mumbled. "The last thing I remember was being with you, Jack. Something's wrong. I feel all numb but like my body's been run over by a truck. Did we get into an accident?" The next several weeks were a nightmare for Samantha and for her parents and friends. She felt depressed and scared because she could tell she had been assaulted, but she had no memory of it. When she met with a sexual assault counselor working with the police and learned that one of the boys had confessed and that she might have to go to court if criminal charges were pressed, she felt terrified and like the whole world would know she was "dirty." The sexual assault counselor got her an appointment with a female therapist who worked with girls and women who have been sexually assaulted. Samantha delayed starting psychotherapy for several weeks by canceling several sessions. Her parents finally insisted that she talk with the therapist and drove her to this, her first, psychotherapy session.

SESSION TRANSCRIPT, ANNOTATIONS, AND COMMENTARY

After the annotated session transcript, I present a summary of Samantha's observations and reflections on her experience in the session. Following this summary is commentary highlighting key themes and take-home points for handling this or similar crises, and questions for reader self-reflection.

THERAPIST: So, Samantha, tell me a little bit about you.

SAMANTHA: (*Stares at her lap*) I'm in school.

THERAPIST: Mm-hmm.

SAMANTHA: (*Still looks down but glances furtively at the therapist*) And I'm into my senior year. I like to play volleyball.

> *Therapist's Inner Reflections:* Samantha seems very withdrawn and in a lot of pain and emotional turmoil. She looks haunted; there's definite fear in her eyes, and she's glazing over and just barely holding it together. Looks like she's heading for an emergency and a breakdown. I want to help her reorient to the present, so I'll engage her in focusing on who she was before the rape with an emphasis on her physical self so that she can become more aware of her body and slow down the flood of ruminations that she appears to be experiencing. By orienting to the strengths and abilities she had—and still has—this can help her do an SOS [as discussed in Chapter 5, SOS refers to slowing down and sweeping her mind clear, orienting to a thought that helps her feel safe, and self-checking stress level and level of personal control] and begin to feel more personal control despite the intense distress she's feeling. I'm not going to introduce the SOS formally to her because that would seem too didactic and intrusive, but I can help her do an SOS and begin to focus herself by showing an interest in her interests and strengths.

THERAPIST: Excellent. I know that you know this—I met with your parents a little bit before you, so they told me that you have been a great athlete for a while. So, volleyball is now your favorite sport?

SAMANTHA: (*Hunches over, looks at her feet, no longer glances at the therapist*) Uh-huh.

THERAPIST: Excellent. Wonderful. Okay. And, um, I also know that things have been rough the past 3½ weeks . . . and that's why you're here today. So, I want you to know that—that we can work on this, that this is actually gonna be, um, a little bit hard at the beginning, but I know that you will—we will figure out ways that you can really overcome this terrible thing that had just happened to you. I'm sorry. So, because you're a good athlete, I know that you work hard . . .

SAMANTHA: (*Relaxes slightly*) Mm-hmm.

Therapist's Inner Reflections: I'm not going to ask her to tell me what's triggering the distress for her because that probably seems obvious to her (even though it's more complicated than she fully recognizes). By acknowledging the trauma in general terms, I've signaled to her that I do recognize what's triggering her but that I'm not going to dredge up what's happened or how she's feeling because she's probably trying very hard to not be aware of the shame and betrayal that I expect she's feeling—and to not think about the rape, even though she probably can't stop having intrusive memories, especially because she was not conscious while the rape happened. For the sake of Samantha's sense of security in talking with me, which is very new and fragile—with this being our first session (and the betrayal she's experienced) and her damaged sense of self and efficacy—I'm going to emphasize her ability to accomplish difficult goals at this point.

THERAPIST: . . . and also your parents told me that you are a very good student, too.

SAMANTHA: (*Looks up tentatively*) Uh-huh.

THERAPIST: You have worked for—for everything that you have now. Right? And you really just have to finish your senior year the same way that you have actually, you know, have worked so hard your whole life to be where you are. So, your parents are telling me that they are concerned because you're not going to school. Hmm. That has been really hard on you.

SAMANTHA: (*Looks at the therapist, then down*) I just don't feel like going to school anymore.

THERAPIST: Mm-hmm. Yeah. So, tell me some of the reasons why you don't want to go to school.

Therapist's Inner Reflections: I'm sure there are many reasons that may seem obvious to Samantha, but I'm asking her to support this shift she's just made from being passive and numb emotionally to being able to actively express her point of view. She's engaging, even though the first signs are anger. Let's see what more specific triggers she recognizes.

SAMANTHA: (*Looks directly at the therapist, eyes blazing*) I don't wanna see certain people. (*She sits back, strokes her ear reflexively with one hand, and sucks on the thumb of her other hand.*)

Therapist's Inner Reflections: The distress she's feeling is intense. I see her doing several forms of reflexive physical self-soothing to tolerate the distress. As she does that automatically, she could put herself into a dissociative trance. I'll support her intention of self-soothing and see if I can gently help her to do it consciously and to access other forms of self-regulation as well so that the self-soothing doesn't lead to a dissociative shutdown. Dissociation could lead the healthy self-protective and self-assertive anger she's understandably feeling to leak into her self-soothing in the form of unconscious or barely conscious self-harm. I'll start by returning to the first part of the SOS: helping her focus on her breathing and being aware of her body.

THERAPIST: Mm-hmm. Mm-hmm. Okay. It's hard to, to see some of the— some of your friends or y—your acquaintances? And now I can see that is really hard, Sam, to just talk about this. And I can also see that your body is telling you that probably right now you need to be soothed. So, one way of doing it, and I bet it's helping you, is by touching your ear—yeah?—and sucking your thumb. We can explore other ways that can also be helpful. Can I show you some other ways? (*Samantha nods.*)

THERAPIST: So, let's try to focus on your breathing, Sam. Can you breathe for me deeply? Can you feel the air coming in from your nostrils? Can you do it maybe one time? Can we try another one? (*Samantha looks down and begins rubbing and then scratching her arm.*) This is too hard. This is painful. Is the scratching helping you? Hmm. Can we explore other ways, too? (*Samantha stops scratching her arm and instead rubs it more slowly and gently. She begins to tap her feet vigorously.*) So, I can see that you're moving your feet. Can you feel your feet on the floor, Sam? Yeah? Can you tell me if your feet are warm or cold? Yeah. Let's try to keep on moving your feet. Keep on moving them. Yeah. Can you move your other foot? Yeah. Alright. Can we breathe a little bit more? Let's do three times this time. Okay? One . . . two . . . three.

SAMANTHA: (*Shifts from rubbing her arm to scratching with increasing intensity; begins to hyperventilate*)

Therapist's Inner Reflections: Samantha's escalating into emotional dysregulation and what looks like a dissociative state. Helping her to relax may be unintentionally leading her to lose track of her ability to self-regulate, I need to stay with the focus on body awareness but step up and gently but firmly guide her with very specific small steps to doing so without hurting herself. I think she needs to see what

I'm talking about, both to be able to cognitively process what I'm saying and to reorient herself to being present and not alone but supported by me. I'll keep the focus on her being in control of herself so that she doesn't experience me as taking control away from her in the way that those boys did by sexually assaulting her when she was unconscious.

THERAPIST: And, instead of scratching, can you touch your other hand and your arm like this? How does that feel? Can you feel your arm? Can you feel your wrist? Yeah? Keep breathing. You're in a safe place, Sam. Nobody's trying to hurt you here. Okay. I like this. Do you feel that your body likes it? When you try to soothe yourself like that? How does it feel?

THERAPIST: (*Samantha gradually breathes more slowly and deeply with a more relaxed torso and legs.*) Nice.

> *Therapist's Inner Reflections:* As Samantha calms down and comes back into the room, I can feel the tension draining out of my body as well. I'm primarily focused on Samantha, but I'm noticing that it helps me personally to self-regulate by doing these simple self-awareness actions along with Samantha. Now I can help Samantha not only feel calmer but also safer and protected. I'd like to give her a hug myself to comfort and reassure her, but I know I'm not her mother (even though I'm thinking about my daughters and wanting to hold them when they're upset or hurt), and she needs to know that no one will intrude on her in this therapy. So even through it seems kind of silly, it makes sense to help Samantha to hug herself, and she'll know that I am contributing to that hug without intruding on her personal space in a physical way that could feel like a replication of the rape (and her brother's murder).

THERAPIST: Nice? Alright. Have you ever given yourself hugs? No? Some-times I give myself some hugs. Sometimes that helps me. Try it—maybe not here but later on. Okay? I'm wondering, you know, how we're gonna find ways that soothing yourself is going to be part of your daily routine, and, at the same time, you can actually soothe yourself and only you will know that you're soothing yourself. Alright? So, we did that sort of breathing a, a little bit of deep breathing, so you know that you're breathing deeply because you want to focus on the here and now, putting your feet on the floor and making sure that you know that you're feeling it, feeling your hands. Right? Feeling different parts of your body and focusing on, you know, where you are.

Therapist's Inner Reflections: If I help Samantha connect these simple breathing and body awareness actions with her athletic skills, that can make this something she can do intentionally both to reduce the intensity of her hyperarousal and to tap into her self-confidence. And I will emphasize the core goal of keeping herself safe, which is what she feels she and her friend (as well as the boys who perpetrated the rape) failed to do. Then I can link the goal of being safe to her withdrawal, which is a problem and a symptom of depression because it keeps her trapped in survival mode but also is an adaptive attempt to protect herself.

THERAPIST: Okay? It's almost like playing volleyball, you know? I bet that you're so good at volleyball because you are actually practicing, and when you practice more and more, you get better and better, right? So, it's the same thing here with our emotions. The more that we try to stay in the here and now, the more that you're gonna feel a little bit safer. Okay? And, so, the more that you feel, you know, that you are in safe environments like—I bet that you're spending a lot of time in your house right now. Is it—is your house a safe place for you? Does it feel safe? (*Samantha nods.*) Okay.

SAMANTHA: (*Continues to visibly relax; makes tentative eye contact with the therapist*) Yeah, it does.

THERAPIST: Okay. Are there any other places that are—make you feel safe? No? Only your house? Okay. Alright. So, tell me a little bit about what would going back to school look like. What do you think that you need in order to feel calm, in order to feel that you can soothe yourself utilizing healthy ways so you can go back?

Therapist's Inner Reflections: Samantha now is associating the main goal of safety with calmer body feelings that represent a main emotion (feeling "nice," which seems to mean that she feels a sense of peacefulness emotionally) and a main thought (that she is not trapped in horrible distress but has active ways to enable herself to feel better). With safety as a main goal that can organize her complicated emotions and thoughts, we can begin to explore her options for achieving the goal of protecting herself (and the related goal of returning to school and resuming her life and progress toward future goals, such as success in school and sports).

SAMANTHA: I have my best friend.

THERAPIST: Mm-hmm. Your best friend. So, tell me, what is your best friend's name?

SAMANTHA: Lily.

THERAPIST: How long have you known Lily?

SAMANTHA: Since high school started.

THERAPIST: Okay. Since freshman? Wonderful. So, you've known her for 3 years now?

SAMANTHA: Yeah.

THERAPIST: Okay. And you can trust Lily? Has she been contacting you? Yeah? So, has she been supporting you these past 3½ weeks? Yeah? How does she support you? What is she doing to help you?

SAMANTHA: (*Smiles shyly*) She'll check up on me like every day or so.

> *Therapist's Inner Reflections:* Samantha is such a resilient young woman! Without my bringing it up, she went right to what's probably the single best way to begin restoring her sense of relational security, which had been shattered by her friend Jack's neglect and the other boys' betrayal and exploitation. Samantha is a little fearful of trusting that her best friend Lily won't also let her down or even reject her, but she can see that her friend is standing by her. The sense of being cared about and valued, and watched over in a helpful and nonintrusive way are clearly crucial for Samantha's recovery. I'll explore that as a potential path forward for her.

THERAPIST: Mm-hmm. Mm-hmm. Wow. So, she actually is contacting you quite often? Yeah. Alright. Have you been able to keep up with some of the work at school? No?

SAMANTHA: (*Shifts back to a tense fetal-like position; withdraws eye contact*) No.

THERAPIST: Alright. Okay. Is that something that you would like to do? Yeah. Okay. So, you're a very brave young woman who has gone through a lot, and your body is very wise and knows how to calm and soothe you. So, I'm wondering if, for next week, maybe you can visit your friend Lily at her house before next week and see how that goes? Would that be something that you are willing to try? Is that something that you think that you can do?

> *Therapist's Inner Reflections:* That was a mistake and a close call. I jumped ahead by implying that I was urging Samantha to go back to school. I got caught up in the relief that Samantha (and I as well) was

feeling when focusing on the security that her friendship provides. I'm glad I caught that by noticing Samantha's nonverbal signaling and stepped back to suggest a much more manageable first step of just going to the friend but not facing the much larger set of stressors and triggers that she'll encounter when she returns to school. One step at a time. I'll help Samantha build a behavioral chain of small steps that can help her reengage with her relationships and her particular areas of strength and success: schoolwork and athletics.

SAMANTHA: (*Looks thoughtful, determined, and then makes eye contact*) Yeah.

THERAPIST: Okay. Alright. And I'm also wondering if you can start talking with Lily about some of the things that you can start doing at home or maybe with her, some of the schoolwork, especially of the good subjects that you really like and enjoy? Is that something that you think that you might want to focus on this week?

SAMANTHA: (*Continues uninterrupted eye contact*) Yeah.

THERAPIST: Alright. And the last thing, Sam. I'm also wondering, since you are an athlete and you got this—right—I'm wondering if there is anything that you can do this week that can help you to maybe jog a little bit or walk fast or—or do something like that around outside—around your house, where you can . . .

SAMANTHA: (*Nods and continues to make eye contact*) Yeah.

THERAPIST: . . . do some exercise?

SAMANTHA: Mm-hmm.

THERAPIST: Is that something that you think that you can do? Yes?

SAMANTHA: Yeah. I can do that. Yeah.

THERAPIST: Alright. Well, I'm really looking forward to seeing you next week. Okay? Thank you.

Samantha's Observations

In a postsession interview, Samantha said that she had been feeling that she didn't recognize herself anymore and that her parents didn't look at her in the same way as before. She was ruminating constantly about the party, berating herself for being so stupid and wishing she had never trusted Jack and his "so-called friends." She had secretly started cutting herself to make the pain and shaking stop, and sucking her thumb to comfort herself. In the session, she initially felt physically tense initially because she didn't want to have to answer more questions from another adult about the assault and about how she was feeling and coping now. She was surprised and reassured when the therapist was very gentle and accepting, but then she felt that she let down her guard and started to space out: "I kind of went somewhere else." She felt extremely embarrassed when she realized that she had begun to suck her thumb in the therapist's presence, but she didn't know how to make herself stop. She felt a strong urge to hurt herself when the therapist brought up the earlier experience of witnessing her brother being killed.

Samantha described having felt a sense of confusion and shock related to witnessing her brother's murder that she realized was very similar to how she had been feeling about being assaulted. That realization helped her to understand why she felt unable to stop thinking about the assault: "It was another time when I was powerless to stop something terrible from happening to someone I cared about, and no one else protected them or me, either."

Samantha emphasized that she found the therapist's guidance to be helpful in enabling her to be "more in my body" and more aware of the present moment and surroundings. She found being able to be more aware gave her a feeling that she wasn't powerless, that she could "take back some control." She also felt calmer and safer, which was very different than the brief feelings of relief that she'd gotten from sucking her thumb or cutting herself—and she also didn't have to deal with feeling ashamed of herself and embarrassed, which had been making things much worse for her emotionally. By the end of the session, Samantha was feeling a small amount of hope that, with the therapist's help, she could talk about the assault and her brother's murder, and figure out how to not feel so terrible that she couldn't stop thinking about those horrifying memories. She also had hopes of figuring out manageable steps she could take to work toward returning to school and "getting back to having a normal life."

Commentary

As the session unfolded, the therapist clearly was focused on three primary goals:

- building an alliance and instilling hope by interacting with Samantha in a way that was nonjudgmental, accepting, nonintrusive, and responsive, and that facilitated a sense of relational security, resilience, active problem solving, and hope for solutions

- assisting Samantha in regulating her emotions and becoming nonjudgmentally aware of the understandable emotional turmoil she was experiencing by identifying and adapting her intuitive ways of coping with memories and emotions, and supporting her by affirming, highlighting, and drawing on Samantha's many personal strengths

- assisting Samantha in setting and emotionally committing to an overarching goal that reflected her current concerns and that enabled her to organize her complicated emotions and thoughts in a manner that provided her with a path forward to restore the parts of her life and the aspects of herself—as an outstanding student and athlete, and as a valued friend—that she had relied on as a source of inner security, pride, and hope for the future

The therapist navigated a number of crucial and challenging choice points in working toward these three goals. As the therapist's inner reflections indicated, a first challenge was to help Samantha to remain sufficiently oriented to be able to self-regulate and benefit from the support and guidance the therapist could provide. Without explicitly teaching the first FREEDOM (focusing, recognizing triggers, emotion awareness, evaluating thoughts, defining goals and options, making a contribution; see the Introduction) step, the SOS for focusing, the therapist helped Samantha begin to be aware of her body and present circumstances for the very beginning of the session (the first "S" in SOS). She also helped Samantha to orient (the "O" in SOS) by highlighting Samantha's ability and interest in sports. And she helped Samantha track not only the intensity of distress she was feeling (using body feelings rather than verbalized emotions as the guide) but also her sense of personal control (again using breathing and tactile self-awareness as a practical way to feel in control).

A common challenge faced when working with clients in or on the verge of crisis is establishing rapport and trust with while determining how—and when—to best help the client disclose the memories and emotions that are causing severe distress. In the postsession interview, the therapist confirmed that she was aware of recent traumatic events that had occurred for Samantha but did not ask Samantha to talk about those events. This signaled to Samantha that she could trust the therapist not to be intrusive, which was crucial in light of the traumatic violation Samantha had experienced and the many questions that she and others were asking her about what happened.

By alluding to the events, the therapist also was communicating indirectly to Samantha that it is important to consciously recognize the triggers that remind her of the traumatic events. In addition to simply being in therapy (which almost inevitably brings up memories), the therapist identified other key triggers, including going to school and Samantha's experiencing distress in her body. Rather than inquiring about the specific triggering stimuli and circumstances, the therapist immediately focused on helping Samantha to respond to triggered distress with body awareness and breathing. Doing so communicated to Samantha that conscious recognition of triggers does not mean that there is any pressure to dwell on or even talk about the traumas, the triggers, or both that elicit trauma-related memories. In this way, the therapist helped Samantha to recognize—rather than simply react to—current triggers for distress as well as the trauma-related memories. Samantha's reaction of increased distress and attempts to withdraw and self-soothe confirmed that Samantha was feeling not just distressed but overwhelmed by reminders—even oblique—of the traumatic assault and the shocking and emotionally painful aftermath. The therapist's shift to helping Samantha self-regulate communicated nonjudgmental acceptance; respect; and support for Samantha's autonomy, privacy, competence, and judgment. The therapist thus clearly let Samantha know that she (the therapist) trusted and respected Samantha and would help Samantha to draw on her strengths to cope with and find a way to overcome what—to Samantha—had seemed to be over-whelming and unmanageable distress.

The therapist initially received little verbal input from Samantha. She therefore had to rely heavily on nonverbal communication and to carefully choose when, how, and how much to engage verbally with Samantha. A challenge with clients in crisis is how to accurately attune to the client's experience when they present as detached, shut down, and dissociative. Each attempt to attune carries the risk of making an assumption with little to no verbal input or feedback. In this case, Samantha had so little to say that the therapist was unable to focus primarily on linguistic distortions, as is evident in their rare appearance in the annotations. It is informative, never-theless, that Samantha's statements toward the end of the session were free from any obvious linguistic distortions; they were brief, terse, and without a great deal of content, but specific and clearly expressed actions with verbs and no presuppositions or mindreading.

The therapist carefully followed Samantha's lead, speaking softly and slowly, and paying close attention to Samantha's nonverbal cues in the moment as a means of attuning and achieving connection. Another chal-lenge for therapists working with a shut down or dissociative client is to be aware of and manage their own internal experience (e.g., doubts, frustrations, sense of urgency) in the absence of consistent or clear feedback from their client. In this session, Samantha involuntarily began coping in what appeared to be a regressive manner (stroking her ear, rocking, sucking her thumb, adopting a fetal position). It was tempting for the therapist to succumb to the pull to take control and tell the client what to do (or not do) to alleviate the client's suffering and also to minimize her own discomfort and concern for the client's vulnerability to social rejection. In this session, the therapist coregulated actively with Samantha by doing the same body and affective awareness exercises that she was guiding Samantha in doing. This provided Samantha with a model she could observe as well as direct experience in ways to attend to her own emotions, thoughts, and, ultimately, goals in the moment.

As Samantha began to suck her thumb and scratch herself, the therapist reframed those behaviors by explicitly highlighting Samantha's adaptive intentions. Rather than asking Samantha to stop the behaviors or to explain why she was doing them (or pedagogically inquire how the coping strategies were helping her), the therapist instead validated for Samantha that her body needed her help to feel better because an injury had occurred, and she acknowledged Samantha's success in attending to her body's needs. The therapist offered ways that Samantha could intentionally adapt the instinctive self-soothing behaviors and experiment with alternative variations of them (e.g., self-hugs) without discounting the usefulness of what might appear to be "regressive" coping strategies in a manner that would have shamed Samantha. In quite the opposite approach, the therapist highlighted Samantha's strengths and skillfulness in helping her body while simultaneously affirming Samantha's core goals (i.e., to care for her body, to calm herself, to be aware of her personal strengths, and to regain a sense of having a life in which she is safe, able to effectively make decisions when faced with important choices, and can trust and rely on the people closest to her or others who should be protective of her).

Another issue to which the therapist paid careful attention in this session was how best to support Samantha in reclaiming areas of her life impacted by the assault and the violation, betrayal, and humiliation she had experienced while also empathizing with Samantha's sense of shock and survival mode dysregulation and disconnection. The therapist was aware that Samantha had not been attending school so that she could avoid seeing the boys who assaulted her as well as other peers who were aware of the traumatic events or related rumors. She affirmed Samantha's judgment in protecting herself from situations, people, or places that are triggers for memories of the assault and betrayal. The therapist also affirmed the accomplishments that have been meaningful to Samantha as a hardworking and talented student and athlete. The therapist noted that, although it has been understandably difficult for Samantha to feel sufficiently safe and focused to fully resume those activities, she also has shown a courageous determination to prepare herself to do so when she feels ready—and highlighted the motivational value for Samantha of those areas of achievement. The therapist affirmed Samantha's personal strengths and commitments, and their importance to her, balancing this with acknowledgment that the emotional and physical shock of the recent trauma and the reopening of emotional wounds from her brother's murder needed to be dealt with as the psychotherapy progressed for Samantha to once again focus her full attention on those sustaining activities.

There are many ways to build a therapeutic alliance, but when a client is in crisis, none is more important than providing coregulation to support the client's emotion regulation. In this case, the therapist provided Samantha with guidance in modifying her instinctive self-soothing behaviors so she could consciously self-regulate and stay grounded (e.g., deep breathing, light touch, hugging herself, moving her feet). In so doing, the therapist provided Samantha with immediate practical ways to shift from dissociatively and automatically withdrawing into and even harming her body to intentionally calming and being aware of her body. Although specific emotions were never discussed—primarily because Samantha needed to regain awareness and self-control of her body before she could meaningfully engage in verbal reflection and dialogue—Samantha was able to experience adaptive emotion regulation on a visceral physiological level in this session, and that was the crucial shift that enabled her to recover from a dissociative crisis.

The therapist also carefully engaged Samantha in collaborative conversation, asking, "What would going back to school look like" and asking permission from Samantha to continue to talk about stressful circumstances and triggers at several points during the session. The therapist also explicitly and repeatedly acknowledged the difficulty of the work to be done while simultaneously communicating that success was not only possible but—given Samantha's strengths and resources—likely. In doing so, the therapist was able to slowly draw Samantha back into the room psychologically and into the relationship conversationally while making sure she felt safe and in control so that she was motivated to return for a next session.

It is not surprising that the therapist felt internal pressure to intervene and rescue a client in crisis, such as we saw in this session with Samantha—or to try to make the client feel better right away or take objectively adaptive steps to assertively confront a problem. This is particularly the case here, considering how Samantha's life has been turned upside down and how much she appeared to have lost and to be suffering in the aftermath of the rape. Therapists understandably often want to jump in and get a client "back on track," but this runs a huge risk of making things worse and disempowering or alienating the client. This therapist's ability to pull back (e.g., "That was a mistake and a close call") and focus on supporting Samantha in pursuing her core goal of safety and regaining control in her life was crucial. The therapist stayed calm and responsive, and did not become frustrated with the Samantha's silence or "regression"; instead, to collaborate with and empower Samantha, she focused on attributing meaning to and guiding her in making largely nonconscious ways of coping conscious and helpful.

Notably, the therapist simultaneously engaged in the same self-regulation techniques she had suggested to Samantha, thus providing Samantha a role model and partner to help her get more settled while also providing support to counteract the sense of powerlessness and abandonment Samantha apparently was experiencing on a continuous basis in her daily life. Intentionally focusing on self-regulation as well as on guiding Samantha in regaining self-regulation had several crucial benefits. By self-regulating, the therapist was joining with Samantha in self-regulation, which is the crux of coregulation. She also provided Samantha with a nonverbal role model for how to take small steps toward self-regulation. The therapist was able to tolerate and nonjudgmentally respond, rather than react reflexively, to Samantha's profound distress by intentionally and nonjudgmentally maintaining awareness of her own bodily and emotional reactions.

The therapist was not simply attempting to shore up Samantha's self-esteem by initially focusing on and subsequently affirming Samantha's strengths as a student and athlete. The strength-based emphasis served as both to a way to help Samantha focus and reorient when she was becoming lost in dissociation, and to envision a path forward to achieving her core goals of restoring her sense of safety and self-efficacy. By helping Samantha to clarify those main goals, the therapist was able to also help Samantha identify immediate steps that Samantha felt willing and able to take to regain hope and a path to recovery. Instead of being trapped in what seemed to be an inescapable emotional prison of shame and irreparable damage, Samantha was able to recognize and commit herself to taking small steps toward resuming her life with the support of a best friend (and, in the background, also a therapist).

The therapist also made the important point that Samantha's past accomplishments were, in large part, a result of Samantha's dedication, determination, hard work, and continuing practice. This provided a framework for the therapy and for Samantha's recovery that emphasized not only Samantha's goals and support system but also her strength, courage, perseverance, and willingness to do the hard work necessary to make slow progress on an ongoing basis. In crisis, all-or-none "solutions" often come to seem to be the only way out of desperate circumstances, and step-by-step solutions can seem too slow, too much work, or too vulnerable to failure. Had the therapist simply suggested a logical set of steps, even with Samantha's apparent endorsement, this would not have engaged Samantha's sense of hope and motivation sufficiently to make success likely. By instead developing small steps based on Samantha's sense of an emotional connection to her best friend, the therapist was able to anchor those steps with Samantha's can-do attitude and also with a strong sense of secure emotional attachment.

Although Samantha initially seemed emotionally shut down and detached, and continued to be hesitant and muted in her communication, she also was insightful and articulate in describing her emotions and the bodily reactions triggered by reminders of the rape. Samantha also was able to accept the therapist's comfort and support, very likely, in large part, as the result of the genuineness and acceptance with which the therapist offered it. However, these auspicious beginnings of a therapeutic alliance were punctuated with moments of intense withdrawal and dissociative detachment. Rather than interpret those peak moments of distress and dissociation as signs of pathology or therapeutic failure, it seemed more likely that the therapist had in fact begun to help Samantha identify and even process some of the traumatic impact of the recent assault while not pushing her to disclose details. Thus, this session demonstrated the possibility that trauma memory processing can be an ongoing process that starts right from the initiation of treatment and that addresses more than the explicit memories of a specific trauma (Ford, 2018).

For Samantha, processing the trauma will not include revisiting the physical rape per se because she was unconscious while it happened. However, her nonverbal reactions as she speaks with the therapist are bodily expressions of the impact that the assaults and the shock, horror, and sense of betrayal in the aftermath have had on her. By demonstrating to Samantha that therapy is a place in which she can safely reflect on anything that is distressing or otherwise important to her, the therapist has laid the therapeutic foundation not only for helping Samantha to recover from episodes of emotional crisis and dissociation but also to resume achieving her life goals. The therapist showed Samantha that she was not interested only or primarily in what happened to her in the rape and its traumatic aftermath but in helping Samantha make sense of those events and her current reactions in relationship to her personal and family history and relationships as well as her goals, aspirations, and hopes. This signaled to Samantha that therapy will not force her to immerse herself in the shock and suffering but instead will enable her to experience that distress in manageable ways with the immediate help and coregulation of the therapist. It also signaled that therapy is an opportunity to decide the meaning (Harvey, 1996) of the recent traumatic assault and its impact—and any other troubling or traumatic event from her life—in the context of her overall life narrative (past, present, and future) and who she is as a person. This was crucial to helping Samantha know that she was not powerless to overcome the intense sense of betrayal, violation, shame, and distrust in both herself and others that she was experiencing in the wake of the recent sexual assault and the betrayal of trust and sense of shame accompanying it.

When the therapist recognized that Samantha had gone beyond the initial stages of stress, distress, and emergency, and was on the verge of the ultimate stage of breakdown, she shifted from emphasizing body awareness and intentional self-calming (i.e., breathing) to active self-soothing. The therapist did so by invoking attachment security—but, importantly, not by violating Samantha's personal boundaries and space by attempting to physically hold Samantha—and suggesting (and modeling) "hugging yourself." This was important on several levels in both resolving the emerging crisis and in preventing future crises. A violation of personal space and boundaries, even though well intended, would have replicated the physical intrusion and violation caused by the sexual assaults. It also would have implied a level of intimacy between the therapist and Samantha that could not have existed in their very new relationship. And even if their therapeutic relationship had been long-standing, it would have implied that the psychotherapy relationship could include physical intimacy that is reserved for close relationships with friends, partners, or immediate family members. By instead suggesting the possibility of "hugging yourself," the therapist was affirming Samantha's intention (and ability) to effectively soothe herself and also Samantha's prerogative of carefully and consensually choosing with whom she would engage in physical intimacy (and not do so to comply to another person's demands, no matter how kind or well-intentioned that person might seem to be).

Thus, this session may seem to have simply involved a therapist helping a client who is experiencing intense posttraumatic distress and dissociation to regain a present-centered focus. That did happen, but the therapist also helped Samantha to begin to recognize that she can recover from the trauma and to acquire some hope. Resuming simple healthy behaviors like exercise, contact with a trusted friend, and nonharmful self-soothing provides Samantha with immediate solutions that are affirming and help her to distance from emotional distress. In the session itself, Samantha experienced how intentionally attending to and guiding her body (and also being guided by her body) could enable her to "come back" and feel a renewed sense of physical strength, confidence, and determination—more like her "old" (i.e., pretrauma) self. With that immediate psychobiological evidence of her self-efficacy and resilience, Samantha had a foundation on which to rebuild the sense of safety, trust (in herself as well as in others), competence, worth, and hope that the traumatic exposure and shock, and posttraumatic anxiety, depression, shame, and dissociation had undermined. That will be a long-term project in therapy and in life, but every journey begins with the first step. This session was that crucial first step, and Samantha's nonverbal shift from dissociation, dysregulation, and disconnection to self-awareness, determination, and hope was evidence that that step had been taken in the right direction and in partnership with (but not dependent on) the therapist.

It's worth noting that the therapist was well aware of, but chose not to explicitly refer to, the additional impact and emotional complications for Samantha of the traumatic events that had occurred when she was a child—that is, witnessing her brother's murder, her mother's inconsolable grief, and the subsequent chronic problems with hypervigilance and depression that her mother experienced and with substance abuse by her father. By focusing instead on helping Samantha to be consciously aware of and take simple familiar steps to care for herself when experiencing bodily distress, the therapist helped Samantha to experience a sense of empowerment and relief. This shift was evident when Samantha was able to relax her body as she breathed more slowly and deeply with the therapist's guidance while remembering and feeling the hurt caused by recent and distant past traumatic events. In this session, it was not clear exactly what intrusive memories or flashbacks to the rape trauma or to earlier traumas that Samantha was experiencing. However, at the moments of crisis in this session, Samantha's nonverbal reactions of dissociation and self-harm appeared consistent with reexperiencing terror, shock, confusion, and helplessness—which are the hallmarks of posttraumatic reexperiencing and that often are not accompanied by an explicit conscious memory of specific event(s). The session thus laid the groundwork for Samantha to process any or all of the traumatic memories that cause her distress at a time when she felt ready to voluntarily choose to undertake that therapeutic work.

Whether it will be therapeutically beneficial or even necessary for Samantha to explicitly retrieve and psychologically process those childhood trauma memories in her current recovery or at some future point in time remains to be determined as she proceeds in this therapy and further into adulthood. What she learned from this initial session is that it is possible, with the guidance of her body, her mind, and the input of a therapist, to intentionally shift from a state of dissociation and depression to feel present physically and emotionally, and to think clearly. This session was a starting point for her in recovering from the depression and anxiety she had been experiencing by drawing on her physical and psychological talents to create safety and achieve her core goals.

One final complexity of this session involves the racial and ethnic background of the client (who is African American) and therapist (who is a Latina). They share the experience of being women of color in a predominantly White culture in which both currently and historically systemic racism and associated traumas and microaggressions are prevalent. Yet, the therapist cannot assume based on these general similarities that she knows how Samantha experienced the racial aspects of the trauma and betrayal related to the assault (or related to her brother's death in the past). Nor can she assume how Samantha will best be able to navigate living in two worlds—her African American family and community, and the primarily White private school and student peer group. These questions require exploration with exquisite sensitivity, and the therapist must draw on her own experience with similar dilemmas but never superimpose that experience on her client.

CONCLUSION

In Samantha's psychotherapy session, the client–therapist dialogue was primarily nonverbal on Samantha's part with verbal guidance and nonverbal coregulation by the therapist. Although Samantha appeared to indeed gain insight, this was not in the form of explicit verbal self-analysis but was based more on joining with the therapist in recognizing and understanding the needs and goals expressed wordlessly by her (Samantha's) body. The therapist did most of the talking, but what they said was largely based on and in response to what they observed Samantha to be communicating nonverbally. By helping Samantha to recognize and put her body's messages into words and to define and develop small steps toward achieving her main goals of safety and self-efficacy, the therapist provided Samantha with a crucial initial experience of how to make the shift from survival mode to self-regulation and renewed hope.

Although the therapist never explicitly alluded to the FREEDOM framework, this session wonderfully illustrates how to apply that framework in a crisis. By focusing, nonjudgmentally recognizing triggers, and incorporating Samantha's reactive and main emotions and thoughts into a personally meaningful set of goals, the therapist was able to de-escalate a client who had gone into a crisis of dissociation and self-harm—and to help Samantha commit to small steps that provided her with a beginning to the longer term therapeutic challenge of restoring her hopes and her life. In so doing, this therapist and client transformed a crisis into a turning point.

QUESTIONS FOR READER SELF-REFLECTION

- What was the most evident moment of crisis in this session, and how do you know it was?

- Was there anything the therapist could have done differently to prevent Samantha from going into a state of crisis in this session?

- What was the most important specific action by this therapist that you believe enabled Samantha to stop self-harming and recover from a pathological state of dissociation?

- Would you have done anything different to resolve this crisis?

- What would you be feeling and thinking if you were in this therapist's place and had a client go into a regressed and unreachable mental state, and begin to engage in self-harm?

- What are the pros and cons focusing on Samantha's present life circumstances versus intensively exploring and processing her recent and past traumas or life-altering events?

- Should the therapist view Samantha's referring to her friend as a defensive way of avoiding talking about what she can do for herself, or can this friendship be added as a complementary, additional way in which Samantha can calm herself and be safe?

- What did the therapist do to calm and regulate their own emotional reactions that you think was most important or most useful for yourself?

- What would be your goal for the next session with Samantha?

- Would you have given Samantha any different or additional suggestions or homework for the time between this and your next session?

- How should the therapist involve Samantha's parents in the therapy, or should the therapist not involve them in the therapy?

- Should the therapist plan on helping Samantha to confront the boys who assaulted her either for legal purposes or to help her feel able to return to school safely?

- Should the therapist plan on helping Samantha decide how to repair the harm done to her relationship with the male friend who encouraged her to get drunk and failed to protect her?

- Should the therapist have helped Samantha take responsibility and deal with feelings of guilt for having placed herself in a risky situation?

- What beliefs about herself should the therapist anticipate and help Samantha deal with as a result of the traumatic violation and shock she has experienced?

- Should the therapist attempt to help Samantha remember what happened in the assault?

8 ENGAGING A SEXUALLY TRAUMATIZED YOUTH IN THERAPY

CASE BACKGROUND[1]

Adam, 15 years old, is beginning the fifth session in his outpatient psychotherapy. He lives in the suburbs of a Midwestern city with his mother, father, and two sisters. His family is well off financially, and he and his siblings attend private school, have personal tutors, and enjoy horseback riding and other sports. For years, Adam excelled in school and was a star soccer athlete. Unbeknownst to his parents, Adam was sexually assaulted a year ago by his female tutor, Alex, who was 19 years old at the time. Following the assault, Adam began to struggle in school and behave in uncharacteristic ways. His pediatrician referred him to the therapist with whom he has met four times and is again meeting in the current session.

---

[1]To view the webinar associated with this case, including a video of the psychotherapy session, go online (https://learn.nctsn.org/course/view.php?id=477). Alternatively, you can go to the main website (https://learn.nctsn.org), click "Clinical Training" in the menu bar at the top of the page, click "Identifying Critical Moments and Healing Complex Trauma," and then click the webinar associated with this case: "Engaging a Sexually Traumatized Youth in Therapy." Although you will need to create an account ID and password, there is no fee to access the webinar.

https://doi.org/10.1037/0000225-009
Crises in the Psychotherapy Session: Transforming Critical Moments Into Turning Points, by J. D. Ford

For all intents and purposes, Adam appears to be a model youth who has had a sheltered and privileged life, and is heading toward a highly successful and rewarding future. What no one but Adam (and the perpetrator) knows is that he was sexually abused by his soccer coach from ages 9 to 12 years old. This escalated from being watched in the shower to being taken into the coach's office and drawn into sexual acts that intensified from fondling to mutual masturbation to fellatio and anal sex. Adam felt caught in an overwhelmingly complicated dilemma. On the one hand, he felt proud that the coach always singled him out for praise in front of the rest of the team, and he wanted to keep his coach's approval. At the same time, he'd seen the coach verbally "tear into" other team members and humiliate them to the point of reducing them to tears and quitting the team in shame, so he feared that if he resisted or protested, the coach would turn on him in that same way. The coach told Adam that this is what real men do, like the legendary Greek athletes who taught boys how to be men by sexually initiating them, and Adam wondered if he should actually feel grateful to his coach. Further complicating the already confusing and traumatic impact of the abuse, the coach was Adam's maternal uncle, Eddie, whom his mother looked up to and adored as her older brother, role model, and protector.

Adam thus felt an unspoken pressure to go along with the sexual acts and to keep them secret as a matter of family loyalty, and from fear that if the secret ever came out, it would "ruin my whole family." He also feared that his parents, especially his mother, wouldn't believe him and would blame him for lying—or if they did believe him, that they'd blame him for it happening.

At first, the coach was very kind and friendly, but, gradually, he became verbally threatening and abusive, and then physically violent (while always careful never to leave easily visible marks, except bruises that he told Adam to lie about and say they were soccer injuries). The coach told Adam that if he ever told anyone what was happening, he'd ruin Adam's life by telling everyone that Adam had propositioned him and was gay. The coach also berated Adam for being a "homo" and being "too weak to be a real man," and he blamed Adam as if the boy were responsible for the abuse by luring the coach into doing things the man never would have done otherwise—and then the coach would punish Adam by forcing him to have sex while physically beating him.

When Adam graduated to a new soccer league, he was extremely relieved to get away from Uncle Eddie, but he felt ashamed that he'd never stood up to the coach and made him stop, and guilty that he had never told anyone so that now Uncle Eddie was probably abusing other boys. Adam felt flooded with those feelings and with anxiety at family get-togethers when Uncle Eddie was present. He made excuses to avoid those family gatherings whenever he could, and when he had to attend, he always stayed as far away from Uncle Eddie as he could. Uncle Eddie never again tried anything sexual with Adam, and whenever he saw Adam, he would act like they were best buddies and give Adam a big bear hug—which made Adam cringe with a feeling of shame and disgust that he was barely able to hide.

Years later, Adam was tutored by a young woman, Alex; he felt close enough to her that he disclosed being confused because he felt a romantic and sexual attraction to males but not to girls or women. Alex told him that these feelings would fade with time and joked about how attractive she found Adam to be, saying that she wished someone like him had been around when she was his age. One evening, while helping Adam prepare for a biology exam, Alex got especially close to Adam and kissed him. Adam pulled away. Alex apologized immediately and said that she didn't know what had come over her. Confused, Adam shrugged it off. During their next exam prep a week later, Alex kissed him again. He pulled away, but Alex told him that the only way to know if he liked guys was to experience being with a woman first. Adam told her that he didn't want to hook up with her. Alex ignored him and started taking off his clothes, justifying her actions by saying that it would help him figure out his sexuality and that he was lucky to have "scored" with someone older. Adam felt dazed and he froze, feeling unable to do anything except just go along with what Alex was doing—much like he had felt when being abused by Uncle Eddie. Alex proceeded to have oral sex and sexual intercourse with him. Adam was confused by what happened and didn't know how to feel about it. He had many consuming questions racing through his head: "Did I lose my virginity?" "Am I disgusting like Uncle Eddie said?" "Did I flirt with Alex too much?" "Did I ask for this?" "Was this my fault?" "Who would believe me anyway?" "Do I like girls now?" "Is this happening because Uncle Eddie did something that made me like a giant neon sign saying, 'I'm just a "sex toy"; anyone can play with me'?" "Is this my punishment for being gay, like Uncle Eddie said, that all 'homos' have to suffer in hell?"

Alex continued to make Adam have sex for their next several sessions. While the sexual abuse by the tutor was occurring, Adam's grades started to slip as did his performance on the athletic field. He started spending increasingly more time alone. His parents were busy—mom, a lawyer; dad, a doctor—and neither really noticed. His little sister Ashley, however, noticed and asked Alex—who also was tutoring her—if something was wrong with Adam. Ashley explained that Adam had been acting weird and asked Alex what she thought about this. Alex brushed it off, saying school has been tougher than usual for Adam lately. Alex then went on to tell Adam that if he dared tell anyone they had sex, she would deny it and tell everyone that he was gay. This made Adam feel even more fearful, ashamed, trapped, and helpless.

Nevertheless, Adam felt he had no choice except to continue to see Alex every week for tutoring sessions. He tried to fake sick so that he could skip, but his parents wouldn't let him. After telling his parents that he felt sick for 5 straight weeks, they decided to send him to see the pediatrician. The pediatrician could tell something was wrong but couldn't get Adam to talk, so she referred him to a therapist. Adam's therapist was a man who reminded him of the positive qualities that had first drawn him to admire and trust his soccer coach, Uncle Eddie. This made Adam understandably very uncomfortable. To avoid looking at his therapist, Adam would pull on the strings of his hoodie and refuse to talk. After a month, Adam asked his parents for a different therapist, but they told him that they were counting on him to get back on the right path, and they liked his therapist and thought he was a good role model for Adam. As they became increasingly frustrated with what they viewed as immature and unappreciative behavior on Adam's part, they also started telling Adam that they were worried he was throwing away his chance to go to a top college, which they had all worked hard to make possible. His parents told him that therapy would help him if he just stuck with it and worked at it like they knew he was capable of. They said that if he really didn't feel comfortable with the current therapist that maybe he should see a female therapist instead. That freaked Adam out more because he did not want to be reminded of Alex's acting nice and caring, and then seducing and threatening him.

Adam decided to continue with the male therapist, but all of these dilemmas and pressures built up over the following month. They culminated in the following psychotherapy session, which was Adam's fifth session with this therapist.

SESSION TRANSCRIPT, ANNOTATIONS, AND COMMENTARY

After the annotated session transcript, I present a summary of Adam's observations and reflections on his experience in the session. Following this summary is commentary highlighting key themes and take-home points for handling this or similar crises, and questions for reader self-reflection.

ADAM: (*Blurts out before the therapist can say anything*) I just feel really done with it. I feel really done with the tutoring, and I feel really done with therapy.

THERAPIST: Okay. So, these things are feeling like ugh. I—I have to go or—or your parents—are your parents making you go to the—the tutor, too, or is it . . .?

ADAM: Yeah.

THERAPIST: Yeah. Okay.

ADAM: Well, because they think that I'm gonna start doing better if I keep going to the tutor, but it's like I started doing a little bit worse, and then I got the tutor, and then the more and more they pressured me to do that, like I just kept doing worse. And like all these things aren't helping. So, I think I might as well just not do them anymore.

Therapist's Inner Reflections: Adam has been very reluctant to reveal anything except a positive superficial facade, so I'm not entirely surprised that he wants to stop therapy. I want to support his sense of autonomy and not make him feel pressured or trapped, but I also want to see if he can let me in on whatever's just happened—or been happening—that is causing him to feel such intense internal turmoil and so apparently helpless to do anything except keep a lid on it. He's clearly on the verge of, if not already in, crisis, and I don't have any idea what's at the root of it. I'll join with his desire to be in control and to do whatever he feels he needs to do in order to protect himself. If I frame this as slowing things down and not just instantly ending it all at once, that might give Adam the space he needs to regain a sense of safety and control without having to entirely give up the potential help that therapy can provide.

THERAPIST: So, you're ready to be (*claps*)—to pull the plug on the—the tutoring for sure and, you know, possibly here, and we'll certainly go with what feels right to you. Uh, I—I want you to have a voice in—in these decisions. You know, not just, you know, your parents saying okay. You have to go down there. So, certainly, if we need to ramp down here, I'm—I'm good with that, and I'm happy to work with you on that.

ADAM: I just wish that I did have a say in all this, you know, because like I can protest all I want, but it's like my parents are just gonna keep making me do these things because they just don't understand that, like, it's just not gonna help because, like, they think that they're helping me, but they really don't know how.

Therapist's Inner Reflections: I need to not make any assumptions here. I know Adam's parents unintentionally put pressure on him, and I don't want to do the same—but I also don't want to "take sides" against them. Now that I'm hearing that the pressure's escalating, I can relate to that based on growing up with parents of my own whose expectations could be a lot of pressure. As a father, however, it's frustrating to hear this bright, talented young man just complain and want to avoid—I did that with my father, too, but I got myself together and didn't just give up. I don't want Adam to give up on therapy or, more importantly, on himself (which is what his attempt to pull the plug on the therapy appears to reflect: He doesn't want to quit; he just seems to feel that nothing and no one can help him, and that he can't help himself either). So, rather than telling Adam how I'm going to help him or what he should do, I'm going to find out what he thinks would be helpful. But first I need to find out what he needs help with: What are the triggers for this intense sense of anxiety and unhappiness that Adam seems to be feeling?

THERAPIST: I respect you c—coming in here and telling me I—I don't want to do this because this is one way to get your voice in. I mean, if you really feel like we—this isn't helping and, you know, uh, and it's adding more stress, then we can certainly ramp down. I don't, you know, I may have to check in with your parents, whatever but . . .

ADAM: (*Sighs*)

THERAPIST: Is it mostly your parents who put this kinda pressure and these expectations? I know they're—the bar is so high with school and with soccer. Is it mostly your parents or . . .?

ADAM: A lot of it is my parents, but I would say like my tutor makes things pretty bad, too.

THERAPIST: How does she do that?

ADAM: She's just kinda like . . . too—too personal.

Therapist's Inner Reflections: That caught me off guard. I thought the tutor might not be the issue, but that tutoring was stressful because Adam is having difficulties in school—maybe encountering academics that were more challenging than he'd faced before, or maybe because anxiety or depression was interfering with his ability to concentrate and do work that he'd otherwise be very able to handle. But Adam's saying that the tutor is "too personal" sounds like he's disclosing some kind of intrusiveness by the tutor that might be more than just putting pressure on Adam to do better or work harder. Maybe this is a serious boundary issue. I need to understand more about what's going on that's triggering for Adam.

THERAPIST: How—how do you mean?

ADAM: Um . . . does stuff that a tutor shouldn't do.

THERAPIST: H—help me a little bit with this. Uh, this is—this is—it's—what's her name, the tutor?

ADAM: My tutor's name?

THERAPIST: Yeah.

ADAM: Alex.

THERAPIST: It's Alex?

ADAM: Yeah.

THERAPIST: Okay. So, she's been getting too close in certain ways?

ADAM: She spends so much time like asking me about like stuff that it just doesn't even have to do with like what—what I'm doing in school and just like—I don't know. She like makes weird remarks that like make me feel so uncomfortable and—and like makes me talk about stuff that—just like—just like a—just annoys me, you know, that I have to deal with her like probing at me. She's always calling me like handsome and like . . . talking about how, you know, if she was my age, like she'd be all over me, and she's not only really talked about how much she wants to, you know, be with me because she thinks I'm so cute or whatever.

Therapist's Inner Reflections: This tutor definitely is overstepping the boundaries by flirting with Adam. I need to clarify what "stuff" she "makes" Adam talk about and what Adam means by saying that she wants to "be with me"; this could be a very serious boundary violation.

ADAM: Um, our last session, she—she actually put her hands on me. I told her to stop (*sighs*), but she kinda took my whole back-pack off my bed, and then she sat down beside me and (*sighs*) started asking how I felt about girls, and then she was rubbing my back (*sighs*), and after that, um, she just like had both of her hands, like one of them was on my leg, and the other was on my back, and she was just rubbing my back, and then she told me that I'd have to see what it was like with her, um, so that I could understand if I liked girls and, um, having sex with girls, and I just shut down, and I told her to stop it, and then I just—I didn't want it anymore, and then I got off the bed, and I walked across the room, and I said I don't like this . . .

Therapist's Inner Reflections: This keeps getting worse and worse. I'm really concerned that the tutor is trying to seduce Adam into a sexual encounter. Her putting her hands on him while sitting on his bed, and talking about having sex with girls, is something I'll have to report, even though Adam did a good job of protecting himself by walking away and telling her to stop.

THERAPIST: Right.

ADAM: . . . but then she told me that it wasn't a weird situation and that I was not allowed to tell anybody about it. Um (*sighs*), and I'm really scared if I do tell anybody about it, she might reveal some other stuff that she's gotten me to say to her that, um, I'm just not ready to be out there, and I feel like she really has me trapped.

Therapist's Inner Reflections: Worse yet: The tutor is being coercive and threatening Adam's privacy. There may be more, but I think it's time to respond to Adam's fear of being exposed and sense of being trapped. I'll focus on the courage it's taken for him to deal with this and now to be willing to tell me and ask for help as well as validate how distressing this is for him by making it clear that this is not a small thing. It's abusive behavior by the tutor.

THERAPIST: Wow. Thank you for sharing that. Um, that—I—I can see why you would feel trapped and confused, and maybe even panicked by what's going on. Does it—is it clear to you that this is—this is an abusive situation? Does that register with you?

ADAM: I know. I know.

THERAPIST: Yeah. This has—this has gone way beyond and has put you in a terrible situation. This is an abusive situation. I'm so glad that you were willing to talk about it here today.

ADAM: Yeah.

Therapist's Inner Reflections: With the confusion and distress this is bringing up for Adam, he needs an orienting thought to focus on. He's feeling unsafe, so his safety should be that focus.

THERAPIST: What is most important is that we have to find a way to safety here because this clearly is not safe. It's not safe for you, this situation. Right?

ADAM: I really don't want to have to do that again.

THERAPIST: Absolutely.

ADAM: It's like (*sighs*) . . . it just makes me feel like violated and uncomfortable . . .

Therapist's Inner Reflections: Adam's doing a great job of breaking this down without my having to do anything but listen and communicate support. The possibility of further exposure is the key trigger, and he's expressing his reactive emotions ("uncomfortable") and thoughts ("violated") very clearly. I think I know what his reactive goal is, but I'll wait for him to say it.

THERAPIST: Yes.

ADAM: . . . and I don't wanna have to have another session because I've just been like—this whole week, I've been really, really panicking about what's gonna happen next week . . .

THERAPIST: Yeah.

ADAM: . . . and what I'm gonna do if that happens again, and I—I just don't want it. Like, it's just too much for me.

Therapist's Inner Reflections: There's a clear goal and a statement of how crucial it is to him. I'm going to make it clear that I understand and support him in making that goal happen without any delay. With that reassurance, he may feel there is hope and that he's not alone with this.

THERAPIST: Right. So, that's where we start. Your starting place is that you are not gonna have another tutoring session. So, I think we can be very careful in terms of who we tell, how we tell, what is told—but minimum, we have to ensure your safety in this really abusive situation. Okay. And how are you doing right now? I mean this is . . .

ADAM: I don't feel so good.

Therapist's Inner Reflections: I think that Adam's starting to go beyond just coping in survival mode, and that can mean becoming aware of distress that he was keeping a lid on. With hope often comes a flood of the feelings that were put aside or that breakthrough when emotional numbing no longer is being relied on for self-protection. I need to help

Adam find the main emotions that can give him a sense of confidence and counterbalance this intense distress. He's struggling with a lot of self-doubt, so I think the best source of main emotions is going to be the reassurance that he's not alone, that I will stand by him through this ordeal, and that I respect his sense of urgency and am committed to helping him without delay. I also think he'll need to feel a sense of closeness and protectiveness from his parents, which will take some work to help them understand and actually do for him—so I'll let him know I will help him with that, too.

THERAPIST: Right. Whew. Yeah. This is very important stuff we're talking about here. I—I'd like us to move quickly on this, um, you know, work with you today and put our heads together so we can find a way to talk about this and, uh, to talk with your parents. Uh, you can share with me your concerns specifically.

ADAM: My biggest concern is probably that at first, they're gonna doubt that it even happened, and then I'm gonna have to, you know, explain it to them. I feel like (*Sighs*) they might think that I initiated it, or, you know, I didn't do enough to stop her or like . . . I caused the problem, and I just don't want them to think of me like as having been in a weird sexual situation.

Therapist's Inner Reflections: Adam's doing a great job of letting me know the potential downside of seeking his parents' support, including what they might mistakenly believe about his deserving blame or thinking of him with less acceptance and respect. Those are important points I'll keep in mind when we talk with his parents. I think we need to move from his goals and concerns to practical options for next steps, and it's crucial that Adam knows that he can retain his privacy and not feel pressured to tell all the details as if he's being interrogated. He needs a model for how to explain this dilemma in a few basic statements that he can use as focal points.

THERAPIST: I—I—I think we can clearly kinda craft in terms of how we— we talk with your parents about this. So, number one, you don't have to go through all the, you know, the details about it. The important message to communicate is that abuse, an abusive situation, has happened in this tutoring and that it needs to stop and that you are not to blame for it, and I'm—I'm—I'm clear on this, that, you know, we have a tutor who had certain responsibilities, and she really treaded way past here.

ADAM: That's all I want—just for it to stop.

THERAPIST: Absolutely. And for, uh, it to be handled in a way that's not gonna blow back on you in ways that you're uncomfortable with. Um, I want to be right at your side with this or to, you know, to help . . .

ADAM: Yeah. If—if, it you could be, I think, here with, um, me and parents, I think they'd have to listen to me.

Therapist's Inner Reflections: That's an important shift from telling me the problem to making a specific request for help—and Adam is starting to visualize a specific positive outcome: being "listened to" by his parents. He's still hurting and scared, but I'm hearing the emergence of not just hope but also some confidence and the beginning of trust in our therapeutic relationship.

THERAPIST: Yes.

ADAM: I think that would help the most.

THERAPIST: Absolutely. Absolutely.

ADAM: I would really—I would like that.

Therapist's Inner Reflections: I see the shift in Adam's nonverbal stance: more upright, making eye contact directly with me, his voice sounding stronger and less detached and hesitant. We have a lot of hard work to do, but he's made the shift from avoidance and survival to facing the problem with a sense that he can get out of the trap and reclaim his life. That will be my focus.

THERAPIST: Okay. That's what we're doing today.

ADAM: Okay. Thank you.

Adam's Observations

After the session, Adam explained that before this session, being in psychotherapy had felt like being "poked" and "probed" about sensitive issues (an unfortunate parallel to the intrusive and violating behavior by the tutor). From his perspective, that only made him feel more upset, helpless, and hopeless. Adam said that he'd decided to stop therapy because he thought this was the only way to avoid having his problems being opened up like an unhealed wound and then "picked at." Adam was surprised, however, to find himself feeling able to reveal the dilemma with the tutor to his therapist. He also was surprised and reassured that, although it was very difficult to talk about the abuse and the deep sense of hopelessness and helplessness he was trying to hide, he actually started to feel relief and a sense of lifting a burden off his shoulders that was heavier than he had even realized. Adam said that he felt especially reassured by the therapist's strong statement that the tutor was abusive and that they could make her behavior stop. However, Adam still worried that telling his parents would make things worse. What helped with this fear was finding that he could handle "putting stuff out there" and that this resulted in the therapist's understanding and actually being helpful. Adam was used to handling life on his own, which he preferred when things were going well. But he'd handled so much so well in his life that he and his parents had come to expect him to never need help. And his goals and approach to life had been a good match with his parents' goals for him and what they thought he should be doing. That mutually agreed on laissez-faire approach of his parents watching from the sidelines was not going to work now that Adam felt trapped in an abusive relationship. Having a therapist "get" this dilemma and be willing to stand beside him while he asked his parents for help gave him hope that therapy could help him get his parents on his side in this immediate crisis.

Commentary

As vividly illustrated by this session, many crises in psychotherapy sessions involve a disclosure of painful, confusing, and often frightening secrets, and the unpacking of the complex dilemmas embedded in those secrets and the burden that keeping secrets can cause. Adam was fearful of revealing the crisis that he was facing—whether consciously or as the unintended result of the confusion and emotional turmoil he was experiencing. So, most of what he expressed to the therapist initially was hopelessness and a wish to escape the pressure he was feeling by avoiding being in therapy. Adam's apparent rejection of therapy was the expression of an unspoken belief. Although unstated, this belief seemed to be something like: "There's nothing I can do except keep this a secret, which I must keep hidden or else I will be found out as a weak and unworthy person, and everything will be ruined in my life and my future as well as for my whole family."

Dealing with the immediate crisis of Adam's declared intent to drop out of both tutoring and therapy was the therapist's first challenge. By identifying pressure from his parents as a trigger, the therapist was able to empathize with Adam consistent with the FREEDOM framework (see the Introduction to this volume):

- recognition of the trigger: parents' decisions about tutoring and therapy for Adam

- reactive emotions: frustration, anxiety, discouragement

- reactive thoughts: therapy and tutoring are making things worse, and my parents aren't helping me by trying to control my choices instead of letting me be in control of myself

- reactive goals: not have to continue in tutoring or therapy

- reactive options: "pull the plug": drop out of tutoring and therapy

With this simple clear formulation, the therapist was able to shift the therapeutic dialogue by refocusing on Adam's largely unspoken "main" emotions, thoughts, goals, and options:

- main emotions: determination, confidence ("you're ready . . . (*claps*) to pull the plug")

- main thoughts: I need to have a "voice" in all of the important decisions about my life based on "what feels right" to me

- main goals: to "do better" (be successful in school, sports, relationships, and so on) and to "have a say in all this" (to be heard and have his views respected)

- reactive options: "ramp down here" (make therapy more helpful and less intrusive) with the therapist's support ("I'm happy to work with you on that")

The therapist summed up his empathic and nonjudgmental acceptance of Adam's perspective and choices, emphasizing Adam's courage and initiative, in a very economical statement: "I respect you coming in here and telling me, 'I don't want do this' because this is one way to get your voice in." Thus, the therapist caught himself suggesting a course of preemptive action ("pull the plug") but was able to pull back and reassert a collaborative perspective (i.e., "ramp down" and "work together") when he noticed Adam's further withdrawal. The therapist used this observation as a cue to step back and reflect on his own internal reactions (i.e., present-centered focusing; see Chapter 5), and then move to Step 4 in crisis management (i.e., explicitly affirming the client–therapist partnership) in which Adam was a full participant. This implicitly addressed Steps 5 and 6 in crisis management by affirming his belief in Adam's resilience and his support of Adam's core values and priorities (i.e., being treated with respect, being in control of his own decisions, and being able to define his own identity on his own terms). This provides a foundation for a brief constructive discussion about potentially ending therapy with Adam and also including his parents in light of their responsibility as his guardians.

However, the therapist's opening as he joined with Adam in support of both his reactive and main perspectives led to an unexpected disclosure. Adam simultaneously reengaged in the therapy and presented the therapist with a second crisis: disclosure of an incident of child abuse that Adam had felt coerced by the perpetrator, the tutor, to keep secret and handle all on his own. At that point, the therapist shifted from making inquiries and responding to Adam's brief or largely nonverbal communications to quietly but actively listening without interrupting as Adam spoke at length. Countertransference reactions can lead any therapist to feel an impulsive wish to rush to the rescue of a client who has been keeping a damaging secret. Although action is of the essence to protect that client, any action needs to be informed by the client's definition of both the problem and the solutions that the client finds acceptable.

The therapist's primary spoken contributions for the next several minutes were largely an affirmation for Adam that the tutor's behavior was abusive, unsafe, and harmful to Adam. This was important both to counteract the intense distress and confusion Adam was experiencing (e.g., "I'm helpless and alone, and there's no way out of this trap." "Am I somehow responsible or to blame for my tutor's sexual advances?" "Will anyone believe this is actually happening, and I'm not just making it up?") and to provide Adam with a new orienting thought as an anchor for him to regain a sense of hope, confidence, and security (e.g., "The therapist believes me and takes what I'm saying seriously, so I can believe in myself and in what I know to be true").

With this foundation, Adam and his therapist were able to work together to identify meaningful options and to develop a collaborative action plan, including deciding what resources (in this case, first of all, Adam's parents) could and should be accessed, and how best to do this (i.e., Steps 7–9 of crisis management; see Chapter 3). Adam began the session with the presupposition that a flight into health or, more simply, a flight to escape from therapy, was the best (or only) option, as is often the case when a toxic secret is being concealed. Respect for the Adam's autonomy and ability to make choices in his own best interests was not only essential to maintaining a therapeutic alliance but also was the polar opposite of the sense of coercion, entrapment, shame, and powerlessness that Adam was feeling. Therefore, at the beginning of this dramatized session, the therapist supported and validated Adam's wish to leave therapy, making this a legitimate option if Adam felt it was the best course. With persistent but cautious nonjudgmental and genuine concern, the therapist was able to help Adam reveal his feelings and their source: the dilemma he experienced as a painful and (from his perspective) inescapable secret. This was particularly important given Adam's description of his tutor as probing and prodding, and of his parents as not caring as much about him as about him living up to their and their community's expectations as a positive reflection on them. The therapist was able to avoid replicating these interpersonal dynamics by respecting Adam's choice of whether to continue in therapy or not and what to share or not. The therapist also clearly made a commitment to Adam to help him achieve goals that he (Adam) felt were his priority and in his best interests.

Language is not only a source of therapeutic and empathic understanding when a therapist carefully listens to and unpacks what a client is (and is not) saying but also is a crucial tool with which the therapist can meta-communicate a nonjudgmental commitment to understand the dilemmas facing a client and their perspectives on them. Note how the therapist in this session consistently used the terminology of "us" and "we" to communicate that Adam was not alone and they could work together. The therapist also repeatedly acknowledged that he believed Adam and took Adam's concerns very seriously—messages that may seem too obvious to require an explicit statement but those that a client in Adam's position (having had repeated experiences of having his concerns either go unrecognized or be rejected) would have reason to doubt. By communicating to Adam that their partnership would be based on helping Adam achieve his own goals (and not placing them second to the goals of the therapist) in ways that he believed were best for him (rather than in ways that were dictated by an external authority), the therapist helped Adam to reflect on and authentically express both the reactive and the main aspects of the crisis of abuse he was facing.

On the basis of what Adam told him about the actions of his tutor and his relationship with his parents, the therapist also made it clear that his intention was in no way to discover flaws or deficits in Adam nor to correct any such defects by "fixing" him. The therapist was not, at that point, aware of the sexual, physical, and emotional abuse that Uncle Eddie had perpetrated in the past nor that Adam had taken away from those abusive experiences a belief that something was fundamentally wrong with him that only an authority figure could fix. However, the therapist recognized Adam's freezing and his description of his paralyzing self-doubt that he felt when abused by his tutor (and while subsequently keeping that secret). The therapist also recognized, but did not comment on, Adam's thinly veiled belief that he was somehow damaged or broken, or in some inherent way deficient and in need of being "fixed." Rather than presenting Adam with this interpretation or challenging him to acknowledge and reappraise those beliefs, the therapist instead communicated to Adam both unconditional positive regard and confidence in his judgment and personal decisions.

To make those messages of respect for and trust in Adam congruent with his apparent attitude of self-doubt and self-devaluation, the therapist provided an explanation of those maladaptive beliefs that located the cause externally to Adam. By unflinchingly and definitively labeling the tutor's behavior as "abuse," the therapist was locating responsibility with the tutor and not Adam, not only for the acts of the tutor but also for those by Adam that were fueling his sense of self-doubt and guilt (including his compliance with the tutor's seduction and coercion; his keeping the incidents a secret; and his subsequent difficulties and withdrawal emotionally from school, from athletics, from his parents, and from peers). At the same time, the therapist was underscoring Adam's ability to recover from and overcome the adverse effects of the tutor's abusive actions by engaging him in a discussion of steps by which the therapist could support Adam to free himself from the coercion by and contact with the tutor. Without attempting to artificially boost Adam's sense of self-esteem or self-efficacy with mere praise, the therapist was metacommunicating confidence in Adam's judgment, ability, and character. The therapist affirmed Adam's courage and strength in both coping with the painful secret and, moreover, in being willing to reveal the secret and, in so doing, taking the large risk of trusting someone who was responsible for helping and protecting him—the therapist—to actually fulfill that responsibility despite having been failed and even exploited by another ostensibly trustworthy and responsible adult—the tutor.

In taking a line of validating Adam's integrity and competence, and placing responsibility on the abuse perpetrator for Adam's reactive emotions of guilt, shame, and fear, the therapist could have unwittingly (or intentionally) implicated Adam's parents as well. The therapist acknowledged and empathically joined with Adam in reflecting on the dilemma Adam felt in relation to his parents. To what extent that dilemma of feeling burdened by his parents' expectations and not appreciated and cared for unconditionally by his parents were the result of emotional nonresponsivity and unavailability by one or both parents, or the result of emotional difficulties on Adam's part in recognizing and accepting their love and appreciation for him, or to other factors, such as a temperamental or personality mismatch between Adam and one or both parents, could not be determined and should not be assumed at that point. Instead, helping Adam to reflect on memories and perceptions of his relationship with each of his parents in greater depth is a goal for future sessions, potentially including conjoint session(s) with him and his parents if that can be done in a manner that is consistent with maintaining the therapeutic priority on the individual psychotherapy with Adam as the primary client.

Engaging immediately with Adam's parents—to inform them of the abuse and enlist their participation in protecting Adam's immediate safety (including by a mandated report to child protective services)—was an ethical and clinical necessity in this case because Adam was a minor. This presented an opportunity and a challenge to the therapist. The opportunity was to offer to help Adam in disclosing the abuse to his parents by doing so in a conjoint session with the therapist. The challenge was to transform the external decision by the therapist that the parents must be informed into a collaborative mutual decision that Adam shared rather than having it simply imposed on him by the therapist. This was critical to not unintentionally replicate the coercion and disempowerment that Adam had experienced in the abuse, and, to a lesser but still problematic extent, in relation to his parents. Here again, by characterizing the tutor's actions as abuse to which Adam must not continue to be subjected, the therapist shifted the frame from Adam's being externally required to have the secret revealed to Adam's having meaningful choices about how to enlist the therapist and his parents in protecting him and supporting his decisions about what was and was not acceptable to him. Although that did not entirely alleviate Adam's under- standable anxiety about involving his parents (because of the sense of shame he felt and his uncertainty about whether they would react in a manner that would be supportive and helpful versus distressed or critical), it is evident that Adam was gradually able to tentatively accept and concur with the therapist's emphatic suggestion that enlisting his parents in support of his safety was essential and could be done successfully—with the assistance of the therapist—so that he did not have to face his parents and make the disclosure all alone.

Making a toxic secret known requires great courage. It is extremely difficult for anyone to disclose experiences of sexual abuse, and—as the therapist noted in his inner thoughts during the session—it is rarer and has some additional gender role-related stigma for males (compared with females) to make disclosures regarding sexual abuse, especially when perpetrated by a female. The stigma attached to sexual abuse of males and gender-restrictive views of how males should handle sexual abuse (e.g., they should be too tough or strong to ever be intimidated or exploited by a sexual aggressor, they should simply turn the tables and become the aggressor them- selves) was given careful attention by the therapist. Both with his words and on a nonverbal level, the therapist also brought a soothing and reassuring sense of calm, undivided attention, and commitment to supporting and empowering Adam throughout the session. When Adam seemed emotionally overwhelmed by memories of sexual abuse and by the effort involved in deciding whether and how to disclose the abuse, the therapist responded to Adam's alternating states of distress and shutting down by "leaning in" with increasing verbal and nonverbal intensity to calmly but assertively affirm confidence in Adam's resilience and core priority of safety, and a clear commitment to developing a collaborative plan to ensure Adam's safety and well-being.

It is apparent that the therapist was shocked to hear that Adam wanted to abruptly stop therapy—and then even more shocked to learn of the tutor's abuse. In both instances, the therapist was actively self-monitoring while responding to both disclosures and then while sitting back in a more relaxed posture and speaking in a quiet and modulated manner, checking to ensure that he was accurately understanding Adam. He also paused to give Adam space to speak and think for himself while the therapist gathered his own thoughts. The therapist responded with genuine concern and nonjudgmental acceptance, avoiding the trap of replicating the pressure that Adam was feeling from his parents (and from his tutor). The therapist communicated validation of Adam's feelings without either endorsing or disagreeing with Adam's parents' position. The therapist offered to explore why the therapy and tutoring "aren't helping" and to respect whatever decisions proved to be in Adam's best interests and that made sense and felt manageable to Adam. Rather than artificially and disingenuously assuring Adam that therapy can help, the therapist acknowledged that the problems that Adam was dealing with might quite possibly be beyond the ability of therapy (or himself as the therapist) to help him overcome or resolve. On the other hand, the therapist expressed confidence through his words and his demeanor that by working together, they could find solutions by taking the problems Adam was facing a step at a time—and by making the first step a definite plan for halting any further exposure by Adam to the tutor and her abusive behavior. Considering Adam's need to have a voice and sense of agency, the therapist acknowledged Adam's expressed desire to terminate therapy while also holding open the possibility they together could "ramp down" and figure out how therapy could be of help, especially if there were concerns in Adam's life for which he would like to have help.

On hearing Adam's disclosure of sexual abuse by his tutor, as a mandated reporter, the therapist was required to report the sexual abuse. He was direct in stating his intent to do so but emphasized that this must be done in a way that was collaborative and considerate of Adam's needs. Adam's expressed need for his tutoring to cease immediately provided the therapist with a natural opportunity to affirm that priority by stating unconditionally that Adam would not have to see the tutor again. Considering Adam's worries and fears regarding both how his parents might perceive the situation and his role in it, and how the tutor had threatened to disclose private information about Adam, the therapist carefully navigated how to make the report regarding the abuse without further threatening Adam's emotional and psychological safety or inadvertently giving Adam the message that the therapist was taking away his control. Instead, the therapist joined with Adam and mirrored and affirmed his determination to be in control of his own life, body, and choices.

To affirm his understanding of the importance to Adam of privacy, the therapist explicitly confirmed that they would, together, carefully decide who was to be told, how the information would be disclosed, and what information would actually be disclosed in an effort to provide Adam with reassurance. The therapist initially took an active stance, labeling the tutor's actions as abusive and unacceptable, and asserting that they would take action to protect Adam from further abuse. He balanced this by stating clearly that how those disclosures would be made would be decided with Adam's full input and assent. The therapist also framed next steps as something they would do together to signal to Adam that he would have the therapist's active support and not have to face this crisis alone—as he had been facing the abuse up to this point.

CONCLUSION

This therapist's response to a crisis of premature termination opened the door to the client's revelation of a more fundamental crisis of abuse. In each instance, the therapist was caught off guard but immediately validated the seriousness of the triggering stressors for the client and expressed acceptance of the client's reactive emotions, thoughts, goals, and options. Although simply quitting therapy or tutoring would not fully resolve the problems Adam was facing, nonjudgmentally accepting those as potential options provided a springboard for helping Adam to see his own more fundamental "main" emotions, thoughts, and goals that could serve as a guide in resolving the essential crisis of disempowerment, entrapment, and abuse.

Adam was able to make a shift from feeling abandoned, betrayed, coerced, exploited, and helpless (and the associated sense of shame, hopelessness, and self-directed anger) to seeing a path to regaining the successful life and the sense of himself as a worthy and competent person with a voice and control of his own choices. That core sense of self-confidence had been shattered when Adam was abused as a child, and now it seemed to him that he would never recover from this second experience of holding the toxic secret of abuse. What he found in therapy, however, was a therapist who had no foolproof answers or solutions but who respected him for his courage, determination, and resilience, and was willing to join with Adam in finding a path, step by step with uncertainty at every step, through the confusing and complex maze involved in the crisis. As such, Adam found a peer (based on their shared humanness) and companion (based on their shared sense of the necessity of preventing any further harm to him), and also a guide (based on the therapist's professional skill, nonjudgmental acceptance, and genuine caring) and role model (an imperfect but dedicated and resilient problem solver and advocate for core sustaining values).

QUESTIONS FOR READER SELF-REFLECTION

- What were the most evident moments of crisis in this session, and how do you know they were?

- At the moments of crisis, what orienting thoughts did the therapist focus on?

- What were the most important things the therapist did to enable Adam to feel safe enough to open up and ask for help in this session?

- What potential countertransference issues should the therapist be aware of? (These might include feeling unappreciated and rejected by Adam, or feeling a fatherly sense of wanting to rescue Adam and punish the tutor, or a thought that Adam was exaggerating the problem and failing to be sufficiently assertive in telling the tutor to stop hitting on him.)

- When Adam began the session by saying he wanted to stop therapy, why didn't the therapist remind him that therapy was a privilege and attempt to persuade Adam to change his mind?

- Should the therapist have focused on making a report to child protective services on behalf of Adam before discussing involving Adam's parents?

- Should the therapist have focused on helping Adam handle his interactions with the tutor more assertively rather than suggesting that Adam tell his parents and ask for their help?

- What are the potential downsides of focusing on involving Adam's parents? What are the potential benefits? Is involving the parents compatible with increasing Adam's sense of self-efficacy and his ability to handle this and other stressors autonomously?

- Should the therapist have focused on helping Adam handle his inter-actions with the tutor more assertively rather than agreeing to help Adam have no further contact with the tutor?

- When, and how, should the therapist ask Adam for more details about the tutor's behavior? Or should the therapist assume that Adam has told him everything that has happened and not "probe" him for more information?

- What changes in Adam's emotional state occurred as he opened up and told the therapist about the tutor's behavior and his reactions? Do you agree with the therapist that Adam's shift in emotion state was a sign of therapeutic progress and not a sign of deterioration?

- How did the therapist communicate authentic compassion for Adam?

- Did you see or hear signs of courage and strength as Adam disclosed the abuse? If so, what were they and how were they different from Adam's words and demeanor earlier in session?

- When, how, and with whom would you report the tutor's behavior to child protective services?

- How might Adam's earlier experience of abuse by his coach/uncle be contributing to Adam's sense of entrapment and helplessness in the current situation with the tutor?

9 UNDERSTANDING AND WORKING WITH DISSOCIATIVE STATES

CASE BACKGROUND[1]

Adam, 16 years old, is meeting for the first time with a therapist on the inpatient hospital unit where he was taken by ambulance after a nearly completed act of suicide. Adam seems detached and confused initially, but he then reveals a dissociative alter that seems to be a voice from his past and is angrily berating and shaming him, and telling him to kill himself.

We met Adam in Chapter 8 as a teenager who came to psychotherapy at his parents' and school's insistence a year earlier because of serious symptoms of depression and anxiety that were severely compromising all areas of his life. Adam had been determined to stop therapy but was able

---

[1]To view the webinar associated with this case, including a video of the psychotherapy session, go online (https://learn.nctsn.org/course/view.php?id=499). Alternatively, you can go to the main website (https://learn.nctsn.org), click "Clinical Training" in the menu bar at the top of the page, click "Identifying Critical Moments and Healing Complex Trauma," and then click the webinar associated with this case: "Understanding and Working With Dissociative States." Although you will need to create an account ID and password, there is no fee to access the webinar.

https://doi.org/10.1037/0000225-010
Crises in the Psychotherapy Session: Transforming Critical Moments Into Turning Points, by J. D. Ford

to trust the therapist sufficiently to disclose a toxic secret: sexual abuse by the young woman who was his tutor. During and after that crisis psychotherapy session, the therapist helped Adam tell his parents about the abuse, and, together, they made a report to child protective services. In the subsequent year, Adam continued in psychotherapy and regained his high levels of achievement in school and sports. However, he continued to struggle with feelings of anxiety, self-criticism, guilt, and shame. Adam started hooking up with other teenage boys and older men in secret, and these brief encounters temporarily helped him feel less alone but ultimately left him even more confused and isolated.

Three months before this first session with the therapist on the inpatient unit, Adam had become attracted to a boy in his class, and they began a sexual relationship that lasted about 2 months. Abruptly, the boy, James, broke up their relationship when James's father learned about the sexual activity and forbade his son from continuing seeing Adam. Adam felt despondent and decided he had to end his life. He went to the roof of the building where he lives with his family and looked down, thinking he should jump. He stopped only when his sister found him on the roof and convinced him not to jump. She also convinced him to call his outpatient therapist, who called 911. Adam was taken by ambulance to a hospital, where he received a psychiatric evaluation and was admitted voluntarily for inpatient psychiatric treatment.

SESSION TRANSCRIPT, ANNOTATIONS, AND COMMENTARY

This session is Adam's first psychotherapy session on the inpatient unit. After the annotated session transcript, I present a summary of Adam's observations and reflections on his experience in the session. Following this summary is commentary highlighting key themes and take-home points for handling this or similar crises, and questions for reader self-reflection.

THERAPIST: I understand that, um, things got pretty dangerous when you were on the roof yesterday.

ADAM: (*Nods*)

THERAPIST: And what happened? Can you tell me about that?

ADAM: I was on a roof.

> *Therapist's Inner Reflections:* Adam seems disoriented as well as deeply depressed. It's crucial to let Adam know that his safety is my main

concern but not in a way that is so clinical that it pushes him away or inadvertently exacerbates the distress he's obviously feeling. I want him to see that we can deal with this tough situation, but we'll go at a pace he's okay with.

THERAPIST: Okay. And, um, what—what were you doing on the roof? Do you know why you went up to the roof?

ADAM: No.

THERAPIST: No. Okay. Was there anything you were thinking while you were on the roof that you remember?

ADAM: Yeah. Um, I was thinking about James.

THERAPIST: Oh. What were you thinking about?

ADAM: Uh, well, we just broke up, so I was thinking about that.

THERAPIST: Okay. You were very close to him I understand.

ADAM: (*Nods*)

Therapist's Inner Reflections: At this point, I could ask Adam more about his relationship with James, but that's likely to bring up a lot of triggering memories and thoughts for him, so I'll bookmark it to return to later. The best way I can help Adam to get oriented and to begin to see some kind of future beyond the pain he's in emotionally now is to help him unpack what he was thinking and feeling when he was at the point of considering suicide. His memory of that episode is likely to be fragmented and confused with some distressing "hot spots" interspersed in a blur of sadness and hopelessness, so helping him get some clarity could be a starting point for then figuring out what he needs to do to carry on and be safe—and maybe have hope—now.

THERAPIST: Okay. And when you began to think about James, what were—what were you thinking about?

ADAM: That we broke up and that it sucked.

Therapist's Inner Reflections: So, there's the obvious trigger and probably an important one: the breakup, the loss of the relationship. Getting some clarity on the specific emotions he was—and still is—feeling can help us move from the triggering event(s) to the dying inner world of Adam's experience. If he's aware of emotions, however painful, he's beginning to revive that inner world.

THERAPIST: Okay. How were you feeling? What were the feelings that you were experiencing on the roof?

ADAM: Sad.

THERAPIST: Okay.

ADAM: Scared.

THERAPIST: Yeah.

ADAM: Um, pathetic.

> *Therapist's Inner Reflections:* Adam shifted rapidly from primary experiential emotions to a self-evaluative emotion that put him outside himself, judging himself like an external critic. And that may echo things important other people may have said to him about their view of him. I need to know more about where that critical voice is coming from; that's the kind of criticism that can signal a sense of worthlessness that can fuel suicidal impulses.

THERAPIST: P—pathetic you said? Okay. W—why did you feel pathetic? What was making you feel that way?

ADAM: He kept calling me pathetic.

THERAPIST: Oh. Who kept calling you pathetic?

ADAM: My Uncle Eddie.

> *Therapist's Inner Reflections:* I didn't expect that! I thought Adam was either alone on the roof or with his sister. No one mentioned an "Uncle Eddie" on the scene. So, I have to assume that Adam imagined hearing someone who he knows as Uncle Eddie when he was in a state of desperation. Could be a psychotic hallucination—or a flashback if there is a real Uncle Eddie. This suddenly got very complicated, I need to just go slowly. I can stay focused and outwardly calm by tracking my breathing, clearing my mind, and orienting myself to understanding Adam's experience as fully as possible so that he's not trapped alone in this inner crisis in which he's found himself.

THERAPIST: Okay. And, um, were you hearing him on the roof?

ADAM: *(Nods)*

THERAPIST: Okay. Was—was he with you, or was it a voice you were hearing?

ADAM: He was with me.

THERAPIST: He was with you. Okay. What was he saying?

ADAM: He was telling me to jump.

> *Therapist's Inner Reflections:* I thought for a moment there that this mystery person may actually have been physically on the roof with Adam when he said, "He was with me." But this sounds like Adam

experiencing the presence of another person who actually isn't there physically and who is saying things that are what Adam actually is thinking to himself. I don't want to inadvertently suggest to Adam that a flashback or a psychotic hallucination was actually happening, but I need to follow his narrative in order to understand what was happening for him.

THERAPIST: I see.

ADAM: And he was calling me pathetic and weak and a fag.

THERAPIST: Hmm. Must have been awful to be hearing that.

Therapist's Inner Reflections: I want Adam to know that I understand that those words are very painful for him to hear—not that I understand all that he's feeling or what he's experiencing but that he's not alone with those feelings when he is courageous enough to share them with me.

ADAM: (*Nods*)

THERAPIST: And so, when he was talking to you in that way, what did you feel like doing?

ADAM: Like, I felt like jumping . . .

Therapist's Inner Reflections: So "jumping" is an attempt to get away from intolerable feelings and thoughts when it seems like there's no other escape than suicide but not a wish to die so much as a wish for a sense of relief, protection, and a little bit of peacefulness in this maelstrom.

THERAPIST: Okay.

ADAM: . . . so I went over to the edge, and he kept tryin' to push me.

Therapist's Inner Reflections: Even though I know how this worked out and Adam's safe now, as he relives the crisis, it's really pretty frightening. He was right at the edge of death. I can imagine standing beside him, looking down, and feeling terrified and dizzy. I want to step back from the edge and pull him back, too, but I can't leave him there alone because he has to be the one to pull himself back, not me. He did step back somehow, and I have to understand how he did that. Then I can step back from the edge *with* him, but not doing it *for* him or making him do it *for* me.

THERAPIST: Hmm.

ADAM: But I fell backwards instead.

Therapist's Inner Reflections: Adam views this as falling backward, and that's probably what it felt like in the daze and depression he was experiencing. But I think it will be important to help him recognize that he actually made an assertive decision to protect himself, which took strength and courage. That's very different from not having the courage to jump, which probably is what he believes now and would be a tragic confirmation of his view of himself as pathetic.

THERAPIST: I see. And then what happened?

Therapist's Inner Reflections: This often is where the episode "ends," when a person's memory is clouded by despair and confusion—with a sense of incompleteness that can lead to a repetition of the unfinished sense of hopelessness and self-loathing that can spur further suicide attempts. So, it's really important to help Adam carry forward the memory to the present and to unpack the emotional pain so that he has a bridge to having a possible future that is not just a repetition of the hopelessness and despair. I'm staying pretty quiet so that I don't intrude on his memory and his inner experience, but I am also staying actively focused internally on walking through this side by side with Adam—one step at a time, starting with what happened next, and next . . .

ADAM: And then my sister came up. I guess she heard us yelling.

THERAPIST: Okay. And this was—this was where you lived?

ADAM: (*Nods*)

THERAPIST: Okay. In your building. You went up there. And so, she—what did she do when she saw you?

ADAM: Um, she grabbed me and she brought me back downstairs, and she called our parents.

THERAPIST: Okay. And what about Eddie? What was he doing or saying at that time?

ADAM: He left.

Therapist: He left. Do you know where he went?

ADAM: No.

THERAPIST: Okay. Tsk, um, what did your sister say to Uncle Eddie? Was he there when she got there?

ADAM: (*Shakes head*) No, he always leaves when my family's around.

Therapist's Inner Reflections: I thought this "Uncle Eddie" might be a dissociative alter identity and that seems very likely now. Hallucinations don't tend to go away when circumstances change, nor do flashbacks. Uncle Eddie is looking like a dissociative alter that is a classic persecutor: a dissociated representation of angry, blaming, and controlling feelings and thoughts that Adam is experiencing but doesn't feel able to own and contain as part of how he is feeling and thinking. Dissociative identity disorder can seem pretty scary and implacable from an outside perspective, and it can be very dangerous when suicidal impulses are essentially let loose in the form of an alter like Uncle Eddie. But I know this means that Adam is feeling a deep sense of shame and terror that he doesn't know how to live with inside himself. It's my job to help him understand how those thoughts and feelings make sense and can be lived with as an expression of himself—and not as a damning condemnation that mean that his life is ruined and worthless. We'll start by getting to know Uncle Eddie and getting "him" on Adam's side instead of as Adam's punisher.

THERAPIST: I see. So, Eddie is with you a lot, is that right?

ADAM: Yeah.

THERAPIST: Okay. And does he always call you pathetic and things like that?

ADAM: Yeah.

THERAPIST: Okay. And does he make you do things like this? Is this the first time he's said you should hurt your . . .

Therapist's Inner Reflections: I'm staying as matter-of-fact and non-judgmental as possible to give Adam the opportunity to reflect on what Uncle Eddie does and says without having to be so distressed that he is in crisis or on the verge of a breakdown. By objectifying Uncle Eddie without making any judgment about whether he is real or either bad or good, Adam may be able to recognize and start to own the thoughts and feelings that he's attributed to Uncle Eddie as his own thoughts and feelings—and to see that he, Adam, is in control of them, not anyone else.

ADAM: (*Covers face with jacket hood, brings knees to chest*)

THERAPIST: You don't like talking about Uncle Eddie. What's going on, Adam?

Therapist's Inner Reflections: Starting the process of reintegration of the split-off alter part was Plan A. Looks like, instead, I have to shift to Plan B, that is, seeing what happens when Uncle Eddie takes over and having a face-to-face talk with Uncle Eddie. I have to be very careful not to indicate that I believe that Uncle Eddie is completely separate from Adam because that would increase Adam's sense of being powerless and dominated by Uncle Eddie. On the other hand, I need to signal to Uncle Eddie that I recognize his voice as valid and important so that Adam won't need to prove Uncle Eddie's reality by slipping further into a state of paralysis and shame or, worse yet, by giving up and letting Uncle Eddie push him to suicide. This is a complex and delicate form of joining and partnering with a client who is not able to be fully present and has learned to escape from overwhelming distress by ceding control to an alter.

ADAM: (*Uncovers face, leans forward on sofa, talks louder*) What the fuck do you think is going on? Adam's not here anymore. That's what's going on.

THERAPIST: Yeah.

ADAM: Who are you?

THERAPIST: I'm the therapist.

ADAM: Doctor, huh?

THERAPIST: Yeah.

ADAM: What are you gonna—you gonna try and get rid of me 'cause you think you know what's best for Adam? You don't know what's best. I know what's best.

THERAPIST: Are you Eddie? Am I talking to Eddie?

Therapist's Inner Reflections: I know this is Eddie, but if I feign ignorance initially, that may give Eddie the sense of having the upper hand. Otherwise, Eddie is signaling he'll have to try to tear me down from my position as an authority so that I don't try to displace him using my status and power as a doctor. I want him to see me as a potential ally and not as threatening or challenging him. I won't agree with Eddie about his emotionally abusive attitude toward Adam, but I will try to find a basis for an alliance with him that can become a basis for Adam to reclaim the thoughts and feelings that he's involuntarily delegated to this alter part of himself.

ADAM: Yeah.

THERAPIST: Okay. Can you tell me, Eddie, what's best for Adam? I—I really wanna get your perspective on this.

ADAM: He needs to be fixed.

THERAPIST: Okay. Tell me what fixing him would be like. Wh—what does he need to be fixed about?

ADAM: Well, he was with that boy, and I thought I had him fixed earlier, but he just kept going back to him.

Therapist's Inner Reflections: Now it's clearer that, at least in part, Uncle Eddie serves as the voice of Adam's ambivalence about homosexuality and feeling attracted romantically to a boy—or possibly Adam's fear of being subjected to heterosexist biases by other people in his life, which may be based on what they've actually said and done or on what Adam fears they'd think. This is an important intersecting complication that I need to keep in mind as I get to know Adam.

THERAPIST: Hmm.

ADAM: And I kept trying to get him to stop, but he wouldn't stop.

THERAPIST: Yeah.

ADAM: So, finally I realized that he was a lost cause, so I brought him up on the roof, and I was gonna start all over again.

THERAPIST: Okay. How would you have started all over?

ADAM: I would'a pushed him.

THERAPIST: Okay. And that would've ended him. Is that what you were thinking?

ADAM: Yeah.

THERAPIST: You felt there was no hope for him, is that right?

Therapist's Inner Reflections: I could try to convince Uncle Eddie that if he succeeds in getting Adam to kill himself, he—Uncle Eddie—also will die and there won't be a "start all over." But I think that would elicit defensive and possibly hostile reaction because Adam (and the alter) would perceive me as trying to take control and dictate his choices, or that I was trying to manipulate him into giving up the option of suicide, which I don't think he'll be ready to do until he doesn't feel trapped with depression and shame, and until he views suicide as not an option based on having better options (as opposed to giving it up with no better option). I think that focusing on Adam's feeling that there's no hope, which Uncle Eddie has reframed as there being "no hope" for "fixing" Adam, is the key. Both Adam and this alter part of him need to find a meaningful hope that they can share and believe in. For Uncle Eddie, I think the hope that may be meaningful is that he can help Adam be a success—that mirrors what Adam's parents have emphasized as their hope for Adam, and it's what Adam wants, too. The bind is that the parents' view of "success" (and Adam's "adultified" translation of it, as expressed by Uncle Eddie) is not fitting with Adam's interests, feelings, and hopes for himself (very possibly including Adam's homosexual feelings and interests). Finding a bridge between those two worlds that honors Adam's hopes and interests, and is accepted by his parents (for whom Uncle Eddie seems to serve as a distorted proxy or spokesperson), is the approach I'll try to take.

ADAM: Yeah.

THERAPIST: Okay. I'll bet you've been with him a long time.

ADAM: Yeah. As long as I can remember.

THERAPIST: Okay. And I'll bet you have a lot of thoughts about what would be good for him, is that right?

ADAM: Oh, yeah.

THERAPIST: Okay. Tell me more about what would be good for him.

ADAM: If he had stayed with that girl, Alex, who he was with for a little while.

THERAPIST: Yeah.

ADAM: He had an older girl slip right through his fingers for some guy.

THERAPIST: Okay.

ADAM: I don't know if there's much fixing we can do anymore, so.

THERAPIST: And you—you helped Adam to be with Alex, is that right?

ADAM: Yeah.

> *Therapist's Inner Reflections:* I've seen from Adam's outpatient thera-
> pist's records that this "girl," Alex, actually was a young adult tutor
> who molested and coerced Adam. I'm not going to say anything about
> that now, but it may help Adam to be aware that Uncle Eddie was
> not "helping" him to be with Alex but instead was reflecting Alex's
> pressure on Adam to meet her needs and to deny his true sexual and
> romantic preferences. Just as Alex apparently said she was pursuing
> Adam for "his own good," so, too, Uncle Eddie is expressing external
> demands and pressure to conform to conventional norms rather than
> Adam's true feelings and values. Adam's relationship with and feelings
> for James, which James apparently did not feel he could stand up to
> his own parents to preserve (paralleling Adam's fear of rejection, for
> which Uncle Eddie is the internal representation), is now associated
> with loss and helplessness. But regaining a sense of the truth and value
> of those feelings despite the external interference that appears to have
> ended that relationship could be a crucial foundation for Adam to
> regain confidence and hope.

THERAPIST: Okay. And tell me what was it about this boy? This was James, is that right?

ADAM: Yeah.

THERAPIST: What was it about Adam's relationship with James that was bothering you or you felt was not good for him?

ADAM: It was faggy.

THERAPIST: I see. Okay. And that's something that you think is very bad for Adam, is that right?

> *Therapist's Inner Reflections:* This is Adam's way of expressing his fear of rejection for being gay. Uncle Eddie vilifies and degrades homosexuality so that Adam can avoid taking the risk of being further hurt by acknowledging being gay and trusting in a gay partner. It also may be an expression of Adam's anger at James for abandoning their relationship and toward himself for not somehow standing up or even fighting to keep that relationship. Being gay, if that's what Adam truly feels, which seems likely, is not the problem; it's the rejection that can occur when other people are heterosexist and degrade or deprive a person because of their sexual orientation. Uncle Eddie is masquerading as Adam's protector while instead entrapping Adam as a victim of an internal struggle between fear, anger, and despair versus self-determination. I wish I could just vanquish Uncle Eddie and rescue Adam, but that would be inadvertently doing harm to Adam rather than helping him take on and master the fear and anger that the alter represents. Instead, I think it's crucial to show Adam how to create an alliance with Uncle Eddie so that he (Adam) can reclaim as his own the feelings that the alter represents.

ADAM: Oh, yeah.

THERAPIST: Okay. Okay. Can you tell me, Eddie, how you tried to help?

ADAM: Well, I would yell at him every night and tell him that it was wrong for him to be with him.

> *Therapist's Inner Reflections:* This tells me that Adam is experiencing ruminations and probably also nightmares that are disrupting his sleep. That's another source of risk that we'll need to address in his therapy. But, first, the focus has to be on their source: the disavowed and avoided feelings and thoughts that Uncle Eddie represents.

THERAPIST: (*Nods*)

ADAM: Um, when I first started thinking that he might be like this, I showed him what it was like and why he wouldn't want it.

THERAPIST: Hmm. How did you show him what it was like?

ADAM: I did it to him . . .

THERAPIST: I see.

ADAM: . . . so he would know.

THERAPIST: Yeah. What did he feel about that?

ADAM: He cried.

> *Therapist's Inner Reflections:* I'm concerned that Adam may be telling me that there is an actual man, maybe even a family relative (for whom Uncle Eddie is a code name), who has sexually molested him. There's nothing about that in any of the records I've seen, but that wouldn't be entirely surprising given how intensely Adam seems to keep any distress bottled up. He may have been afraid, like so many kids are, of reporting abuse, especially if it was someone trusted by the family like a coach or teacher or religious official, or an actual member of the family. This is something I will need to talk about with Adam when he's not in this acute phase of crisis.

THERAPIST: Okay.

ADAM: I thought that was a good thing that he would understand that this is how he would feel afterwards.

THERAPIST: Yeah. Yeah. And then you saw he kept doing it.

ADAM: Yeah.

THERAPIST: Okay. When did you think that he should jump off the roof? When did you decide that that was what was right?

ADAM: Uh, yesterday, when he was crying over the fact that he wasn't with James anymore. I thought, well, if this is how he's gonna act about boys instead of girls . . .

THERAPIST: Mm-hmm.

ADAM: . . . there's no hope.

THERAPIST: Okay. Yeah. Was that the first time you ever wanted him to die or hurt himself?

ADAM: Yeah. I always wanted him to just get fixed instead.

THERAPIST: I see. So, you had worked pretty hard it sounds like . . .

ADAM: Yeah.

THERAPIST: . . . and you felt it was, like, the end of the line, is that right?

ADAM: Yeah.

THERAPIST: There was no hope for him? Okay. What do you think about being here in the hospital now?

Therapist's Inner Reflections: So, we've established that the impulse to suicide was a last resort. That opens the door to other options if there is some meaningful hope that things can be worked out so that Adam feels able to pursue his true hopes and to handle the fears, anger, and shame that have led him to find an alter to handle in his place. The hospital represents that sense of life-and-death urgency, but it also can represent the beginning of regaining hope. Although Uncle Eddie doesn't seem interested in hope, he's an expression of Adam's not having given up—so even though the alter represents hopelessness and coercion, finding how that aspect of Adam's feelings can also experience a sense of genuine hope seems like the crucial shift.

ADAM: I don't really like it.

THERAPIST: Okay. Say more.

ADAM: Uh, I know that you guys here try and tend to tell people that all their problems are okay and that they can be happy with who they are, but I know that that's not okay for Adam, and he needs to be fixed, and I don't feel like you guys are gonna fix him here.

THERAPIST: Would you be, like you're doing now, part of talking with me and helping us to understand your perspective?

ADAM: Absolutely. I'm not gonna let you be alone with Adam.

THERAPIST: Okay. And you're with him it sounds like all the time.

ADAM: Yeah. I never go away.

Therapist's Inner Reflections: Uncle Eddie is Adam's inner watchdog and tormentor, but he also represents Adam's desire for support, guidance, and genuine protection. Those adaptive goals could be a basis for a partnership between me and Uncle Eddie on behalf of Adam's safety. Uncle Eddie's statement that he's always present also provides an opening for me to help Adam understand that upsetting feelings don't disappear when he tries to not think about or feel them. When distress is avoided, it can become a constant downer like Uncle Eddie. But when painful feelings are acknowledged, they can be scaled down and made manageable. So, by offering to partner with Uncle Eddie, I'm modeling for Adam how to acknowledge and make peace with— but *not* give in to—his (Adam's) most distressing feelings and beliefs about himself. I'll begin by exploring how the dialogue goes between Adam and Uncle Eddie; in other words, I'll explore how Adam reacts to the distressing feelings and thoughts that he's trying to shut out.

THERAPIST: Okay. So, you're listening always. Okay. What does Adam say when you talk to him? What does he—how does he respond to you?

ADAM: Um. He usually cries. Asks me to leave him alone, and I tell him it's for his own good.

THERAPIST: What does he think of you being here talking with me?

ADAM: Uh, right now, he doesn't really like it, but I think he'll realize that in the long run, it's a good thing that I'm talking to you instead of him.

THERAPIST: Hmm. Do you think he doesn't want to talk with me?

ADAM: I don't know what he wants, but I don't think it's good for him to talk to you.

THERAPIST: Okay. W—why is that?

ADAM: Because you're gonna try and tell him he's okay just the way he is, and he's not. He needs help.

THERAPIST: Okay.

ADAM: And I'm the only one who really knows how to help him.

> *Therapist's Inner Reflections:* I can agree with Uncle Eddie that Adam is not fine and needs help, but I'll redefine what this means. From Adam's perspective currently, as expressed by Uncle Eddie, Adam is not fine because he's a failure and he needs help to be "fixed" because he is struggling with homosexual feelings and a sense of loss and grief. From my perspective, Adam is not fine because he's understandably fearful of and hurt by rejection and loss, and he needs help being safe, which will involve restoring a well-deserved sense of self-confidence and pride, security in primary relationships, and hope and enjoyment in his life. For Adam to have that safety and to achieve those goals, Uncle Eddie definitely needs to participate so that Adam can be more active in dialoging with and ultimately reversing the balance of power, such that the alter becomes part of Adam's inner voice and not an external entity. But the first priority now is getting Adam back in the conversation so that I can begin to help him see that he is my priority and Uncle Eddie is expressing concerns that I can help Adam deal with.

THERAPIST: Yeah. So, I think it's clear to me that you need to be involved for sure. I need to understand your perspective. I need to understand Adam's perspective, too, and part of it is working together to figure out what to do. I mean, you're stuck here in the hospital. I know you don't like it. I wanna know more about how Adam feels about being in the hospital, but part of it is you're together all the time, and it doesn't seem like Adam's very happy. I know you're not happy with how it's going. Part of it is figuring it out together.

ADAM: Yeah.

THERAPIST: So, I would like to be—to talk to Adam now if you think that would be okay with you, Eddie. Would that?

ADAM: Yeah, but if things go poorly, I'll be back.

THERAPIST: Yeah. I know you will.

ADAM: Okay.

Therapist's Inner Reflections: To proactively circumvent the suspicions that Adam has about therapy, which he's expressed through Uncle Eddie, I'm going to invite the alter to join in if he (actually Adam) feels that I'm saying or doing anything that triggers feelings of fear or anger at a level at which (Adam) doesn't feel safe or is unable to cope with. Instead of attempting to keep the alter out, inviting him in signals to Adam that those feelings can be voiced and dealt with.

THERAPIST: And s—Eddie, one more thing before you go. If ever you're feeling it's going poorly, if ever you're feeling I'm saying or doing something you would prefer me not to, I think it is important to let me know. I have one more question.

ADAM: Okay.

Therapist's Inner Reflections: I just realized that I need to leave Adam and the alter with a focal point that we can agree on as an overarching goal. Adam's safety is a key place to start.

THERAPIST: Um. How safe are things now in the hospital?

ADAM: Well, you guys are watching him, so he's not gonna do anything.

THERAPIST: Is that okay by you for now?

ADAM: Yeah.

THERAPIST: Okay. And you'll work with me on that.

Therapist's Inner Reflections: I'm not going to let the alter go without a commitment to work with me. That begins to shift the alter's role from a persecutor to a protector.

ADAM: Yeah.

THERAPIST: Okay. I really appreciate hearing what you have to say, Eddie, for sure. If Adam wants to talk with me, I want to speak with him for sure.

ADAM: Okay.

THERAPIST: Okay. See if you can get him.

> *Therapist's Inner Reflections:* By asking the alter to "get" Adam, I'm communicating to Adam that I recognize that the alter must be taken seriously as a part of Adam's reality. I know that even if Adam is completely dissociated and amnesic for the conversation I've had with Uncle Eddie, Adam is listening to me and is making his own decision to be fully present again. This can help him to learn that by paying attention to—but not being intimidated or controlled by—the alter, it is possible to move the alter to the background and regain a sense of self-determination. The alter represents Adam's sense that he's lost control of his own thoughts and feelings, as if the internal distress he feels has become so overwhelming that it's now an abusive external force that is torturing and trying to control him. Helping Adam to feel sufficiently safe and supported to be able to experience those distressing feelings and thoughts as manageable is a long-term goal and the first step is letting him know I can help him with Uncle Eddie.

ADAM: (*Sits back into sofa*)

THERAPIST: Were you listening?

ADAM: (*Nods*)

THERAPIST: What did you think about what Eddie was saying?

ADAM: (*Shrugs shoulders*) I don't know. It—kinda scary, but . . .

THERAPIST: Yeah.

ADAM: . . . it could be good.

THERAPIST: So, can you tell me what's scary and then what could be good?

ADAM: Um. You could take his side because he's not gonna let you take my side.

THERAPIST: Hmm. And if I were to do that, what would that mean?

ADAM: I don't know. I guess it means I really do need fixing.

> *Therapist's Inner Reflections:* Adam is asking whether I think he needs "fixing." Instead of giving him generic reassurance, I can help him

by explaining that I see Uncle Eddie as a part of Adam, not a separate external person or force, that is expressing feelings and thoughts that are actually Adam's but that are confusing or troubling for him. And that I view Adam as the person who's actually in control and knows what's best for himself. That way I'm taking seriously the distress that Uncle Eddie represents, but I'm also empowering Adam as the one in control.

THERAPIST: Well, what I think about it is there's a part of you called Eddie and there's Adam, and you have very different ideas and thoughts and feelings about what needs to happen, and the solution is to figure it out together. I wanna help by understanding, and that's hearing from you, hearing from Eddie, and any—anyone else, any other part who could help me help you. Um, that's my job. My job isn't to tell you what to do. One of the things Eddie said is that he's been around for a long time. I—is that true?

ADAM: (*Nods*)

THERAPIST: And the sense I get from him is that he tries to help, and I know it got really scary and dangerous yesterday, but what do you feel about him helping? I know again it wasn't good, but is there any way he's tried to help that you felt was helpful?

ADAM: No.

THERAPIST: Okay.

ADAM: All he does is hurt me more.

Therapist's Inner Reflections: Adam is making it clear that he is phobic of feelings or thoughts that are distressing. That doesn't mean that he can't face and come to terms with distressing thoughts and feelings but that we have to start by carefully examining those a little at a time—only as much and with as much intensity as Adam can tolerate without abdicating to the alter.

THERAPIST: Okay. Okay. That's very painful because you and he interact so much. So, my job, again, is to help by understanding, and we need—I'm hoping we could work together to figure out how things will be better. Do you think you can work with me to try and figure this out 'cause I really, really want to understand?

Therapist's Inner Reflections: I'm focusing on helping Adam by "understanding" and "figuring out" the dilemmas Adam is facing from his perspective because I think that will feel safer and more manageable to Adam than a more conventional therapeutic agenda of exploring and reworking his feelings and memories. He can tell me what he thinks I need to "understand" and what he wants to "figure out" so that he's in control of how intense the therapy becomes.

ADAM: Okay.

THERAPIST: Okay. Are you feeling safe now?

ADAM: (*Shrugs shoulders*)

THERAPIST: Okay.

ADAM: I mean, I don't know. I feel safer, I guess, because I know you guys won't let Eddie do anything to me, but it's hard to feel safe because he's always here.

Therapist's Inner Reflections: From Adam's perspective, distressing thoughts and feelings—as personified by Uncle Eddie—are a danger and not a part of his inner experience that he can handle. By offering to hear Uncle Eddie's views and work with them, I'm communicating to Adam that it's possible to acknowledge rather than avoid distressing thoughts and feelings, and to work with them to develop solutions to problems that otherwise seem unsolvable—and that that is the way to achieve safety, not by trying to make the thoughts or feelings go away.

THERAPIST: And you—you should know that you—if you heard or didn't hear that he did say that he would work with me to help keep things safe and that things are safe now and that he would let me know. What do you feel about that? Either when you heard it or now that I'm repeating it?

ADAM: I don't know if I trust him because I don't know what he means by keeping me safe.

THERAPIST: Okay. Is there anything in particular you're worried about?

ADAM: I'm worried that he's gonna pretend and he's gonna keep lying. Then you're gonna say it's okay for me to go home, and then as soon as I go home, he's gonna turn back into the old Uncle Eddie.

Therapist's Inner Reflections: I get it. Adam doesn't want to be left alone with the inner turmoil that he's experiencing. He wants to be sure he knows how to deal with those feelings, thoughts, and the impulses (including suicide) that he's has when he can't tolerate the distress. That is an excellent practical benchmark for assessing when

Adam is safe enough to leave the hospital. It won't be just that he has a new understanding and coping skills to face and deal with distress—that is important—but also we need to be certain that he has reliable and available support in relationships that he trusts and in which he feels he can be open and is accepted for who he is (including but not limited to his sexual orientation and his goals for himself). That's a lot to accomplish and will take work well beyond what can be fully completed in this hospitalization. However, we have to lay a solid foundation before Adam is discharged so that he doesn't find himself on the roof feeling helpless to prevent Uncle Eddie from pushing him off the edge.

THERAPIST: I see. So, there's a real trust issue here. Okay. Trust is so important. So, again, just to repeat myself, I need to hear from you and Eddie, and we need to figure out how to make this better, okay? I'll be here every day. We'll be meeting every day, and let's work together to figure out how to make things better and safer for you and all parts of you, okay?

ADAM: Okay.

Adam's Observations

Adam came into this session with apprehension about meeting a new therapist consistent with his past experiences with authority figures who proved to be abusive: "In the past, when adults say they want to help me, they usually ignore me or even hurt me, like my soccer coach Uncle Eddie, and my tutor." When the therapist said he was here to understand, that was both surprising and a relief: "As a teenager, it seems no one really wants to understand me, only getting me to do what they want or what they say is best for me." It also was very important to Adam that the therapist said things that helped Uncle Eddie calm down: "When Uncle Eddie is calmer, I am calmer." By the end of session, Adam felt able to actually listen to his own feelings without being overrun by Uncle Eddie, and that gave him a faint, but distinct, sense of hope that he could find a way to free himself from Uncle Eddie and get on with his life.

Commentary

In this initial therapeutic session with Adam, the therapist was quickly confronted with not only a complex clinical presentation but also a high-stakes series of decisions as he began to understand that Adam's developmental trauma history had resulted in the development of dissociated parts of self. While Adam presented as the primary client, on learning of and then observing Adam shift into the persona of Uncle Eddie (a dissociated alter/part self within Adam), the therapist endeavored to establish a therapeutic alliance with both Adam and Uncle Eddie. This approach, similar to that taken in conjoint family therapy with actual family members present, was particularly important because Adam and Uncle Eddie appeared diametrically opposed in their views and needs. As if working with a couple experiencing severe discord or with an angry adult caregiver and a child who is the identified patient, the therapist carefully worked to build a relationship with both Adam and Uncle Eddie, recognizing that this was actually helping Adam to begin the process of coming to terms with distressing thoughts and feelings that he had been attempting to suppress or get rid of. This experiential avoidance had the unintended adverse effect of pushing those thoughts and feelings out of awareness but not eliminating, let alone resolving, them. Thus, the inner voice of Uncle Eddie appeared to represent a dissociated part "self" who was separate from Adam but always present within Adam's mind.

To ensure Adam's safety and to develop a therapeutic alliance with Adam, the therapist needed to understand both Adam's and Uncle Eddie's perspectives—because both actually were what Adam was thinking and feeling but were artificially separated because Adam did not feel able to cope with the profound dysphoria for which Uncle Eddie had become the voice. By aligning with Uncle Eddie as if he were a separate person, the therapist created an opportunity to reduce Adam's level of risk by beginning to redefine the alter as a protective presence who had Adam's best interests at heart. This was not based on a mistaken presumption that the feelings and thoughts that Adam attributed to Uncle Eddie were benign. The therapist recognized that shame, loneliness, anger, impatience, and hopelessness are a volatile and painful emotional mix that can lead to self-harm, suicidality, or other dangerous impulses. However, for Adam to be able to tolerate and make peace with those feelings and thoughts, both Adam and Uncle Eddie needed to be engaged collaboratively in developing an alliance. That was the foundation for then developing a plan for therapy that would shift the relationship between Adam and Uncle Eddie from one of victim and persecutor to one in which Adam was able to differentiate himself from the actual Uncle Eddie (and other abusers he has faced) and own the distress that Uncle Eddie represented as an affirmation of his right to make choices in his life based on his true self without paralyzing shame or guilt.

From the perspective of the FREEDOM framework (i.e., focusing, recognizing triggers, emotion awareness, evaluating thoughts, defining goals and options, making a contribution; see the Introduction to this volume), the therapist established a focus for himself as well as for Adam by emphasizing that Adam's safety was the paramount priority. With this orienting thought as a guide, the therapist engaged Adam and Uncle Eddie in a dialogue that he consistently described as serving two main goals: creating a respectful partnership and gaining understanding. Those goals were a down-to-earth way of communicating to Adam that therapy is a process in which the therapist works as a partner—not as an external controller or authority like Uncle Eddie—alongside (and not above) the client to gain an understanding of what is most important and will be most helpful for the client's safety— not to "fix" or find fault with the client. Thus, from the outset and throughout the session, the therapist modeled for Adam how it was possible to use the orienting thought of safety and the main goals of partnership and understanding as ways to focus, calm oneself (i.e., to experience main emotions), and begin to find hope and think clearly (i.e., to draw on main thoughts) in the midst of a crisis. In so doing, the therapist enabled Adam (and Uncle Eddie) to genuinely consider therapy as a viable option because, as the therapist demonstrated, therapy could make a contribution to what Adam and Eddie both valued—Adam's safety and success in life—despite their apparently antithetical positions.

At the same time that the therapist modeled how to focus and draw on core values, he also modeled and helped Adam actually engage in a safe and tolerable examination of the reactive side of the FREEDOM paradigm. The triggers identified included Adam's loss of the relationship with James, the social rejection that Adam had experienced (or fears will occur) as a result of being out with his gay sexual orientation, and the rejection by significant others that Uncle Eddie represents. By cautiously exploring Uncle Eddie's views and Adam's reactions to Uncle Eddie, the therapist was able to help Adam identify and nonjudgmentally reflect on the distress he was feeling with greater clarity and less confusion. This gentle but thorough exploration revealed a number of reactive emotions (e.g., anger, disgust, shame, fear, grief), reactive thoughts (e.g., that Adam needs to be but can't be "fixed," that homosexuality is bad but also something Adam does not feel he wants to or can change, that Adam is helpless to deal with distress—aka Uncle Eddie), reactive goals (i.e., to give up, to end his life, to "fix" him, to make him obey Uncle Eddie, to make Uncle Eddie go away), and reactive options (e.g., commit suicide; delegate all negative feelings to Uncle Eddie; give Uncle Eddie total authority; drop out of relationships; stop going to school or participating in activities, such as athletics). As a result, without subjecting Adam to an interview that might have felt like an impersonal evaluation or an intrusive and emotionally overwhelming interrogation, the therapist was able to help Adam express (and begin to reflect on but not feel pressured to go deeply into) the internal turmoil he was coping with.

This session illustrated the calming effect that intensive listening, non-judgmental openness and curiosity, and consistent offering of a collaborative working relationship can have with a client who is feeling confused and hopeless, and who is literally psychologically falling apart. The therapist paid exquisite attention to every word and phrase that the client used, following up on every statement (verbal and nonverbal) from the client with an open-ended question or paraphrase that expressed an unwavering interest in understanding what the client meant from the perspective of the client (i.e., nonjudgmental acceptance, active empathy). While the transcript does not show the therapist's nonverbal modes of communication, his pacing, vocal tone and inflection, and body language were consistent with his words in expressing calmness, openness, genuine interest, compassion, and a firm commitment to preserving Adam's safety.

In the session, Adam made several significant shifts in psychological state. This was most evident in the sudden emergence of a dissociative alter, which appears as if the client (Adam) had become an entirely different person who acts and views himself as an entirely different person separate from the client (Uncle Eddie). The therapist had to make a rapid determination whether the client was experiencing a psychotic auditory hallucination— a disembodied voice in his mind—or a dissociative fragmentation of the client's self—a shift in identity to that of an alternative self (hence the term, "alter"). The client's nonverbal mannerisms made it clear that this was not simply a psychotically hallucinated inner voice (as complex as that is) but a dissociative alter. To avoid escalating the situation in the session by challenging or confronting Adam or attempting to dismiss the alter, the therapist nonjudgmentally accepted Adam's definition of Uncle Eddie as someone he needed help dealing with and respectfully engaged in a dialogue with the alter to understand what led Adam to the brink of suicide and how the alter is expressing feelings, thoughts, and impulses of Adam's that Adam has attempted to disavow.

The interaction between the therapist and Adam or the alter appeared on the surface to be quite straightforward as conversations in which they were getting to know each other. However, under that surface was a great deal of nuance. The therapist recognized that the alter was serving a complex set of functions for Adam, including voicing internalizations of

- criticisms he had received or expected to receive from other people, such as his parents, who had expectations that the client (Adam) found intrusive and unempathic;

- intimidation, exploitation, and devaluing he had experienced from adults who had sexually abused him (including the real Uncle Eddie, who also was Adam's athletics coach, and a tutor); and

- condemnation, harassment, and microaggressions that he had experienced directly or vicariously as a result of identifying his sexual orientation as gay and seeking sexual and intimate relationships with male peers or men.

The alter also represented several aspects of the client's emotional distress and dysregulation, including

- a shame related to both confusion about his sexual identity and a sense of being weak, passive, and unworthy of being respected or loved in relationships;

- grief resulting from having lost or having been rejected in important relationships, including a recent romantic relationship;

- anxiety about being unable to have meaningful and trustworthy intimate relationships and friendships;

- frustration at being unable to succeed in pursuing and achieving creative expressions of his interests and talents; and

- despair and hopelessness.

Moreover, the alter expressed the client's adaptive qualities in several respects, including a determination to

- assertively stand up for himself;

- take control of his own life and decisions; and

- resolve the emotional turmoil that he was experiencing, and achieve success in meaningful relationships and creative pursuits of his own choice.

The therapist unobtrusively yet precisely and seamlessly guided the discussion with Adam and the alter through this set of three domains. First, the therapist invited a description of Adam's concerns about himself. This led to an outpouring of criticism, intimidation, and condemnation from Uncle Eddie, which the therapist did not directly challenge but instead used as a segue to reframe the alter's intent as a desire to help Adam. That shift defused some of the emotional intensity and suspiciousness expressed by the alter followed by declamations by the alter of his disappointments in the client (i.e., indirect expressions of the client's shame and grief), and his worries, frustrations, and hopelessness for Adam. The therapist responded to this with compassion and empathy, and then shifted the focus again to emphasize the client/alter's desire to "help" Adam and invited the alter to join with him in working toward the goals of making Adam safe. Most of this was implied rather than explicitly stated to avoid overloading Adam emotionally while laying the groundwork for therapy that would follow over the next days in the hospital and into the future, after Adam leaves the hospital and returns to his family and community.

From a crisis management and prevention perspective, the therapist had taken crucial steps to begin to neutralize, or at least diminish, the two primary risk factors that could lead to further and more severe suicidal crises. The first risk factor was the client's dissociative fragmentation and the continued presence of the alter that was amplifying Adam's distress and dysregulation while also providing Adam with an impetus and a psychological structure for enacting self-harming or self-destructive avoidant impulses. Making that alter and its relationship to Adam an explicit party to the therapeutic interaction, and explaining to Adam that the alter was a part of himself that needed to be understood and brought into a cooperative partnership (with the help of the therapist) were essential first steps in enabling Adam to regain a position of primary agency in relation to the alter instead of feeling and acting as if the alter were in control of him.

This agenda of restoring self-determination to Adam was done, and needed to be done, without engaging in a power struggle or an attempt to simply eradicate the alter. Despite the toxicity of the alter, it was a part of his experience and self that could not be excised and that would become less toxic and more manageable only when Adam was able to accept the voice of the alter as an expression of part of who he is—but also as a distortion of himself that was a reaction to difficulties in formative relationships (e.g., with parents, with friends and intimate partners) as well as to the hurt and injury caused by abusive experiences. By aligning with the alter as a potential helpful contributor to, and beneficiary of, psychotherapy, the therapist began what would be a complicated but now potentially feasible therapeutic process. This involved helping Adam to own what is himself in the alter and accept but not internalize the reactions expressed by the alter as the result of relational injuries and abuse that were caused by the acts of others but for which he was not to blame and that did not define who he is as a person or what his life would be in the future.

The second primary risk factor was the impulse to self-harm or suicide. By unconsciously bifurcating his will to live (located in his ordinary self, Adam) and his desire to escape or punish himself through suicide (located in the alter), Adam reduced his ability to be in control of his choices about self-harm or suicide. The result was a scenario in which the alter appeared to be in a position to make the choice to suicide for him instead of Adam's having to make the choice for himself. By framing the next steps in therapy as helping Adam and the alter to understand and work with one another on behalf of Adam's safety, the therapist began building a bridge linking Adam's will to live with his disavowed and transferred (to the alter) impulse to die, and this increased Adam's awareness and ability to assume control of decisions about his own safety. Adam had abdicated the responsibility for managing those impulses, but he divested them to an alter who was still part of him and therefore shared the desire to live even if that was obscured by the toxicity and the intimidating presentation of the alter. So, in fostering a partnership between Adam and the alter while making it clear to Adam (and indirectly therefore, also to the alter) that it was Adam as a whole person who was the client and whose safety and ability to make his own decisions was the priority, the therapist began the process of helping Adam to reclaim his authority over his own life and his responsibility to manage impulses to self-harm or die. Without this pseudo-partnership of Adam and the alter as a starting point, Adam would have no way to understand how, or why, he should and could take on that responsibility. He would be too mired in despair and burdened by a reexperiencing of abuse to feel willing or able to exert the physical and psychological energy required to inhibit intense avoidant or self-punitive impulses. With that partnership as a metaphor, Adam could get support from not only the therapist but also from the healthy aspects of the alter and could envision and undertake the reclamation project. Adam implied as much by saying that he felt safer in the hospital because there were people there who wouldn't allow the alter to push him to self-harm. A therapeutic goal would be to enable Adam to recognize himself as a person who, with support from the kinds of relationships that he chooses for himself, could accept the alter as part of himself and take on the protective role for himself.

By relentlessly and nonjudgmentally siding with Adam in each state of mind—depressed, dissociated, angry, hopeless—the therapist also helped Adam to experience the sense of secure attachment and partnership that he had longed for. This was highlighted when the therapist affirmed that he was aware of Adam's presence even when it seemed that Uncle Eddie had taken over. This helped Adam to realize that he was able to remain present, if only as an observer, when he felt completely preempted by Uncle Eddie, which opened the door to Adam's asserting himself and negotiating as an equal (and ultimately as the dominant self) with the feelings and thoughts that Uncle Eddie expressed. As Adam eventually becomes able to observe what seem to be the thoughts and reactions of an entirely separate self—with his therapist's help in reframing Uncle Eddie's intent in nontoxic, non-abusive ways—he can recognize that these are an expression of important feelings and thoughts of his own that have become mixed up—because of past traumas—but can be, and need to be, unscrambled so that he can take ownership of his healthy ability to be self-assertive.

Uncle Eddie was a complex psychological phenomenon that may have served several functions for Adam but at a great cost that included the degradation or loss of a coherent sense of self and a sense of hopelessness and worthlessness that proved to be potentially life-threatening for him. By adopting Uncle Eddie as a voice within himself, Adam may have been attempting to contain and cope with the dysregulation triggered by flashbacks or other intrusive memories of the abuse perpetrated on him by the actual Uncle Eddie. By introjecting this external figure, Adam may have been able to gain a sense of control over the memories and associated distress that he could not achieve when he was a child in thrall to his abusive adult uncle and coach. Just as the actual Uncle Eddie/coach initially presented himself as an ally and source of caring and approval, Adam may have initially internalized Uncle Eddie as a helpful protector who only wanted what was best for Adam (which Uncle Eddie now claimed as his attitude). However, the internalized Uncle Eddie was inevitably associated with abuse, devaluation, and ultimately threats of violence because those aspects of Adam's actual interactions with his uncle/coach were probably indelibly emotionally imprinted in his memory as the most distressing and recent capstone to the abuse. As a result, Uncle Eddie's initially soothing function as a transitional object (Gaddini, 1975) and as a source of security in a primitive twinship transference (Kohut & Wolf, 1978), appeared to have devolved into a source of psychological threat and damage that exacerbated Adam's shame, depression, and hopelessness, and left him struggling with escalating dysregulation that now posed a serious threat to his life as well as a source of major psychosocial impairment.

By joining and offering to partner with Uncle Eddie, the therapist undertook several complex therapeutic maneuvers to reduce the likelihood that Adam would continue to experience suicidal crises and to increase Adam's sense that he could take ownership of the troubling emotions, conflictual and self-critical beliefs, and disturbing memories that Uncle Eddie was now expressing for him. In terms of motivational enhancement, engaging as an ally with Uncle Eddie on behalf of Adam's safety and well-being reduced the potential adversarial power struggle (and escalation of hostility and threats by Uncle Eddie as a result of Adam's fear of being annihilated if he confronted

Uncle Eddie) that would likely result if the therapist confronted or attempted to dismiss Uncle Eddie. Having a reasonable and friendly conversation with Uncle Eddie also provided a model for Adam of how it was possible to use his intellectual and interpersonal skills (which had increased substantially in the years since he was a younger child entrapped by his uncle/coach) to both negotiate a reasonable accommodation with the internal doubts, fears, shame, and anger that Uncle Eddie voiced and change the definition of the problem from some deficit or flaw in himself to finding a way to create a life that would express his best qualities and strengths and that would best serve his well-being as he transitions into adulthood.

The conversation with Uncle Eddie also confirmed that the therapist accepted Adam without judgment and with unconditional positive regard: If the therapist could treat the obviously obnoxious and maleficent Uncle Eddie in a respectful manner with nonjudgmental acceptance, then the shame that Uncle Eddie might seem to deserve (and that he accused Adam of deserving) might not be valid. Because the therapist spoke of Adam with clear respect and positive regard, this further demonstrated that Adam was worthy of such positive valuation without directly challenging Uncle Eddie by arguing the point explicitly. The therapist also pointedly but by implication rather than confrontation did not accept Uncle Eddie's criticisms of Adam or the ways in which Uncle Eddie insisted Adam must be changed and reformed. Instead, he aligned with and shifted the fundamental focus of Uncle Eddie by defining a shared goal of promoting Adam's safety and well-being.

It's important to note that at the point of this interview, the therapist was unaware that there was in fact an actual Uncle Eddie who had sexually abused Adam. By continuing to explore Adam's views on his relationship with the alter whom Adam knew as Uncle Eddie in a nonjudgmental manner with a focus on Adam's safety and self-determination, the therapist was opening a door for Adam to disclose that burdensome secret for the first time. In addition, the dialogue that the therapist undertook with Uncle Eddie would provide opportunities for Adam to indirectly reveal the abuse that Uncle Eddie had perpetrated. For example, when the therapist asked how Uncle Eddie had tried to help Adam, the alter replied, "When I first started thinking that he might be like this, I showed him what it was like and why he wouldn't want it. . . . I did it to him so he would know." While this could have meant that Adam mentally berated himself or otherwise symbolically subjected himself to emotional abuse delivered by Uncle Eddie, there was a clear hint that something abusive may literally have been "done to" Adam. Thus, this session highlighted the importance of handling crises that involve dissociative fragmentation—or any other potential indicators of traumatic abuse or violence—of being open to the possibility that what appear to be symbolic representations of a client's distress also may represent an actual past (or current) experience (or perpetrator) of violence or abuse. This therapist, and the therapist whom Adam saw on an ongoing outpatient basis, would carefully follow up on any potentially relevant information from Adam or other credible sources that could reveal past or current adversities that may have contributed to the current crisis or that could lead to future crises.

CONCLUSION

This case demonstrated how what seemed to be a routine inpatient psychotherapy session in the aftermath of a patient's close brush with suicide rapidly morphed into an in-session crisis with the emergence of a malevolent and controlling dissociative alter. By maintaining a focus on the patient's safety and the development of a partnership aimed at gaining understanding, the therapist was able to foster a sense of security and hope for a profoundly depressed young man.

The session illustrated the importance of nonjudgmentally accepting the most toxically reactive and even self-loathing aspects of the client's experience, while never losing sight of the client's essential integrity, resilience, and core strengths. This empathic and validating acceptance is a model for the client as to how it is possible to acknowledge rather than avoid inner conflicts and distress, and transform them into hope and a commitment to self-awareness. By shifting the focus from Adam's view of himself as worthless, helpless, and deserving to die to a view of Adam as deserving respect, caring, and confidence, the therapist enabled Adam to transform a crisis of abuse, abandonment, and despair into an alliance in which Adam could face and resolve his internal conflicts by drawing on his internal strengths with the guidance of trustworthy allies.

QUESTIONS FOR READER SELF-REFLECTION

- Would you have asked Adam about yesterday's experience when he contemplated suicide in any way differently than the therapist did? What are the pros and cons of starting immediately with questions about that high-risk event as opposed to starting on lower intensity topics?

- How did the therapist use the focusing skill from the FREEDOM framework to ground himself as the session become more stressful and intense, and to develop a partnership with Adam (including with the alter) based on a shared goal?

- What were the most important things the therapist did to develop an alliance with Adam's alter part, Uncle Eddie?

- What mistakes would you be concerned about making if you were the therapist and were attempting to balance your responsibility to your client, Adam, while also demonstrating to the critical alter, Uncle Eddie, that you could work together on behalf of Adam's well-being?

- When Adam shifted and it seemed that Uncle Eddie was speaking through him, should the therapist have persisted in speaking to Adam and refused to talk to this alter?

- Should the therapist have accepted the alter's views of what is "good for Adam" to win over the alter? How could that have compromised Adam's trust in the therapist?

- What personal reactions might you have if you talked with Uncle Eddie? Would your feelings about the judgmental and shaming attitude that he expressed toward Adam make it difficult for you to engage in the kind of alliance-building conversation we saw in this session?

- What are the pros and cons of the therapist's decision to directly ask Uncle Eddie about urging Adam to commit suicide?

- Should the therapist have attempted to convince Uncle Eddie to leave Adam alone and to let Adam make choices without intervening? Should the therapist have attempted to convince Adam to be assertive and set limits with Uncle Eddie so that he (Adam) did not give up control?

- Should the therapist have told Adam/Uncle Eddie that suicide was not an acceptable option? How might this have paradoxically decreased Adam's safety?

- If you were this therapist, how would you decide when Adam was safe to go home again? How would you involve Adam in that decision? Would you involve the alter in it?

- What potential countertransference issues should the therapist be aware of? (These might include feeling as helpless to deal with the alter Uncle Eddie as Adam seems to feel or feeling a fatherly sense of wanting to rescue Adam and argue with or even eliminate Uncle Eddie, or feeling critical of Adam for not taking on and getting rid of Uncle Eddie himself.)

10 CONFRONTING A CRISIS OF TRAUMA AND DISTRESS ACROSS GENERATIONS

CASE BACKGROUND[1]

Rose, a 17-year-old young woman, is outraged because her therapist made a report to Rose's school of sexting of photos exposing her that Rose's former boyfriend took and posted. Although Rose had objected, the therapist felt ethically and legally responsible to mobilize school and law enforcement personnel to take action so they could protect Rose and prevent this from happening to other youth. Rose had been deeply ambivalent but reluctantly went along with the therapist's decision to make a report—never affirmatively agreeing but also not adamantly objecting to the decision. A week later, Rose is meeting for her next session with her therapist.

---

[1]To view the webinar associated with this case, including a video of the psychotherapy session, go online (https://learn.nctsn.org/enrol/index.php?id=498). Alternatively, you can go to the main website (https://learn.nctsn.org), click "Clinical Training" in the menu bar at the top of the page, click "Identifying Critical Moments and Healing Complex Trauma," and then click the webinar associated with this case: "Trauma and Distress Across Generations." Although you will need to create an account ID and password, there is no fee to access the webinar.

https://doi.org/10.1037/0000225-011
Crises in the Psychotherapy Session: Transforming Critical Moments Into Turning Points, by J. D. Ford

Rose was born in Latin America. Following the murder of her father, 5-year-old Rose fled with her mother to the United States. The murder, which Rose didn't understand at the time, nevertheless was frightening for her because she had never seen her mother so distraught and she didn't understand why her father wasn't there to help. Rose was afraid to leave her home because she had witnessed numerous shootings and violent altercations by gangs and police in her neighborhood. Those fears were compounded by the sudden loss of her father, which was never explained to her but which she imagined vividly as the result of a brutal assault or shooting. Then, the journey to this country was even more frightening for Rose: It involved long walks and bus and train rides that were exhausting and that exposed her to unfamiliar people, many of whom seemed very frightened or harsh and angry. She saw people get into fights and shoot guns, and she felt terrified that her mother would be attacked and killed, leaving her all alone.

Rose and her mother were able to get across the border into the United States after several sleepless and frightening weeks, and they met relatives who lived in California. Rose missed her grandparents, who were like "angels—always protecting me and making me happy," so she began feeling very close to an older relative who reminded her of her grandfather. Rose's mother needed to work to pay for their food and to help with the rent, so she began leaving Rose with anybody who was around in the house they were staying in—and Rose was happy that that older man often volunteered to look after her. However, when they were alone, the older man forced Rose to have sex with him, and this went on for more than a year until he left to find work in another community. Rose was 7 years old at the time, and never told anyone about those experiences. Her mother was working two full-time jobs and relied on relatives to take care of Rose until she was 11 years old. Then, Rose and her mother moved to an apartment in a nicer neighborhood. Rose stayed at home on her own after school most evenings, but she felt safe and comfortable because the neighborhood was safe and she had learned to cook for herself. Rose also became friends with girls in her new school, spending most afternoons after school with them once she was in middle school at age 13.

However, as she entered adolescence, Rose began having nightmares. She would wake up sweating and felt terrified to sleep on her own. She also began having panic attacks and begged her mother not to leave her alone in the apartment. Her mother didn't understand what was so upsetting for Rose: In her mother's view, things were much better for them now that they had their own place to live in a safe neighborhood, where people were friendly. A neighbor advised Rose's mother to take Rose to see a therapist.

Her mother didn't think this was necessary, but after Rose wet the bed on a several occasions, her mother decided to take her to the clinic. Rose and her mother didn't know what a therapist was or how seeing a therapist could help them. However, over time, as she met with the therapist, Rose realized that it helped to have someone to talk to who was a good listener and who pointed out qualities and abilities that Rose had that she had not recognized or believed could be true about herself. Rose's mother was happy to see Rose feeling better about herself and more confident and happy in her life.

A few months after beginning therapy, Rose met, John, one of her best friend's brothers. At the beginning, John was sweet and very caring. Rose liked his company. When he told her how beautiful and smart she was, Rose felt as if she finally could like herself again like she had before the abuse. She also felt less lonely because now she didn't have to spend afternoons and evenings on her own in the apartment. Rose felt more at ease and free from the bad memories. She also noticed that she was able to have sex with John without this triggering any nightmares or bad memories from her childhood. However, there was a turn for the worse in her relationship with John. He began to do drugs with Rose when she stayed with him at his apartment, and he asked her to do things sexually that she didn't feel comfortable with, including taking pictures of her unclothed after they had sex. John became demanding and controlling, Rose began feeling uneasy and isolated. According to John, she was only allowed to spend time with him and nobody else. She decided that she needed a break from the relationship and told John. He was furious and called her all sorts of awful names, but she stood her ground and told him that was exactly why she wanted a break: because she deserved to be treated better in relationship. Rose felt scared of John's anger but proud of herself for calmly standing up to him. Then she had a terrible shock that felt like she was being abused all over again. At lunch a few days after the breakup, Rose walked in on her friend showing other girls and boys at school the pictures John had taken of her undressed. The kids were laughing like this was a big joke, and they looked at Rose in a way that made her feel "like garbage." She felt deeply betrayed and humiliated, and ran home to her room in tears.

Rose tried to act like everything was normal for the next couple days, but at night, she fell asleep sobbing. Finally, in her next session with her therapist, she revealed the sexting and John's betrayal. She described trying to reach out to her girlfriends, but nobody would talk to her. Even her best friend wouldn't have anything to do with her as if she were embarrassed to even be seen with Rose. Rose couldn't stop thinking that her classmates were looking at pictures of her naked body and mocking her. Other kids posted nasty words, such as "slut," "whore," "easy," and "skank" on Rose's Facebook page. Every day when she got home, Rose ran to her room and cried until she had no more tears. She explained to her therapist that she had started cutting herself to make the pain more bearable. She also told her therapist that she wanted to kill herself. She had no set plan yet, but she didn't see the point in living anymore.

From Rose's perspective, she had no friends and her mother was too busy to care. She was afraid to tell her mother because she was sure her mother would blame her and then she'd feel even more ashamed and alone. Walking down the halls during school was especially difficult. When she tried to get her mother to listen and help her, her mother said Rose was to blame for acting like a slut, and she wished Rose had never been born. It was at that point, Rose said, when she began to think her life was over. She said she didn't want to kill herself, but she didn't know how to go on with her life feeling so exposed, criticized, and humiliated.

Rose's therapist realized that Rose was in crisis, even though she wasn't imminently intending or planning to suicide. To help Rose feel less alone and powerless, her therapist said that the school needed to know that Rose was being subjected to cyberbullying and that she (the therapist) would talk with someone in authority at the school so that the school could help Rose. She also told Rose that she wanted to hold a family session to talk with her mother to make sure she was aware of what was going on in school and to develop a plan for Rose's safety. Rose was reluctant to have the school informed and to talk with her mother, but she agreed that it was only right that the school should stop the bullying and that she really wanted her mother's support.

During the conjoint session with Rose and her mother, Rose shared how she felt hurt and ostracized because of the sexting and cyberbullying. The therapist supported Rose for her honesty and courage. The therapist also acknowledged how hard this must be for Rose's mother and how much the mother was taking on with her work and being a single parent without the kind of support from parents or other family members that had been the norm when living in their country of origin. As the therapist empathized with her, Rose's mother began to express anger at Rose for making her life difficult. She screamed that Rose was ungrateful and didn't appreciate the hard work and the new home. "I will *not* quit my job to babysit for you, Rose," her mother yelled. Her mother then began sobbing and said she couldn't do anything else for Rose and that she also wanted to die so that other people would have to figure out what to do for Rose. The therapist asked what she meant by wanting to die, and mother stated, "I just want to kill myself. Nothing is getting better. No matter what I do, it's wrong!" While the therapist talked with her mother about this, Rose sat frozen—as if paralyzed by mother's reaction. Rose's mother said she had been praying and fasting as a means of warding off bad spirits and bad thoughts so she wouldn't kill herself.

The therapist helped Rose and her mother to see how similar they were feeling because each of them was trying so hard to make a good life for herself—and for each other—because they cared so much about each other and were trying so hard to protect each other from being hurt or mistreated. The mood in the session shifted dramatically as Rose and her mother refocused on how important they were to each other and on their ability to support each other during upsetting and painful times. In this way, the therapist helped them de-escalate the distress and feel the emotional bond between them. She helped Rose and her mother remember how they had used the strength of their relationship to get through tough times in the past. Rose's mother was able to reassure Rose, saying: "I'm your mother. Rose, you don't have to take care of me. I'm strong enough to handle this and to help you get through this." She continued, "As a girl, I had the same thoughts that you are having, but I made it through that, so I know we can make it through this. I forget sometimes, like you forget, but I know we can make it through this." Rose tearfully thanked her mother: "That's all I need, mama, just to know that you're going to be okay and that we'll get through this together."

Rose and her mother agreed that each would be sure to keep themselves safe and to not keep secrets or let resentments build up and come between them. Rose said that she felt "like a giant weight just got off my shoulders, like I can breathe again and I'm strong enough to get through this. And like I finally got my mom back again, and she still loves me." Rose's mother agreed to let the therapist know if she had any further thoughts of actually ending her life or harming herself, and said she'd be willing to talk with a therapist if that happened "as long as she's as good and kind a person as you are." Rose also said she would keep working in therapy on getting through "this mess I got myself into, so my mother doesn't have to worry about me."

At that point, the therapist raised the issue of making a report to the school to protect Rose. Rose's mother agreed that a report was necessary. Rose initially protested that a report would only expose her to more humiliation and ostracism, and remained opposed despite the therapist's efforts to develop a plan together with Rose that would minimize the possibility of further exposure. Rose said she really didn't like it, but if a report had to be made, the therapist had to be sure that the adults at her school understood how hurtful the exposure had been for her as well as to make sure the school didn't do anything to draw further attention by students to Rose. "They better not put my stuff out there and make me even more a target," said Rose. "I don't want any more of the drama than what John has already caused, and I need to get my friends back not turn them against me!" The therapist agreed that this was essential and that she'd make sure the school understood.

Despite making sure that the school administrators and Rose's teachers understood Rose's legitimate need to be provided with support and not exposed to more harm, Rose's therapist was aware that the social contagion triggered by the sexting was likely to continue and possibly temporarily increase. Any actions by the school personnel, regardless of how well-intended and couched in privacy, would most likely be discovered by some students. Her therapist planned to be open to and supportive of Rose's reactions to this outcome and to other emotional reverberations that Rose was experiencing. The therapist also realized that the betrayal and violation that Rose had experienced by her boyfriend's actions, and via the reactions by her friends and other peers as well as by her mother, were going to continue to create emotional shock waves for Rose that would need careful attention and empathic support in therapy. While feeling prepared for Rose to be in emotional turmoil, the therapist expected that the positive work they had done in therapy would enable Rose to rely on the security and trust she was developing in their therapeutic relationship as a stable foundation. Rose's situation, however, was so fluid and complex that a major crack in that foundation occurred in the intervening week, and Rose once again felt in the midst of a crisis.

SESSION TRANSCRIPT, ANNOTATIONS, AND COMMENTARY

This is Rose's next psychotherapy session with her therapist after the conjoint session in which she and her mother were able to regain a sense of being together emotionally—and in which they and the therapist were able to establish a plan for the therapist to make a report to Rose's school.

ROSE: (*Sounds and looks outraged*) I feel like I'm at the beginning now!

> *Therapist's Inner Reflections:* Rose really is starting all over in some important way, and the message she's sending nonverbally is that she's very upset, so something must've happened.

THERAPIST: Like you're starting over.

ROSE: (*Glowers*) Yeah.

THERAPIST: S—so tell what happened in this last week. What's—what's different?

ROSE: I have no one. I still have no one. I came to you because you were the one supposed to help me, right? But you didn't help at all.

Therapist's Inner Reflections: This is very different from Rose's positive outlook after she and her mother were able to reconcile in our last session, but a lot can happen in a short time in the chaotic life of a teenager. And Rose has had many terrifying experiences in which she had reason to feel alone and fear being abandoned. I'll see if that's what's coming up for her now.

THERAPIST: Okay. Tell me a little bit more about what—what feels like it's not helpful. I'm just hearing that something is different. Something has happened, and I just . . .

ROSE: Well, first off, no one's talking to me. I have no friends. Not even Natalie.

THERAPIST: Okay.

ROSE: She walked right out. I tried to talk to her here and there but nothing. Everyone's looking at me still, calling me names like I'm just somebody. Actually, a nobody!

THERAPIST: So, Natalie stopped talking in this last week, or did something new happen? Did you have an argument?

ROSE: Well, she just got distant from me.

Therapist's Inner Reflections: Natalie's her best friend, so a rupture there could be devastating. Is this Natalie actually shunning Rose, or is Rose expecting that and interpreting Natalie's behavior (confusion? worry or embarrassment for Rose?) to mean that Natalie is "distant?"

THERAPIST: Okay. And the other friends?

ROSE: They just left. Since John, they just left me.

THERAPIST: Okay. So, it sounds like that's been going on for a few weeks (*sighs*). And the situation with John is the same? He's . . .?

ROSE: He's still ignoring me. Still calling me names. But it all happened because of you. I said everything to you. I trusted you, and I can't stop thinking that it was your fault.

Therapist's Inner Reflections: A loss of support from and possible rejection by her friends are important problems to keep track of, and they're going to amplify Rose's fears about trusting me. I know the most likely specific trigger, so let's get that right out on the table immediately.

THERAPIST: *(Nods)* Because I contacted the school to let them know what happened.

ROSE: Yeah. And now everyone knows. I had a teacher I used to talk to—you know, to help me out, and now everyone's walking around like they can't talk to me. Like I'm some kinda child and don't know what I'm doing.

THERAPIST: And that includes the teacher who you were talking to before?

ROSE: Yeah. So now I'm completely alone.

Therapist's Inner Reflections: To clarify the problem, it's critical to know if any positive actions have been taken by the school since I notified them. If not, that makes my reporting seem like a complete failure to Rose—that I'm just another person who lets her down (and as a woman in a quasimaternal caregiving role, this lumps me in with her mother)—but also a person who exposes her to public shaming (so I'm also like John and a reminder of his exposure of her). If they did do anything to help, that could be a foothold for helping Rose distinguish between abuse and betrayal versus true caring and support.

THERAPIST: I'm—I'm wondering what the school has done. So, since I alerted the school that you were being picked on, that you were being bullied, has anything different—did the school . . .?

ROSE: I mean, they tried to put me in some group, but I'm not gonna be seen with those kids. My reputation is ruined already. How is that gonna make anything better?

THERAPIST: I hear you saying that you're feeling really alone at school. Natalie is not around. The teacher—the support that you were looking for—that it's not there right now. I'm wondering, too, about home. Has the school talked with Mom? Has Mom had any conversations with your teacher?

ROSE: Oh, yeah. She knows everything. My mom, she told me everything was gonna be okay, she was gonna support me, and it changed. Completely. After that talk with me and her, it didn't—it didn't do anything.

Therapist's Inner Reflections: Mom and I both promised to help, but from Rose's perspective, we're both letting her down—or making things worse. Is that what's happening with her mom?

THERAPIST: What do you think happened? So, Mom was supportive . . .

ROSE: Well, what happened is that I brought her in here with you.

THERAPIST: Yeah.

ROSE: That's what happened.

THERAPIST: Yeah. And so, Mom was supportive. She was in shock.

ROSE: At first. At first, she was supportive.

THERAPIST: I'm sorry. I'm really tryin' to understand what changed and— but I hear how frustrating this is for you, and I see that you're angry and angry with me for . . .

ROSE: Well, I want you to take responsibility.

Therapist's Inner Reflections: I'm still not clear if something has changed between Rose and her mother, but the first order of business is for me to step up to the plate and show Rose that an adult is willing to take the burden off of her by taking responsibility for actions she views as hurtful.

THERAPIST: I am responsible. I feel that the discussion with your mom was certainly a decision that was made here. The discussion with school was made here.

ROSE: I brought her here to make everything better, but it hasn't gotten better. And I just want you to take responsibility in fixing that.

THERAPIST: Okay. Can we talk about fixing that and what do you think we could do together to make—make that better? I'm certainly responsible for talking to the school and letting them know that you were being bullied and harassed, and, you know, as we talked about that, that seemed to me a very important thing for your safety. And now what—what should we do about what's happening at school? What—what can I do?

Therapist's Inner Reflections: By accepting responsibility, I can remind Rose that my actions were based on the goal of making her safer, the opposite of exposing her. And I can invite her to partner with me in defining what needs to be changed and what I can do to help with that.

ROSE: To be honest, I don't know what to do at school. I just wanna stop going to school. Having to deal with all of that and on top of that, my mom? I don't know how to put up with that.

Therapist's Inner Reflections: We'll bookmark the school situation and focus on the primary relationship with her mother because that clearly is her emotional foundation. And if that has developed new cracks or reopened old ones, Rose won't feel confident enough to face school.

THERAPIST: Tell me about your mom.

ROSE: She's just not being there. We spoke on how we were gonna get through this, we were gonna talk about it, and she was supportive at a point. And now it's just turned to nothing. She doesn't wanna deal with that anymore. It's not her problem. She doesn't wanna babysit me.

Therapist's Inner Reflections: I wonder at exactly what "point"—from Rose's perspective—mom stopped being supportive? What actually changed? Was there a trigger for mom or Rose? Or is this a resumption of an old pattern in which mom is working all the time and exhausted?

THERAPIST: So, that means that she's still working the long hours?

ROSE: Yep.

THERAPIST: She's not home?

ROSE: And then now everyone's picking at my mom, questioning her, and I guess it's all this pressure that she can't handle. She's just not her. She doesn't wanna take responsibility as a mother, and that's what I need her to do. After finding out what I did to myself, yeah, she was supportive, but it wasn't really there. I didn't really feel it at all. And now, all of a sudden, she wants to end her life like I did and all of this extra stuff. Like, why? For what? Knowing I need you here at this time—now you want to leave. That makes no sense to me. All because I got exposed. Got exposed by John, and then you put me out there like John. Put my business out there.

Therapist's Inner Reflections: I think the crisis may be that mom's depression has escalated, and she's directly or indirectly telling Rose she wants to escape by ending it all. That's very serious. Rose veered away from that very quickly, and while I don't want to avoid the issue that is really between Rose and me, I'm very concerned that Rose is burdened by her mother's depression—and that depression could actually lead her mother to attempt suicide. That would be a devastating loss for Rose, and I have to check on Rose's mother's safety for her own sake as well.

THERAPIST: By telling the school about the bullying that was happening.

ROSE: Yeah. I guess she can't handle the pressure that I've been receiving. She was supposed to be the rock of the family. Since it's only me and her, she was my backbone. And I don't know what to do with her.

THERAPIST: She is overwhelmed, it sounds like. Am I right about that?

ROSE: I guess she is.

THERAPIST: You're certainly overwhelmed. There's a lot going on at school. There's a lot for you to manage and together you're—it seems like you're moving apart. And it sounds like Mom is saying something pretty similar. She's not sure right now about whether she can manage all of this. Am I hearing that correctly?

ROSE: Yeah.

THERAPIST: And I remember when Mom was here, she talked about her work schedule. The multiple jobs, the high expectations, and that sounds like there's a lot to manage, and now it feels like it's all overwhelming, so I'm wondering how can we work together to figure out how to make this feel more manageable for both of you or how to bring you together in a way that the support is felt. So, I'm not suggesting that the support isn't there, but you're not feeling her support right now.

Therapist's Inner Reflections: The best, and probably only, way I can protect the safety of both Rose and her mother is to join with Rose in developing a plan to reduce her worry about losing her mother and to reinstate some of the seeds of support for Rose by her mother that we started to plant in our last session. Rose feels that she has to do this all alone, so the key first step is to help her see how I can actually do something, more than just talking about her feelings, to help her with her mother. Usually talk that promotes self-reflection is the way therapy heals, but in this kind of crisis, I need to use talking more strategically to define actions that can make a difference.

ROSE: Well, how am I supposed to do that? How am I supposed to bring her back in here or try to explain to her this all over again if she doesn't even wanna hear it anymore?

THERAPIST: I think it's important for you to have her support given all that you're going through in school, and I'm wondering whether whatever's changed in the last week, whether that is something we can try to mend because that's still important for you to have your mom. So, so let's talk about that. The mention of taking her life. Does she talk about having a plan to hurt herself? Does she seem like she's in danger right now?

ROSE: I don't see it, but I don't wanna risk it.

THERAPIST: Yeah.

ROSE: 'Cause I know I hit that point, and I can't imagine my mom hitting that point.

Therapist: So, it sounds like—I'm just wondering for your mom, like, she's had this week to kinda digest all the things that we've talked about, which was a lot. Right? There's—there's a lot to—to sort of say to her and inform her about. So now, what do you think we might be able to do for Mom? What do you think she might find helpful or useful? Just some ideas. It's certainly not your responsibility to do that for her.

Therapist's Inner Reflections: I'm aligning with Rose almost as if she's a cotherapist, because I think she's carrying the burden of being her mother's primary support person. But it's crucial to emphasize that this really shouldn't be Rose's responsibility so that she can begin to shift and allow herself to be the daughter and not the primary partner or therapist for her mother.

ROSE: I don't know, because if I'm taking these things in, she should also, and it's not her in this position.

THERAPIST: Yeah.

ROSE: It's me. She was supposed to protect me, and now I feel like I have to protect her.

THERAPIST: Yeah. What do you think Mom thinks about this idea that she was supposed to protect you?

ROSE: Clearly, she's not thinking about it at all.

Therapist's Inner Reflections: Rose is making the crucial shift in her mind, but it's hard for her to view herself as a daughter when she views her mother as not taking care of or protecting her. I realize that there are major gaps and things that Rose's mother does that are triggering or hurtful for Rose, but I think that Rose knows that her mother loves her and that Rose's distress is more based on believing that her mother isn't strong enough to keep herself safe, let alone Rose.

THERAPIST: I'm gonna offer maybe another idea, and this might not be correct. Just stop me if it seems just not your mom. If I remember correctly, when you came in the first time, it was pretty hard for you. It was hard even speaking the words to tell me what had happened and what was going on for you, and then we were talking about cutting, thoughts about killing yourself, and that was the first week. Last week, for Mom, that was her first week. That was her first week hearing all that you've been though, all that you're going through, and so I want to keep that perspective of where she is right now and really keep some attention to her strengths. So, I hear what she said in the heat of the moment, but you've described her in ways that it sounds like she is pretty tough. So, help me understand what we might be able to do to provide some support for her.

Therapist's Inner Reflections: Here again, I don't want to inadvertently increase Rose's sense of responsibility for her mother, but if she believes she can do something actively, with my help, to be supportive of her mother, that could give Rose a greater sense of control where she's feeling helpless (not just with her mother but in her life generally and her relationships). I think Rose has been emphasizing her need for her mother's support because she doesn't believe she can make things better in her life, and she wants her mother to do that for her. It's an understandable wish but one that conflates support with being rescued, and it undermines Rose's self-confidence.

ROSE: I mean, I'm trying to see about it, to not go back and forth with her anymore because it's just gonna continue on and on, and I want her to support me so I'm able to feel more supportive towards her.

THERAPIST: You're sort of here together, right? You need her. She needs you. You've relied on each other your whole life and—and you're going through quite a bit. I'm not sure if she knows how to be supportive to you. She might need some help with that just as you're asking how to be supportive to her.

ROSE: So, I should bring her back here?

Therapist's Inner Reflections: Yes, but not with the idea that talking in therapy will magically make Rose's mother less stressed and more able to empathically support Rose. Giving Rose's mother help in accessing resources so that she doesn't try to just get through this alone (and inadvertently rely on Rose as her sole or primary source of support) could show Rose that her mother is capable of finding solutions without relying on Rose if she has help from resource people who, like me, have her best interests at heart. That would communicate to Rose that she—Rose—can do the same thing for herself, with this therapy as the base, instead of trying to get through her dilemmas all on her own or making her mother responsible for rescuing her.

THERAPIST: I—I think we have to figure out together how to give her some resources. Whether it's that she comes here and you talk together, or whether she might wanna talk to someone by herself, or whether there are other things that she might wanna do for support. Right? There—there might be things in the community. There might be church. There—I don't know what her—her form of support will be, and I have no way of knowing that unless we talk to her.

ROSE: I mean, I could try to get her to open up to the church because she's really into that. That's what she relied on.

THERAPIST: Okay. And do you think that that's a conversation you can have with Mom about? Given what she said to you, right, and your concern for her about where she can find some support for herself right now while you try to support each other? If there's ever a point where she seems unsafe or you're really worried about her safety, then that's an immediate, you know, call for help. Emergency. But for her, this is Week 1, and you've made it through a lot of weeks yourself and might be able to talk with her about going forward, for her, what that could be like.

ROSE: Yeah, I could try again.

THERAPIST: Okay.

ROSE: I know I could start somewhere with my mom.

Therapist's Inner Reflections: Better yet, Rose is remembering resources that provide a new option that she can discuss with her mother— so now Rose is recognizing her own strengths as a creative problem solver and thinking of ways to support her mother without being burdened. Now let's leverage that increase in self-efficacy as a basis for looking afresh at the school situation.

THERAPIST: Anything that you wanna talk about with school?

ROSE: Everyone talks about it. Rumors. Not knowing anything, they still talk about me.

THERAPIST: And before the pictures, you were doing things after school with friends.

Therapist's Inner Reflections: What past successes might be a starting point for making the current situation more manageable as a set of solvable problems rather than a hopeless disaster?

ROSE: Yeah.

THERAPIST: And doing activities after school or . . .? What kind of things were you doing at school?

ROSE: I mean, we would go out, like, movies, mall, and stuff, but it all stopped.

THERAPIST: So, I'm wondering about—so, when I ask about Natalie, you said she hasn't really said she doesn't wanna hang out. You just get that feeling, and I'm wondering about other friends or the activities after school. Have you gone to any of them?

ROSE: No.

THERAPIST: Have you been told you shouldn't?

ROSE: Everyone's just gonna look at me, stare at me, talk about me. I'm not gonna put myself in that anymore.

THERAPIST: Are you feeling embarrassed around Natalie? I know—I hear you saying that Natalie isn't responding.

ROSE: I expected her to understand that I made a mistake, and everyone makes mistakes.

THERAPIST: Okay.

ROSE: So, that's why her just being distant, it doesn't make sense to me.

Therapist's Inner Reflections: Rose makes a very good point, but I think she may be projecting on to Natalie her own self-blame for having made a "mistake." Although there may be a real issue with that friend, it will be more helpful to Rose if she can become more empathic with herself.

THERAPIST: So, what I heard you say was, "I made a mistake. Everyone makes mistakes." But mistakes happen, and it seems like since this has come out, you've sort of moved back to that space where you're by yourself and maybe a little less sure about reaching out to other people or even being around them.

ROSE: Yeah, I just—I don't know how to trust people because—it's like everyone I come across, they ruin it some way or another.

THERAPIST: What are the things that you're hearing or worried about hearing?

ROSE: I don't need them judging me anymore not knowing where I come from, not knowing the struggles I've been through, and them thinkin' they know everything. Especially they talk about my mom sometimes.

THERAPIST: So, they don't know you. They don't know your struggles. They don't know your mom. But it sounds like it still hurts when you hear the things that they have to say.

Therapist's Inner Reflections: I'm saying this to communicate indirectly to Rose that she knows not just what she and her mother have been through but, more importantly, their strength and courage in having faced and come through the past "struggles." Those are the key to Rose feeling able to trust herself and her mother to be able to get through the current struggles.

ROSE: Well, yeah. Like, they shouldn't talk about something they don't know.

THERAPIST: How do we work together on maybe not being in a space where things are said that are not pleasant and by people who don't know you, don't understand where you've come from? Like, what can we come up with to give you more than that? More after school? More in your weekends? Because being alone is sort of what made you so sad.

ROSE: I mean, I thought about clubs, something that would keep me going. Something that I could find that would keep me going.

Therapist's Inner Reflections: Rose's response highlights her resilience. She took that invitation and went straight to creative and practical brainstorming, and the seeds of a solution: returning to her core interests and finding or reclaiming a peer group with whom to share those interests.

THERAPIST: Okay. So, is there any club that you might get some enjoyment out of if you were—if you're showing up once a week, every now and again?

ROSE: I mean, I found this book club. I like to read, you know, like, the stories that there's always like a happy ending or something like that.

THERAPIST: And book clubs have their own characters and things that people really focus on, and I hear part of your concern about doing anything with other teenagers right now. This idea that after the pictures were out, you're showing up, but they're not seeing you. They're seen the pictures. They're seeing you without your clothes on.

Therapist's Inner Reflections: With the nonthreatening context of the stories in books, I can go back to help Rose face the unresolved stressor that's troubling her, the public exposure. But if people who look at those pictures just see a body, they're not seeing Rose, the whole person. So those are not the people, the peer group, that Rose is seeking. She wants to be with, and be seen by, people who see her with respect and appreciation—that's a story that could be a fresh start.

ROSE: Yeah. They're not actually seeing me for what I can be, and that's just all I need.

THERAPIST: So, I'm hearing that, like, the more time you spend by yourself and alone, the longer that continues. Maybe joining one club. Might not go back to doing everything you were doing with your friends, but maybe one thing, um, gives them an opportunity to get to know you all over again. The way you think, the way you feel, you know, all the things you say they don't know about you even though they're judging. What are your thoughts about maybe that one thing?

ROSE: I mean, I don't think it would be horrible, but if it's like a fresh start, I mean, it could make a difference.

THERAPIST: I don't wanna lead you to believe that there won't be moments where you feel embarrassed or wonder what they're thinking, but we can work on that together. Like, what's the plan for when you start feeling a little unsure or embarrassed?

Therapist's Inner Reflections: Tempering Rose's renewed optimism with some caution about the reality that there will be additional triggers and difficult times ahead is essential so that she isn't caught off guard—so she is proactively prepared to handle the inevitable but not always easily predictable stress reactions that she'll experience without being maladaptively hypervigilant.

ROSE: I wouldn't know where to go with that. I just usually shut down when it comes to that.

Therapist's Inner Reflections: I can help Rose by reflecting back my observations of her healthy assertiveness. And that by doing something for herself, she can also know that she's making a contribution to her mother's peace of mind—providing support by living her own life fully.

THERAPIST: There are things that you've said to me, like really standing up to me and saying you have done this and you need to be responsible, and I'm wondering whether that's a voice we can work on with you or your friends. How to indicate to them that you're willing to stand up for yourself if they're not treating you well. And certainly, with Mom, I'm wondering if you join one activity, the book club or another activity if you find something else, whether she might then start, you know, not feeling what you said she said about babysitting. She'll know you have an activity that you're doing.

ROSE: I mean, I could check on the book club and maybe introduce her into something. Something that relaxes me. Maybe she could get into it.

THERAPIST: So, one of the things that we can do is, like, build in a time that we can check in with each other.

ROSE: Yeah, that—that's fine.

THERAPIST: You think of anything else that we can work on together that would be helpful, I'm really wanting to hear about it. Let's talk about it.

ROSE: Alright.

Therapist's Inner Reflections: Rose has made a crucial shift in this session by regaining her trust in herself and in her therapeutic partnership with me. That hasn't solved the many difficult problems she's facing, but it has provided her with a sense of hopefulness and a commitment to taking action to resume her own life while also supporting her mother in more manageable ways. This is a valuable template that I can help Rose return to in future sessions when current stressors or reminders of past traumas trigger her into intense stress reactions and the state of emotion dysregulation in which she began this session. Each time that happens, my goal will be to help her learn again that by choosing whom to trust and by drawing on her strengths, she can overcome.

Rose's Observations

In a postsession interview, Rose had the following comments about her experience during and after the session:

In this session, I felt angry and wanted my therapist to figure out everything that she has done. Her advice did not turn out well for me, and I wanted her to fix it. It was easier to be angry at my therapist because John isn't around and my mother is already struggling. She was the only one I could blame for everything. When my therapist suggested that we might do something together, it gave me some hope. Initially, I was distrusting, but with some thought, it seemed like the best option. I have been feeling guilty and responsible for my mother's struggles; maybe my speaking up about what has been happening made my mom feel worse, although, it may have also allowed for things to be dealt with. That's what I hope.

Commentary

Rose's anger directed at her therapist was understandable as an immediate reaction to feeling unsupported, unprotected, and even rejected by her mother; other adults (her teacher and "the school"); and her friends and peers. The anger also was understandable as a reaction to the outgrowth of the developmental trauma that has occurred both to Rose personally (i.e., sudden loss of her father and vicarious trauma in reaction to her mother's response, loss of community ties and violence because of the need to flee to the United States, sexual abuse as a child, betrayal and cyberbullying by her boyfriend, and the threat of losing her mother to suicide) and to Rose's mother intergenerationally (i.e., unspecified events in her childhood that led her to feel suicidal, murder of her husband, loss of community ties and violence because of the need to flee to the United States, and vicarious trauma resulting from learning of Rose's past and current traumatic experiences that triggered a resurgence of suicidal thoughts). Rose's therapist recognized that Rose's anger was an expression (and transference to her) of the impact of both the recent obvious experiences and those historical adversities, and of the adaptation Rose has made to protect herself and survive the emotional (and, at times, physical) injuries that they have caused her. The therapist also was aware that Rose's mother's difficulty in managing her own emotional reactions in her relationship with her daughter—and therefore in being able to be unconditionally accepting, supportive, protective, and empathically responsive and available to Rose—also had as much to do with her own complex trauma history, emotional injuries, and survival adaptations as with her fears for or frustrations with Rose. The emotion dysregulation that Rose's mother experiences has made it very difficult for her to stay focused on, let alone to communicate to her daughter, the love she feels for Rose and her appreciation of her daughter's worth and strengths. Helping Rose to find a way to help her mother cope with severe emotion dysregulation, both to reduce the secondary traumatic stress reactions Rose experiences as a result and to prevent the potential primary trauma of the loss of her mother because of complete emotional breakdown or suicide, was an essential immediate priority in the current crisis in their psychotherapy session.

At that critical point, however, an even more immediate question was how to repair the therapeutic alliance. Rose's therapist focused on validating Rose's sense of betrayal and modeling how it is possible to accept responsibility honestly when one's actions have inadvertently led to emotional hurt or distress without taking on blame or becoming defensive because of feeling guilty or unfairly blamed. The therapist thus demonstrated to Rose that trust and safety in a relationship are based on a willingness to understand and support the other person's hurt and anger, and to join with them in making things right again—not on words or hopes alone, no matter how comforting those may be in the short run, but on a combination of words and actions that empower and support her (Rose) in safely achieving her goals This directly paralleled what the therapist had helped Rose and her mother recognize in their relationship, and the therapist realized that now Rose needed to test this way of looking at life and relationships by applying it to her relationship with the therapist. Rose's anger was a way of testing the therapist and their relationship to be able to reaffirm that she could trust that her therapist genuinely cared about her, to share and support her core goals and values, and to act accordingly.

From the perspective of the FREEDOM framework (i.e., focusing, recognizing triggers, emotion awareness, evaluating thoughts, defining goals and options, making a contribution; see the Introduction), the therapist did her own SOS (i.e., slowing down and sweeping the mind clear, orienting to a thought that provides a sense of confidence and purpose, and self-checking stress level and level of personal control). She nonjudgmentally noticed her own bodily, cognitive, and emotional reactions when faced with the triggers posed when Rose angrily pointed blame at her (the first "S" in SOS); then focused on the main thought of being determined to understand and find a path to helping Rose (the "O" in SOS); and then observed that, with that goal, it was possible to listen nonjudgmentally and think clearly about the dilemmas that Rose was dealing with (the second "S" in SOS). With that grounding, the therapist was able to help Rose to walk through the FREEDOM steps in a spontaneous conversational manner, processing two dilemmas that were driving Rose's sense of desperation. First, she helped Rose to clarify the dilemma of the hurt and fear she was experiencing in relation to her mother, and then the dilemma of feeling rejected and abandoned by her peers and, in particular, her best friend.

In addressing each dilemma, the therapist helped Rose find a core orienting thought that enabled her to regain a sense of control, confidence, and hope (e.g., the unbreakable bond of love between Rose and her mother; Rose's competence when she sets her mind to achieving a goal). This was not done as a formal artificial exercise but by following Rose's train of thought and modeling self-reflection with questions that helped Rose to recognize the triggers that were of most concern to her and to feel a sense of nonjudgmental acceptance of her (Rose's) reactive emotions, thoughts, goals, and response options. This is an example of helping a client to walk through the "EEDO" steps in the FREEDOM framework in a seamless manner that communicates empathy while also helps the client to self-reflect rather than simply react. In so doing, the therapist demonstrated to Rose that the therapist could be trusted to take Rose's feelings and concerns seriously, which provided Rose with the emotional safety she needed to reengage in the therapy.

The therapist also was able to use the FREEDOM framework to help Rose access her capacities for adaptive emotion regulation. This was done by highlighting examples that Rose provided of core "main" emotions (e.g., determination, love), thoughts (e.g., self-confidence, self-esteem), and goals (e.g., to stand up for herself while also restoring relationships that had become frayed). With this counterbalance to the reactive distress that Rose was experiencing, Rose spontaneously considered response options based on a sense of self-confidence and self-worth as well those that were consistent with her core values and life goals (e.g., letting the therapist help her get out of the bind of being her mother's keeper; finding ways to be involved with potentially supportive peers that tapped into her interests and enabled her to be open to restoring key relationships). Thus, without giving Rose advice or directives, the therapist was able to help Rose to develop plans for practical next steps that could restore a sense of control and hope.

Protecting the Client and Preserving the Alliance

Rose expressed an overwhelming sense of feeling abandoned by those who matter most in her life, claiming "I have no one." It was immediately clear that Rose's sense of abandonment and betrayal extended beyond her mother and close friends to include feeling betrayed by her therapist. The therapist's report of the cyberbullying to school officials was dictated by a unilateral professional and ethical duty to report that illegal activity to both the protect Rose and to enable legal authorities to take any required actions to protect the community from such actions. However, Rose was strongly against and ultimately deeply ambivalent about this decision and action, fearing that it would expose her to further humiliation, shaming, and potentially additional bullying and harassment by peers. Although it is most likely that Rose's peers found out about and circulated the sexting pictures independently of the therapist's notification of the school, in Rose's view, that disclosure widened the field of those who were seeing her "exposed" (whether they actually ever saw the sexting pictures or only knew of their existence).

It was the lack of having a say in the decision that was the core betrayal by the therapist, in Rose's view, because this seemed to her to be yet another instance in which someone made a decisions for her that took control of her life and privacy away from her and exposed her to harm. The additional "betrayal" was essentially guilt by association because, while the therapist's actions were intended to protect Rose's safety and privacy, parallel actions by others (e.g., the abuse perpetrator, her ex-boyfriend, peers who were ostracizing her) that violated Rose's safety and privacy also involved malicious (or at least selfish) intent to exploit or even injure Rose. Those other people, including Rose's mother, also overtly denied having any responsibility for hurting Rose and instead blamed her as a victim who ostensibly had caused her own victimization—an accusation that Rose directed toward herself as well.

The therapist therefore explicitly and nondefensively acknowledged that this difficult but—from her position—necessary decision to intervene further on Rose's behalf was in some important ways not fully collaborative and did reveal Rose's private matter to other adults whom Rose did now want to be privy to the sexting. The therapist also demonstrated a meaningful interest in helping Rose figure out what they could do together to help Rose cope with and regain a sense of safety and control in light of what was actually happening when people were doing things that were directly hurtful to Rose. This established the therapist's intention to be fully collaborative with Rose and separated their therapeutic relationship as a source of support rather than a source of additional hurt or harm for Rose. In so doing, the therapist was able to increase her empathic understanding— and ability to empathically express this understanding—of the dilemmas that were most intensely distressing for Rose. Rather than focusing first on the situation at school, which was where Rose had started in her initial comments, this instead led to a discussion that focused on the fraying of Rose's relationship with her mother. That focus was consistent with Rose's initial statements that her therapist had failed her, which directly paralleled her expression of similar concerns with her mother in their prior session and therefore was an expectable transference reaction by Rose.

It's important to note that, although most likely Rose's anger and sense of betrayal in relation to her therapist included a transference to the therapist of the hurt, frustration, and sense of abandonment Rose was experiencing in relation to her mother, this does not imply that her reaction to the therapist was not legitimate. Rose was reacting to what she experienced as an empathic failure by her therapist: a failure to accept her (Rose's) perspective as definitive and adopt it as her (the therapist's) own, and to act accordingly. That the therapist was acting on behalf of Rose's best interests insofar as the therapist could discern them and that this involved taking a perspective that was broader than the defensive viewpoint that Rose was adopting did not invalidate Rose's reaction. The therapist did usurp Rose's authority to make a decision that affected Rose and ideally would be a collaborative mutual decision fully endorsed by Rose as well as the therapist.

This is an example of a situation in which that ideal is overridden by the legal, ethical, and clinical imperatives to protect Rose (and other potentially vulnerable youth) from harm. That choice was not endorsed by Rose, and as a result, the scenario replicated, in part, Rose's other experiences in which she had been subject to another person's decisions and had been preempted from being able to have control of her own destiny. This crisis could not be resolved until Rose had been fully reassured by her therapist's actions that her therapist understood and supported Rose in asserting her right to not be preempted in that way. The shift to focusing on Rose and her mother did not obviate the need for that closure.

Striking a Delicate Balance in Parent–Child Relationships

The therapist helped Rose to explore and give voice to the hurts and fears she was experiencing in her relationship with her mother while not defending or blaming Rose's mother. This involved supporting Rose in describing how she was experiencing her mother as being emotionally overwrought and overwhelmed, and how frightening this was for Rose—rephrasing this as feeling burdened by worry about her mother and feeling responsible for protecting and not upsetting her mother when she herself was in need of care and support that she wished her mother could provide (and felt keenly disappointed, and angry—as she did with her therapist—that she was not experiencing her mother as providing). In this session, a delicate balance was found as the therapist collaborated with Rose to better understand her mother's distress, particularly as the mother had recently expressed some suicidal ideation, while also recognizing the mother's resilience (based on years of working hard and keeping Rose and her together as a family) and working toward potential reciprocally beneficial solutions that involved mutual support between daughter and mother. Rather than explicitly or implicitly directing Rose to be understanding and appreciative of her mother, the therapist offered to help Rose to come to her own understanding of her mother's strengths and weaknesses, and to distinguish between what her mother's actions expressed about her (the mother's) emotional state versus what they said about her mother's love for and appreciation of Rose. This did not falsely promise Rose that her mother would be able to meet her (Rose's) emotional needs and expectations. Instead, the therapist focused on what Rose most fundamentally wanted from her mother: love, recognition, and support. The therapist helped Rose to consider how those needs might be met if Rose could separate her mother's emotional reactions from her mother's deeper feelings about Rose, while also understanding that her mother might be unable to express those feelings in a way that would meet Rose's needs when her mother was preoccupied with distress.

Given the objective precariousness of Rose's mother's emotional state, the therapist also did not suggest that Rose look only, or primarily, to her mother for support and assistance in dealing with the many stressors Rose was facing. Instead, the therapist proposed to collaboratively work together with Rose to establish sources of support such that Rose could think of her therapist as one of the people who could and would support her—further repairing the therapeutic alliance—while also helping Rose to extricate herself from the risky position of viewing any one person as her sole source of support. The therapist was aware that this view was imprinted for Rose through no one's fault by the traumas she and her mother had experienced and the two-against-the-world view that they had needed to rely on when it objectively seemed like they were the only ones to care for and protect one another. In addition, this "all my eggs in one basket" view had made Rose vulnerable to exploitation by her ex-boyfriend (who coopted Rose by acting as though he was the only one who really cared about her or protected her, only to turn this into coercive control of Rose).

The therapist viewed Rose's ability to disengage from the toxic relationship with the ex-boyfriend and to assert her disappointment with her mother, her best friend, and the therapist as signs that Rose had the strength and good judgment to not accept less than mutual relationships, and that those qualities could be a foundation on which Rose could build a revised view of herself (as someone who is a "somebody" and not a "nobody") and of how to acquire support in relationships (by choosing people and activities that matched her values and interests). This naturally opened the session dialogue to considering Rose's dilemmas—and opportunities—at school and with friends.

Rose was able to consider that she brought value to her friendships and to consider how reaching out to her best friend—even though doing so might lead to further hurt if her friend was not willing or able to reciprocate—

was an important contribution to that friend and to their strained relationship. Rose also recognized how she was making a contribution (the final FREEDOM step) to her mother through her steadfast caring despite her mother's emotional dysregulation—and that this was a contribution she could make without sacrificing her own well-being to attempt to rescue or protect her mother as if she had to be her mother's caretaker. That realization could reduce the role reversal and parentification that Rose had been experiencing in relation to her mother as well as help Rose to understand that the therapist's actions on behalf of her (Rose's) safety also were not a betrayal but a vote of confidence in Rose.

Building Social Support and a Sense of Self

Rose faced very real stressors with her peers and friends at school and in her personal life. Thus, the therapist did not conclude the session with the discussion of Rose's relationship with her mother. Despite the historical primacy and centrality of the mother–daughter relationship, especially given their mutual loss of father/husband and their extended family and community, going forward as a young adult, Rose would naturally expand her support system and focus increasingly on peers. As was evident in her premature overattachment and enmeshment with her ex-boyfriend, this could put Rose at risk of exploitation or, at the very least, of relationships that are hurtful, conflicted, or simply a bad fit for her as a person. Rose also was used to seeking connection with the people who were available—rather than based on shared values or interests. She also was used to being appreciated for her kindness and willingness to give of herself to emotionally support others but also exploited for those qualities when she was not equally cared for, and recognized and valued for her intelligence and creativity.

The therapist therefore nonjudgmentally inquired about how Rose viewed the actions of peers, especially her best friend, and helped Rose to consider how to approach those relationships based on what Rose believed to be right for herself—while also not assuming the worst about others (such as the best friend) when there was history in the relationship of genuine caring and respect. This helped Rose to replace her projection of her own self-criticism onto her best friend while also preparing her to think of that (and other important) relationship(s) as an opportunity to learn whether there was a "fit" among the people involved rather than a test of whether other people could accept her and whether she was, in fact, acceptable as a person.

The therapist also was concerned that "next week [should] be better than this past week" to prevent Rose from dropping out. Although psychotherapy cannot guarantee immediate benefits in vivo in clients' lives, all talk and no action is a formula for premature termination when clients experience their day-to-day lives as intolerable or completely unmanageable. This also does not mean that it is necessary, or even possible, to find no-fault solutions to the problems facing the client that protect the therapist or the therapy from being to blame—whether in the client's perception or in actuality, or both— if the client's choices and actions out in the world have results that are disappointing or adverse consequences. However, of course, it is important to always carefully consider potential adverse consequences that could occur when helping clients develop plans for extending what they are learning in therapy into their daily lives. Most new choices in life, or modifications of long-standing behavior patterns, have complicated outcomes that are rarely unequivocally positive. The key is that the therapist helped Rose identify potential actions and activities that originated with Rose and were based on her interests and preferences.

Moving From Confusion to Clarity

Initially, Rose's communications were replete with linguistic distortions. She was not failing to communicate a strong message, and her thoughts had a definite logic that was not fundamentally irrational (given the emotions she was experiencing and her adverse experiences). However, what she was saying was incomplete and based on assumptions that she was accepting without an explicit definition and test of their veracity; for example: "I came to you because you were the one supposed to help me, right?" The deletion includes an omission of how and why Rose "came to" therapy, what it meant for a therapist to "help" a client, and according to what authority a therapist was "supposed" to help. Rose implied that having sought therapy from this therapist that the therapist must do what she (Rose) defined as "helping." The generalization is the implication that all therapists would act according to Rose's wishes, and therefore this therapist was violating that universal rule. The implied causative is that by violating Rose's rule about how therapists should help, this therapist was causing Rose to experience the intense distress she was feeling. The lack of referential index is an omission of the distress that Rose was experiencing, which was implied but not stated, and which was in reference to events outside of the therapy that went unmentioned here (as well as to the actions or lack of action by the therapist). The mindreading is an assumption that the therapist knew how she was "supposed to help" and an implied assumption that the therapist didn't care enough about Rose or her (the therapist's) responsibilities and therefore was failing to help Rose. The nominalization is treating the act of helping as a fixed entity rather than a process that can be (re-)started and modified at any time. The presuppositions include all the aforementioned assumptions that Rose was making about the therapist's responsibilities, failures, thoughts, and actions as well as about what this implied about herself (i.e., that she had been abandoned; that she was or was not deserving of help, that she depended on the therapist to enable her to solve the problems she was facing and to overcome or eliminate the distress she was feeling).

Thus, in a single sentence, Rose communicated a vast amount of information but without the clarity that she needed to understand her own feelings and thoughts, and to determine how to define and solve the problems that she was facing. This is entirely understandable given the distress that Rose was feeling. This does not imply that Rose was unintelligent. Quite the opposite: Rose was highly intelligent and was trying to think through some very complex dilemmas despite feeling emotionally dysregulated. Linguistic distortions are the product and expression of emotional dysregulation, not an inherent deficit or weakness in the person. As Rose's therapist modeled self-regulation by interacting calmly and thoughtfully in an effort to empathically understand and collaboratively partner with Rose, Rose's responses became progressively freer of distortions—that is, coregulation provided her with the scaffolding necessary to think and express herself with greater clarity. For example, as the discussion of Rose's relationship with her mother progressed, she was able to say quite clearly:

> I mean, I'm trying to see about it, to not go back and forth with her anymore because it's just gonna continue on and on, and I want her to support me so I'm able to feel more supportive towards her. . . . I mean, I could try to get her to open up to the church because she's really into that. That's what she relied on.

In the first sentence, two deletions are evident (i.e., "see about *it*" and "*it's* just gonna continue"). However, she's described what happened and what she wants to feel (i.e., no nominalization) with her mother specifically (i.e., no generalization and a definite referential index) without assuming anything about what her mother was thinking or feeling (i.e., no mind reading) or how she or her mother should act or how their relationship should be structured (i.e., no presuppositions). She linked what she wanted from her mother with what she was "able to feel . . . towards her," but she did not make her mother's actions responsible for her feelings (i.e., no implied causative). In the second sentence, there are no deletions or other evident distortions; instead, Rose described a complex set of linked possibilities quite specifically, showing impressive insight into the role that "the church," as a supportive community, a respite from stress and worry and a source of spiritual faith, could play when a person was faced with adversity.

CONCLUSION

In this session, Rose's therapist was able to help her to regain trust and self-regulation in the face of desperate aloneness and shame by providing validation, respect, comfort, clarification, and practical help that Rose had not found in key relationships. The therapist did not fault those relationships nor did she encourage Rose to adopt an attitude of dependence on her therapist as a "rescuer." Instead, she affirmed Rose's judgment, resilience, and worth, and helped her to empathically understand both the dilemmas and the options she had in relationships that involved emotional disconnection, disappointment, and, at times, rejection, betrayal, and exploitation. This session showed how a client in a crisis state of shame and fear related to betrayal and abandonment could be guided toward reflection and understanding if her therapist attended to her own self-regulation and provided her client with emotional attunement that was calming and restored genuine security.

The session also illustrated how the arc from dysregulation to regulation is not a single smooth trajectory. Rose moved in her affect and her linguistic communication from dysregulated toward greater balance and clarity but not without bumps in the road. When reminders of her core conflictual relationship themes (i.e., exploitation, coercion, neglect, and betrayal) emerged in the therapeutic dialogue, Rose's affect became more labile, and her thinking and communication became more subject to confusion and distortions. Her therapist remained a steady influence, a north star to whom Rose could turn and find direction when resurgences of dysregulation occurred. Repetition of this pattern of dysregulation followed by coregulation and understanding, and then a return to dysregulation before again restoring regulation and understanding, is the complex arc when a client in crisis is guided toward increasing stability in sustaining emotion regulation.

Rose still faced a great deal of uncertainty about how to navigate the complicated relationship with her mother and how to find in that relationship what she needed without asking for more than her mother could provide. But she was facing that challenge with a greater sense of clarity and emotional resolution, and the linguistic structure of her communication reflected that clarity. As such, this case is a good illustration of how, as a therapist helps a client in crisis regain emotional regulation—in large part by self-regulating internally while guiding the client toward greater self-understanding and understanding of a key caregiver—the evidence of progression can be found not just in the client's increasing degree of outward calm and acceptance of the therapist as a person whom the client can trust and with whom they can collaborate (i.e., the therapeutic "alliance") but also in the way that the client is thinking and expressing their thoughts linguistically.

QUESTIONS FOR READER SELF-REFLECTION

- What response from the therapist seemed to most help Rose shift from angry blaming to reflecting on and seeking help with her feelings of loss and aloneness?

- What potential countertransference issues should the therapist be aware of? (These might include feeling defensive in reaction to Rose's displacement of blame, feeling angry with Rose's mother for letting Rose down, or feeling helpless to protect Rose from the violation of her privacy that has been caused by the ex-boyfriend's sexting.)

- Should the therapist have challenged Rose to recognize that the blame she was placing on the therapist really belonged to Rose's mother for burdening and not protecting Rose? Why would that have been counter-therapeutic and have potentially worsened the crisis?

- What are the pros and cons of focusing on problem solving about Rose's mother's depression and potential suicidality? Did this encourage Rose to avoid her own issues, or did it help her to reflect on her feelings and fears related to her relationship with her mother, or both?

- Should the therapist have been more assertive in validating Rose's feeling of rejection in relation to her best friend to show Rose she was on her side as an ally? Or might that have intensified Rose's feeling of abandonment and aloneness, and encouraged her to isolate herself?

- What is the significance of the church and faith-based communities for a family such as Rose's and her mother?

- Was the therapist too quick to support Rose's idea of joining an activity group at school, or could that have provided Rose with a tangible first step toward restoring her sense of community and competence? How would you follow up with Rose in future sessions to determine whether that involvement was helpful, or was a source of additional stressors, or was just not happening?

- What was the turning point (or turning points) in this session when Rose was able to shift from dysregulation to resuming self-regulation, and what specific behaviors by Rose were the evidence of that shift?

- Was the therapist too apologetic—or not enough—for having taken the action to protect Rose despite Rose's fear that this had left her more exposed? Did the reporting actually leave Rose more exposed, or did it protect her, or both?

- What were your first thoughts when you saw how angry Rose was at the outset, and how would you have focused yourself at that moment if you were in the therapist's position?

- What approaches to self-regulation and recognition of countertransference can you see in the therapist's self-reflections, and how did this help the therapist maintain her focus on Rose's welfare and her empathic attunement with Rose?

11

HELPING A FAMILY COPE WITH THE THREAT OF REVICTIMIZATION

CASE BACKGROUND[1]

A mother (Monica) is bringing her teenage daughter (Trish) and 11-year-old son (Michael) to meet with her individual psychotherapist to break some very bad news. Michael and Trish's father, Neil, from whom Monica is divorced, has been incarcerated for 5 years after being physically abusive toward Michael, Trish, and Monica. Trish says she was never seriously physically hurt by her father and that she "just puts the bad memories out of my mind, where they can't bother me." Trish met with a therapist after her mother filed domestic battering charges against Neil and took the children to a shelter so that they wouldn't have to live with Neil anymore. She says

---

[1]To view the webinar associated with this case, including a video of the psychotherapy session, go online (https://learn.nctsn.org/course/view.php?id=481). Alternatively, you can go to the main website (https://learn.nctsn.org), click "Clinical Training" in the menu bar at the top of the page, click "Identifying Critical Moments and Healing Complex Trauma," and then click the webinar associated with this case: "Helping a Family Cope With the Threat of Revictimization." Although you will need to create an account ID and password, there is no fee to access the webinar.

https://doi.org/10.1037/0000225-012
Crises in the Psychotherapy Session: Transforming Critical Moments Into Turning Points, by J. D. Ford

that the therapy was "okay—mostly a bunch of drawing and games. I don't remember what we talked about." Monica views Trish as "really resilient." She says that Trish "won't let anything or anyone stop her when she sets a goal, which can be quite a handful" but adds that she thinks "it's a sign that she's strong and healthy, that the violence by her father hasn't left her with any emotional baggage." Monica has noticed, however, that Trish has intense nightmares almost every week in which she's screaming and sounds like she's fighting some kind of attacker, "but when she wakes up, she's totally fine, so it seems more like adolescent hormones and brain farts than anything to worry about."

Monica worries a lot about Michael. Michael still has a subtle scar on his cheek from a time when he was 6 and his father was strangling his sister for back talking him. When Michael tried to stop Neil, his father lashed out, and his ring caught Michael's cheek. No report was made to child protective services at that time. Michael often witnessed his father abuse his mother and sister, and was the target of abuse as well, although less often because he was younger, small for his age, and a boy. He also avoided his father and would hide when his father became violent. Monica describes Michael as "my little duckling: He's shy and sweet but also nervous and a worrier." Michael had problems with bed-wetting when the domestic abuse was occurring, and that continued until he met with a therapist after his father was incarcerated. The therapist taught Michael the coping cat anxiety management skills and showed him how to use those and other sleep hygiene techniques to be able to feel safe and listen to his body's signals when he needed to urinate even while he was asleep. Michael continues to be mildly anxious about school and peers, and he has occasional panic attacks when he sees or hears someone being angry or physically aggressive. But, for the past several years, he has done very well academically and has been active in sports and social activities with peers.

On the night that resulted in Neil's incarceration, Monica had returned home from work early and was going to surprise Neil with his favorite bottle of Irish whiskey before dinner. When she pulled into the liquor store lot, she saw what she thought was Neil's car. When she looked through the window, she saw Neil kissing a woman. She couldn't make out who it was, but she was furious. Not sure what to do, she went home. When Neil arrived, Monica greeted him with a slap and was cursing at him, calling him "useless" and "trash." Neil threw back some profanities of his own, and the verbal abuse quickly escalated, becoming physical. Hearing the shattering of glass, Trish and Michael rushed downstairs. They found Monica lying on the floor atop a shattered glass table with their father's hands around her neck; she was kicking her feet in an effort to get him off her. Neil was screaming, "I'll kill you for this," and yelled at both children to leave. Trish raced to Monica to try to help, but her father pushed her away. Michael was frozen in fear. He couldn't speak, move, or react. Neighbors had heard the fight and called the police, who arrived and pulled Neil off of Monica. Neil was taken away in handcuffs, and an ambulance took Monica and the children to the hospital. While there, a domestic violence counselor spoke with Monica, and she decided that she had to get help for herself and her children. Monica was in individual therapy for 2 years with the therapist with whom she and her children will meet in this session. She also made sure both Trish and Michael saw individual therapists until each of them seemed fully recovered.

Fast forward to 5 years later, when Monica learned from the prosecutor's office that Neil was being released early from prison. This news triggered panic attacks and nightmares for her, so she resumed seeing the psychotherapist she had seen for a couple of years after the trial. Trish or Michael could see that their mother was upset but had no idea why. They were glad she started in therapy again because they felt as if they knew the therapist (although they had never met him in person) because Monica would comment occasionally on things she had learned in therapy and found helpful. For example, she had shared this with them:

> The doctor told me that we all have an alarm in our brain that goes off when we get stressed and showed me a way to focus the thinking center in my brain so I can turn down the alarm and be the "calm Monica" instead of the "angry, nagging Monica" when you guys are stressed out or do things that used to get stressed out.

The children would just laugh and tell Monica to save the therapy talk for her therapist, but they secretly felt reassured that therapy was helpful to their mother.

Although the police reassured Monica that a condition of Neil's parole was that he could have no contact with her, they advised her that Neil could petition for visitation with their children if he continued in therapy, and the department of children and families might grant him supervised visitation in the future. Monica felt like her world was falling apart and asked her therapist if he would help her break the news to the children in a family session. After discussing the pros and cons of this approach, they agreed to go ahead with a family session. The therapist advised more than a single session might be required and that, because his goal would be to support Monica in helping her children cope with the emotions this news brought up, this would be different than their individual sessions. Monica said she understood and wanted him to pay as much attention to how her children were doing as to her because what mattered most to her was ensuring that her children saw that they all had support in handling this together as a family. Monica and the therapist also developed a plan for helping either or both of her children to subsequently meet with another therapist of their own or all together in family therapy, if that proved to be necessary or helpful.

SESSION TRANSCRIPT, ANNOTATIONS, AND COMMENTARY

In this psychotherapy session a mother, Monica, discloses to her two children, Trish and Michael, that their previously domestically violent father is being released early from prison.

(*The family members sit on a couch with mother and son close together and daughter sitting pointedly as far away from the other two as possible.*)

> *Therapist's Inner Reflections*: I see immediately an intergenerational coalition, with Monica and Michael strongly emotionally tied together and Trish separating herself from both of them. This seems developmentally expectable with a younger child closer to his mother than an adolescent daughter asserting her independence. But it may be amplified by the trauma they've experienced.

THERAPIST: I'm glad to meet you in person, Trish and Michael. I'm the therapist your mother met with a few years ago, and we've been meeting again recently. I've heard a lot of things—mostly good by the way (*smiles*)—about you from your mother. I'm sure you've heard some things about me, too—I hope also mostly good even though I am a "shrink." Your mother and I have talked a lot about handling stress.

(*Monica nods nervously. Michael stares intently at the therapist. Trish pointedly looks at her lap.*)

THERAPIST: We've also talked about positive experiences, including a number involving you two, so that therapy can be a place to build on the good things in life as well as deal with stress. So, that's what I expect we'll do today.

MONICA: We need to have a family meeting to talk about something important.

TRISH: (*Sighs deeply and rolls her eyes*) Okay, so what *are* we here to talk about?

MICHAEL: (*Looks down, silently taps and shakes one leg rapidly*)

MONICA: (*Sighs heavily, looks at the therapist, then at her children*) There's something you need to know. Your father is going to be released from jail in a month. It's earlier than we thought, but the social worker told me said that he can't have anything to do with any of us unless we say it's all right. And you can just say no.

MICHAEL: (*Looks up at his mother in horror, then stares at the floor and seems in a daze*)

MONICA: I know this is a shock, but we're going to be okay. We'll get through this together. It won't be like it was before.

TRISH: (*Speaks loudly in a shrill voice*) Whaddaya mean he's getting out? You said it would be years before he'd ever be out!

MONICA: (*Slumps back as if slapped, closes her eyes momentarily and grimaces, then looks pleadingly at Trish*) We have to pull together now, I'm sorry, but we can get through this . . .

Therapist's Inner Reflections: This is very difficult for all of them, but Monica's the family leader, and she's showing them that despite feeling distressed, she can help them face this challenge. I don't want to inadvertently undercut her authority or her competence, so I'll stay silent.

MICHAEL: (*Looks at the floor, his upper torso shaking, and taps one leg furiously while breathing rapidly and shallowly*)

MONICA: (*Sits forward, looks intently at Trish, speaks in a pressured but determined manner*) I am *not* going to let him, or any person, hurt any of us. We'll get through this together.

MICHAEL: (*Looks around dazedly and in a panic, eyes go wide as if seeing a threat, lunges for the floor at the edge of the office, rolls up in fetal position whimpering softly with eyes closed and hands over his ears*)

Therapist's Inner Reflections: Michael's escalated into an emergency state. This is where I can help Monica so that she doesn't have to try to be the crisis therapist for Michael.

THERAPIST: (*Makes eye contact with Monica, then Trish*) Michael's having a hard time with this. I'm going to just move over beside Michael to see if I can help him while he's doing some hard work.

(*Therapist gradually leaves his chair and lowers himself onto the floor. He approaches Michael slowly but without touching him, speaking both to him and to Monica and Trish.*)

MICHAEL: (*Stays in fetal position, shakes, lips move soundlessly, has eyes closed and hands over his ears, rubs his ears vigorously*)

Therapist's Inner Reflections: I think Michael's having a flashback, hearing scary things that are likely to be intrusive memories of the past violence—but that's just a guess, so I'll reframe his reaction as not just having a bad memory but also making it go away. Also, I'm focused on moving close enough but without touching him, so that he can feel my presence and hear me, to reduce the feeling of isolation but without feeling physically or psychologically assaulted.

THERAPIST: (*Sits on the floor with arms around bent legs; he's next to Michael, where Michael can see him but doesn't touch Michael and still speaks both to him and to Monica and Trish*) I know you're feeling very scared, Michael, but no matter what you're remembering, you're safe right here and now. Just take your time. You're doing a really good job of figuring out how to make the bad memory stop and go away.

MICHAEL: (*Looks intently at the therapist while he speaks and for several seconds after the therapist pauses, then looks off in the direction where he'd looked in terror before, looks puzzled, silently mouths some indistinct words*)

THERAPIST: (*Speaks softly*) There you go. I'm right here, and you're doing it—you're doing a great job of figuring out how to make the memory go away.

MICHAEL: (*Looks calmer, more present and focused, then looks beyond the therapist and sees his mother and sister, looks around in panic, and then covers his face*)

Therapist's Inner Reflections: Seeing his mother and sister triggered Michael back into the state of fear—for Michael, probably because they're associated with the violence since they were targets of the abusive ex-husband/father. It's not just as simple as reassuring Michael that he's safe with me; I also have to help him recognize that his mother and sister are safe, too, and they weren't when the violence was happening, so he's probably reexperiencing the fear of witnessing harm to them.

MONICA: (*Abruptly leans forward toward Michael, voice tense and shrill*) Mikey, come on. You can do this.

Therapist's Inner Reflections: I was hoping that Monica would be reassured by my helping Michael, but when she saw the look of horror on his face, that understandably triggered her. Now her terror is escalating Michael's distress and disorientation. I'll speak directly to Michael to help him regain a sense of safety and indirectly to Monica to help her feel more secure that Michael is going to be okay and that she can help him by letting me guide him through this.

MICHAEL: (*Jumps with startle, rolls back into fetal position, starts rubbing his arms vigorously*)

THERAPIST: Mike, do you know where you are right now because I think maybe it's—you're having a hard time remembering that you're sitting with your mom . . ., and I'm not somebody you know very well, but I'm a therapist, and your mom and I are gonna make sure that you're safe.

MONICA: We're just here to make plans, okay? (*Reaches over and rubs Michael's back*)

Therapist's Inner Reflections: Monica is taking a calmer tone and reassuring Michael, but I'm concerned that her touch will inadvertently increase his sense of physical danger because he can't distinguish good from bad touching in this state of dissociation. I'll suggest gently to Monica to step back, and then I can focus on helping Michael to know that he's not alone and what he's experiencing are scary memories that his mother and I can help him put away like closing a book.

THERAPIST: (*Speaks to Monica*) We'll just give Michael a little bit of time to adjust. It was very scary for him when things got bad in your family years ago, and I think he's remembering some of those times. And, Trish, that's what sometimes happens. You probably have memories at times, too. And, Michael, we can help you with those memories. That's why we're talking right now. Are you hearing things that are scary?

MICHAEL: (*Nods several times in staccato*)

THERAPIST: Yeah. Okay. But you can hear me, too, and you can hear your mom, and when your mom is rubbing your back, she's safe, and you're doing a really good job. That's great. You're doing a really good job of breathing, and your mom is safe right now, and so are you.

MONICA: That's right, you're okay now, Mikey. (*Stops rubbing Michael's back, sits back on the couch, more relaxed but still tense*)

MICHAEL: Okay. (*Looks at Monica, gradually unfolds and leans on one arm, still on the floor*)

THERAPIST: Yeah.

MONICA: Okay. That's better. We're all fine.

MICHAEL: (*Looks at Monica again, startles and has a look of shock, first rubs and then scratches his arms vigorously*)

Therapist's Inner Reflections: Monica could see that giving Michael physical space helps him to feel calmer and to listen to my guidance and reassurance. So, it's a shock to her that he's had another triggered stress reaction, probably seeing the look of anxiety on Monica's face. Now I'm going to have to coregulate with both Monica and Michael so they don't keep escalating one another. They both need reassurance that Michael is not losing it so Monica doesn't lose it. Grounding Michael so he doesn't hurt himself is priority one and Monica also so she doesn't try to physically or verbally restrain Michael—which I see she's on the verge of doing.

THERAPIST: Michael's doing some more very hard work now, Monica, and that's really good. I think you just figured something out, Michael. That's really great. I know that the memory isn't gone completely, but you came right back here. Sometimes it helps . . .

MONICA: (*Leans forward as if to lunge at Michael*) Mikey, you have to stop it. Stop it.

THERAPIST: (*Moves between Monica and Michael*) Sometimes it helps just to feel your arm. Are your arms itchy? That's okay. That's alright.

MONICA: (*Speaks shrilly*) No, it's—that—it's not.

THERAPIST: If you need to scratch a little bit . . .

Therapist's Inner Reflections: Helping Michael gain control of the self-scratching and shift to a milder version as if he has a simple physical itch can shift his perspective from terror to feeling safe enough to feel some normal bodily and emotional tension. This gives him permission to feel afraid and to try to release the extreme tension he's feeling by scratching but less violently as he feels safer with my guidance and the reframing of his goal not as survival but as figuring out what to do with a bad memory. That communicates that what he's experiencing is real and he's not going crazy or is totally vulnerable because it's not happening now—it's a memory that we can deal with. I hope Monica can hear that and also shift from panic to feeling a sense of relief and security. Because Monica is so strongly triggered by Michael's behavior, it may be harder for her than for Michael to make that shift until she sees evidence in Michael's behavior that he has recovered.

MONICA: It's too much. He'll hurt himself.

THERAPIST: I understand. Yeah. Yeah. Okay. There you go. Just take your time. I think Michael will not need to scratch when he knows that he's figured out what to do about the bad memories.

MICHAEL: (*Slows down the scratching, then resumes gentler rubbing of his arms*)

MONICA: That was not okay. He'll hurt himself.

Therapist's Inner Reflections: I'm not going to try to reason with Monica right now because words alone won't reassure her. Staying the course with Michael, helping him psychologically come back from the abuse memories and know that his mother and he are safe now, is the key.

THERAPIST: Well, that's where we're starting right now. Michael, whatever— whatever you're remembering, do you know where mom is? She's right there. Okay. She's safe now, and so are you.

MONICA: (*Leans forward tensely, reaches out to Michael with her hand*) Mikey, can you hold my hand, please, instead?

MICHAEL: (*Rolls back up, resumes scratching, faster and harder*)

MONICA: (*Reaches more intensely toward Michael*) Can you hold my hand, please, instead of doing that? Mikey, *please*! Okay?

THERAPIST: Okay. Just . . .

MONICA: Stop it! You can't hurt yourself!

THERAPIST: (*Leans to Monica*) Just take your time, Monica. You're doing a great job, and so is Michael.

Therapist's Inner Reflections: Monica is trying so hard to help Michael, but instead of helping, she's communicating that she needs him to reassure her. I need to gently interpose myself between her and Michael while communicating reassurance to her that I've got this handled.

MONICA: (*Sits back on the couch*)

MICHAEL: (*Slows the scratching and again resumes rubbing his arms*)

Therapist's Inner Reflections: That's better. Now we can get back to trauma memory processing that needs to focus on helping Michael have a different way of understanding the terror that he's feeling—some main thoughts like that he's here now and doesn't have to go back, and that when he hears my voice, he can use it like a tuner for a musical instrument to regain a calm tone.

THERAPIST: (*Speaks softly to Michael*) You're doing a really great job just figuring out how to make sure that you don't have to go back to those terrible memories. If you're hearing something really scary, that's okay. We're right here now. Can you hear me, Michael? Just a little bit? It's okay

MICHAEL: (*Stops rubbing his arms, unfolds more, and starts to lie down on his side with hands under his head, as if going to sleep*)

Therapist's Inner Reflections: Ever so slowly, Michael needs to feel safe enough to sleep, so the memories probably were of times he felt terrified and couldn't sleep. He doesn't literally need to sleep now, although it would be fine if he fell asleep; he needs to feel the sense of safety and calm that enables a child to sleep but that's been shattered by violence. Now, I'll keep talking with him and modeling for Monica how to do this, almost like a lullaby . . .

THERAPIST: Nobody's gonna do anything. If you wanna lie down, that's okay. Would you feel better that way? (*Pauses*) Okay. There we go. That's good. See, Monica, Michael is really very smart about this. Sometimes when you're scared, you need to just kind of get down on the ground and make sure that everything is okay. There you go. And he doesn't know me very well, so it's kinda scary for him to have a—a guy here 'cause . . .

MONICA: I just don't understand, how this is appropriate?

Therapist's Inner Reflections: That rhetorical question deserves a direct answer. Monica sees Michael's scratching himself and now going into a fetal position as regression. I need to help her understand that it's a child's healthy way of putting away an upsetting memory, so it makes sense.

THERAPIST: It's appropriate because Michael is figuring out how to put the memory away. He has some very scary memories, and he's figuring something out right now. That's why you're here to make things better.

MONICA: How do I know? He won't talk! What if he's internalizing all of this?

Therapist's Inner Reflections: I recognize Monica's anxious and frustrated reactions as her own posttraumatic stress reactions. She was directly

traumatized by the domestic violence, so it's completely understandable that she'd be reacting with a desperate attempt to rescue Michael
both because of her concern for him as a parent and to feel rescued
herself when she wasn't—when the violence was being directed at her
by her ex-husband. Monica's posttraumatic stress disorder is triggering for Michael, and she needs reassurance that this is going to work
out okay and not just be what she probably most dreads: that Michael
(or she herself) is falling apart and can't be "fixed."

MICHAEL: (*Tenses up, starts scratching his arms again, rolls back into a ball*)

THERAPIST: Oh, no. He's—he—he's hearing you, and he's hearing me, and he knows that we're here.

MONICA: (*Speaks shrilly, leans and reaches out*) Mikey, please stop. Mikey, please. Mikey, stop it. Mikey, stop it. Mikey, please stop. Mikey, please, please. Come on. We're okay. You're okay.

Therapist's Inner Reflections: I hear a terrified mother and a terrified little girl, crying for help. I need to signal Monica nonverbally that I've got this handled, and that she doesn't have to stay in survival mode to protect Michael or herself—as she no doubt did when the violence happened.

THERAPIST: (*Reaches out, palm down, to Monica, as if to signal "Slow down; it's okay"*) Okay, Monica.

MONICA: (*Sits back, softly*) He can't do this.

MICHAEL: (*Relaxes, stops scratching, starts rubbing his arms more gently, stretches out*)

THERAPIST: Good job. Good job. Okay. I think you just helped him to calm down and slow down. That's great. Michael. Your mom is right here.

MICHAEL: (*Looks through his fingers at Monica, then looks at the therapist, gradually unfolds, and leans on one arm, still on the floor in the corner*)

Therapist's Inner Reflections: I'm going to attribute Michael's calming down to Monica's becoming calmer. She's having a real struggle to disengage from panicking and trust that I can help Michael—and her—be safe and get through the traumatic memories they're both experiencing, so she needs an affirmation from me that she's making a crucial difference and helping Michael.

THERAPIST: Whenever, whenever you're ready, if you want to, you can just kinda take a peek and see who's here. There you go. There's mom.

MONICA: (*Speaks to Michael*) Can you talk about this?

Therapist's Inner Reflections: Not yet, Mom. Slow down. We'll get there but don't rush; be calm.

THERAPIST: There you go. It may be a little soon to talk about it. Okay, Monica? But I—I know it's something that we will talk about, but right now, I think Michael just needs to know you're here and his sister (*Michael scratches.*) is here, and you're all safe because it was a scary memory. . . .

MONICA: But he's so quiet. I don't know what's going on with him ever.

THERAPIST: Mm-hmm. Well, that's probably because a lot's going on. Right, Mike?

MICHAEL: (*Sits up, rubs his arms*) Mm-hmm.

Therapist's Inner Reflections: It's important that Monica gradually understands that Michael is working hard internally in ways that he, of course, doesn't understand but that make it hard for him to express what he's feeling and thinking. And he's only a kid, so he's not going to be able to explain to his mother, or even to himself, that he's having flashbacks. That would be much too clinical a way to explain it to Michael, or to Monica, anyway. The message is that he's been upset by scary memories, but now he's learning that he can put those memories away and not have to feel trapped and helpless when he recalls them because he's putting them away where they belong— like closing a book when he's done reading a chapter and wants to put the book away.

THERAPIST: Yeah. You got a lot going on. And just do whatever you need to do but be careful with your body. Okay? Yeah. That's good. Just don't—don't do anything that hurts yourself even though I know you're trying to kind of get rid of all those memories, and you're doing a good job with that, and they're gonna go away. It takes time, but they are gonna go away. And right now, you and your mom and your sister are safe right here. That a—that's great, Mike, so just take your time. Okay? See Mom? There you go. She's right there. Trish is right there too. Okay. There you go. Alright. So, it's okay if I sit back up in my chair for a moment? (*Therapist lowly gets up and sits in his chair.*)

MICHAEL: Mm-hmm.

Therapist's Inner Reflections: Now Michael, and also Monica and Trish, can see that the way to put away bad memories is to know they're not happening right now and that everyone's okay and here together now—so what happened in the memory isn't happening now. The idea is not at all complicated, but the key is that he's getting that idea paired with feeling more secure and present. That's a shift in his body that tells him he really is doing something to make things better, and it's also a shift in his thinking so that he knows what to think to help his body feel calmer.

THERAPIST: I'll come back and join you if that's—if you'd like. If it's helpful, just let me know. Okay? Okay. I know you don't know me that well, but thank you for trusting me this much. I really appreciate it. So, this is why we're meeting. This is exactly right, Monica, so you can help your daughter and your son carry on with the good life that you've made for each other and helped each other make for one another. You've done a great job on that, and this is not going to change that, but some adjustments are necessary to make sure everybody's safe. And am I right in—in recalling that you have made some arrangements so that their dad can't make any contact with them unless they say it's okay?

Therapist's Inner Reflections: This affirmation for Monica of her success in protecting and caring for her children despite the violence in the past and the distressing reminder of that now with the early release of her ex-husband from prison can help her to retain a memory of this session as a success with Michael's getting help (including from her) in learning how to protect himself by figuring out that he can get through—and put away—memories that have been scaring him. So, the session is consistent with Monica's core goal of ensuring her family's safety.

MONICA: Yes.

THERAPIST: Okay. That's really good. Did you know that your mom had done that?

TRISH: If she's done that, why can't I go to the mall with my friends?

Therapist's Inner Reflections: I'm glad to hear from Trish. I don't want her to be the neglected third wheel. She's stayed aloof, but that shows a lot of composure in this high-stress situation.

THERAPIST: That's a good point; we'll have to talk about that. Maybe, maybe there is a way, Trish. Let's not give up on that. Okay? Have you ever been able to negotiate and come up with a— a plan together?

MONICA: She usually does what she wants anyway.

> *Therapist's Inner Reflections*: Trish needs her mother to signal a willingness to find a mutually agreeable plan. To be able to do that, I think Monica needs to hear that her efforts to protect her children are appreciated—and that will have to come from me, not Trish. By affirming Trish's goal of autonomy and Monica's goal of being recognized as the family leader, I may be able to be the bridge between them as well as serve temporarily as the observing ego for each of them.

THERAPIST: Well, that's one way of doing it. So, maybe this would be a good time to be able to come up with a plan together so you can do what you want, but you can know that (*looks at Monica*) your daughter is safe and (*looks at Michael*) you can know that your sister is safe, too. Alright. (*Looks at Trish and Michael*) Now your mom is doing a really good job. She's making sure everybody's together, and she's been planning so you two wouldn't be surprised by this. Of course, it's—it's a surprise because you didn't know, but your mom didn't wait. She decided to tell you right away so that would know exactly what's happening, and you would know how to be able to handle this together as a family.

MONICA: We just need to all be on board with this. Okay?

> *Therapist's Inner Reflections*: Monica's understandably impatient to "close the deal" by getting Trish to sign on to her plan, but Trish thinks this means curtailing her social life, and she won't agree to that—or if she says she agrees, it will be only words, and more conflict will ensue. This is an important time to help them get more specific and operationalize what they're agreeing to.

THERAPIST: But we need to talk about what being on board means. That's a good point. 'Cause see, I think it might mean something different for Trish or for Michael. I know that's challenging, Monica. I know you don't want to let them out of your sight, but I also know that you've encouraged them to be independent. (*Looks at Trish and Michael*) But I guess you can see how important it is to your mom that she knows where you are—not to keep track of you in a bad way but so that she can always be there if you need her.

MONICA: I'm afraid of him taking them—just abducting them or somebody picking them up off the street, and I won't know where they are.

THERAPIST: So, you wanna know where both of your kids are no matter what so that . . .

MONICA: Yes. I do.

THERAPIST: That would never happen? Fair enough.

MONICA: And I also wanna make sure they're not hurting themselves so that I don't get calls from the school and then, all the sudden, I have social workers at my door. You know?

Therapist's Inner Reflections: Monica is shifting to her unresolved concern that Michael is losing it and that this could lead to losing him if the "social workers" decide she's not a fit parent. Seeing Michael dissociate and hurt himself is understandably distressing for her, but I hadn't realized how much that is amplified by her fear of losing Michael entirely.

THERAPIST: Of course. And did you notice how well Michael did at putting that memory away? The more that we help him do that, he won't need to hurt himself at all. I think those memories have been bothering Michael, but this is a chance to help him put them away, but we've gotta do that carefully and gradually and not put pressure on. You can't pretend everything's exactly the same. But the good things don't have to go away. So, I'm thinking maybe we could meet again a couple a times? Would that be alright with you, Monica?

MONICA: Yes.

THERAPIST: I don't wanna take away from your time, and you've done great work in therapy.

Therapist's Inner Reflections: The first part was for Trish more than for Monica—to acknowledge that this is not how she wants to be spending her time. The second part was to support Monica so that she remembers this session with a sense of hope and confidence, and as evidence that therapy can enable Michael to recover from trauma by facing bad memories with a therapist's guidance.

MONICA: Hmm.

THERAPIST: Okay. Trish, would you be willing to meet once or twice again just to iron out some of these issues around the mall and stuff so that you can have your freedom?

TRISH: Whatever.

THERAPIST: Okay. Well, I'll take that as a "you're considering," and that's fair enough. I don't blame you. Michael, would you be willing to come back?

MICHAEL: (*Nods rapidly affirmatively*) Yeah.

THERAPIST: Okay. We'll figure out how you can put those bad memories away and make sure that your mom's safe 'cause I see how important that is to you. Okay. Would you like to go over and sit by her or are you comfortable where you are? (*Michael moves to his mom and sits close to her.*) Okay.

MONICA: Okay. (*Chuckles*)

THERAPIST: There you go. The good thing about that is now you can keep an eye on her. (*Chuckles*)

Monica's, Trish's, and Michael's Observations

Monica found the therapist's way of describing what she viewed as Michael's "obviously very disturbed" behavior confusing. As Monica explained,

> I didn't know why he kept saying Michael was working hard and figuring out how to make the memories go away when it just looked like Michael was freaking out. I wanted him to do something to calm Mikey down and make him stop scratching himself, and when nothing he was doing seemed to make things any better, I had to step in and tell Mikey to just stop. I felt really helpless and frustrated, and worried because it was like Mikey was having a seizure, and he was hurting himself. His teachers say he sometimes has panic attacks, and they have to take him to a quiet room until he calms down, and they think he should be seeing a therapist, or maybe I should be doing something so he isn't so stressed at home that he can't handle school. I'm really worried that that is going to get worse now that their father is out, and who knows what he'll do to upset them or maybe even to get back at me by hurting them.
>
> The session really didn't go the way I wanted at first, with Mikey freaking out and Trish giving me the attitude. I have to say that I was disappointed that the doctor didn't seem to see how serious these problems are and acted like Trish could just do whatever she wanted and Mikey could totally lose it, and it was no problem. So, I guess I was really surprised that Mikey actually calmed down so fast at the end, like he almost felt he'd done something good to get over the bad memories—if that even was what was actually happening. But, whatever. Michael seemed better and more relaxed than I've seen him for a long time at the end of the session, so the doctor must know what he's doing, even if I don't see how it works.
>
> Trish didn't really come out of her shell, so that's gonna be a problem. I wish I could have had more time to set her straight about why she has to be more careful to not get in with the wrong crowd or just go off on her own and

not watch out that she's safe. At least she said she'd come back for another session; that's more than I expected. I hope we can talk all of this out and get together as a family. Maybe this rocky start is just the way it has to go. I do trust the doc; he's been a big help to me with my anxieties and depression and self-esteem, so I hope he can see what we need to do to get through this together and that he can get Michael and Trish to see that so they're on board and we're all pulling together.

Trish's comments about the session were:

It was okay. It could've been worse. It was weird that Mikey spazzed out. I worry about him; he gets so freaked out. I mean he's a good kid—really sweet, unlike most boys his age, who are little monsters. But he just gets so upset, actually a lot like our mother. She was on his case like a fly on you-know-what. I wanted to tell her to just shut up and leave him alone when she was freaking out and that was freaking him out even more. That's the way she gets: She goes from being all fine and acting like she's got her stuff in control to just totally losing it. Like about me and my friends, or going to the mall. She must have zero memory about what it was like when she was a kid, or she just remembers the bad parts, like how she ended up with the jerk, my father. I doubt she'll lighten up and see that I need to have a life, and she can't always be watching everything I do and criticizing me and my friends and telling me I can't do this and I can't go there. But she seemed to back off some when the therapist called her out for yelling at Michael. He did get her to back off, I'll say that. I'll show up for another session if there's a slight chance he might get her to cut me some slack and back off my case.

Michael said that it was scary at first in the session

because they were talking about my dad, and all of a sudden, I just started shaking, and then I had to try to hide. I don't know why. I was really scared. I heard scary noises, and I couldn't see anything. It was like it was all dark at night. I wanted to run away or hide until the yelling stopped and I could see again, but I was shaking so much I couldn't get up. So then my arms started itching, and the more I scratched them, the more they itched, until all of a sudden, it stopped and I felt okay again. I sort of remember the doctor sitting beside me on the floor. That was okay because when he was talking, the noise wasn't so bad. And he said I was doing a good job, that I was doing something to make bad memories go away. I don't know what I did, but I felt better, so that's good. And he didn't yell at me, so that's good, too. I don't like it when people yell, so I hope I don't have to see my father because he yells a lot. Maybe the doctor can make him stop yelling or make him not bother me 'cause I don't want him around. He scares me and he scares mom. I just want us all to be safe.

Commentary

Each person and family carries with them the stories, feelings, and beliefs that help them to make sense of what's happened to them and how they were changed by those experiences, including flashbacks that involve fragmentary, confusing, and overwhelming feelings without a clear memory (as Michael was experiencing in this session) as well as clear memories that they're trying to not think about (but that, when suppressed, can lead to intense distress, as Monica was experiencing). When past experiences influence how someone views a present-day situation, it can be a particular challenge to untangle what is historical and what is relevant in the here and now. Monica's experience of being a survivor of past domestic violence and abuse understandably led her to rely on survival mode to cope by being hyperaware and hypervigilant to any potential threat to her children or to her. The children also experienced the traumatic shock of witnessing their father's violence, which deprived them of a sense of security on multiple levels. Instead of having a father whom they could trust to care for and protect them and their mother, their father was a threat. Despite their mother's efforts to protect them and herself, she couldn't ensure that either she or they were safe. With their mother's safety in jeopardy, the children faced the possibility of losing her as well and being without any parental caregiving or protection. Thus, both because of the direct harm that occurred in the domestic violence and the loss or threatened loss of security with their primary caregivers, the children experienced the kind of developmental trauma that can lead to the severe problems with terror, dissociation, and emotional dysregulation that Michael displayed in this session (Ford, 2017a; Ford, Grasso, Levine, & Tennen, 2018).

The first priority when severe emotion dysregulation emerges in a crisis is safety. There are two aspects to safety that I had to consider simultaneously as the therapist in this session. The first is the objective safety of the clients in their lives outside the therapy setting. Both children emphatically said they didn't want any contact with/by their father at this time. Therefore, I first emphasized my support for Monica's efforts to ensure that no harm would come to her children (and by implication, to her as well). I affirmed the value of setting realistic limits so that Monica would be able to keep track of her children's whereabouts while they determined whether the ex-husband/father's release to the community would lead to any unwanted encounters. Several times during the session, I also expressed respect for Monica's efforts over many years to ensure her children's safety to communicate to her that I see her as courageous and successful as a protector and role model for her children (emotionally as well as physically).

The close second priority was the emotional (and physical) safety of each client in the session itself. This was most evident in relation to Michael's dissociative flashback and self-harm. But it also was evident in Monica's desperate attempts to stop Michael from "losing it," which were reflections of her unresolved posttraumatic stress issues, which ironically had the effect of exacerbating rather than relieving Michael's terror and dissociation. The crisis in this session was not primarily about present or future danger (although that, understandably, as just described, was Monica's focus). From a therapeutic perspective, the crisis was about the triggering of unresolved aftereffects of the past domestic violence and abuse. This was most evidently the case for Michael. After Monica revealed that the ex-husband/father was going to be released imminently from prison, earlier than expected, Michael became increasingly agitated physically and detached and uncommunicative psychologically. When he crawled down to the floor and scrunched up into a ball, eyes closed, and shaking all over and appearing to attempt to ward off an attacker, my focus narrowed rapidly from interacting with all of the family members to communicating directly to Michael with a message intended to quietly and calmly reassure him and help him reorient to the present place and moment. To do this, I moved from my usual position in the therapist's chair to be closer and literally at the same level as Michael—but with care to not intrude on his personal space and definitely not to touch or attempt to hold him because Michael would probably have interpreted those actions as an assault. I made that judgment because, although I couldn't be sure what Michael was experiencing internally— that these were in fact intrusive memories of past violence based on the history of domestic violence and the immediate trigger of learning from his anxious mother that his father (the perpetrator) was imminently being release from prison—it seemed likely that Michael was reexperiencing some threat of violence in the form of a dissociative flashback. Helping him to feel the nonthreatening presence and to hear the calm voice of a protective adult who was close enough to help but not too close seemed to be the crucial focus at that crisis point.

However, Monica had become progressively more agitated and continued to repeatedly and forcefully tell Michael to get up and stop acting strangely. As she did this, Michael understandably became increasingly agitated and detached, and began to scratch himself. Monica and Michael then mutually escalated their own and each other's agitation in a vicious cycle until I attempted to help by supporting Monica while simultaneously providing her with role modeling for how to quietly let Michael know that he was safe and that it was okay for him to do whatever he needed to do to feel safe and make the bad memories go away—as long as he was careful not to hurt his body. That gave Michael permission to cope in a way that initially was maladaptive but that he could change to become adaptive by simply remembering one main thought: to keep his body safe. That was one of Monica's primary goals as well, so I was attempting to help her recognize that she had a different option for achieving that goal than being passive (which is how she saw me, although I think that was largely based on her fear and transference) or aggressive (which was what she was doing by forcefully ordering Michael to stop and describing his behavior as "bad" and "inappropriate"). Although I did not interrupt the flow of the session to make this explicit, my approach in the session followed the FREEDOM steps (see the Introduction to this volume). I was helping both Michael and Monica be aware of (rather than just diffusely reacting to) their alarm reactions without judging or feeling ashamed of or attempting to suppress or avoid those reactions:

- **F**ocus: The orienting thought that I suggested repeatedly to both Monica and Michael is that each of them was doing a very good job of making things safe.

- **R**ecognizing triggers: The ex-husband/father's release was the obvious trigger, but Monica's reactive behavior was the most crucial and proximate trigger for Michael just as Michael's reactive behavior was a trigger for Monica.

- **E**motion awareness: Both Michael and Monica were experiencing terror as a primary reactive emotion, and Monica also expressed sadness while acknowledging those feelings I highlighted as main emotions that were a bond between them: the love and caring that they felt for each other, and strong feelings of determination and courage.

- **E**valuating cognitions: Monica's reactive thoughts that Michael was losing it and I (the therapist) wasn't helping were clear. Michael's reactive thoughts were only expressed nonverbally, so I attempted to put them into words in a way that helped him make sense of the confusion he was experiencing: He thought that he was trapped back in a terrible scary situation. These reactive thoughts might be judged to be "irrational" on a superficial level, but from a nonjudgmental and empathic perspective, they are reflections of Monica and Michael's resilient attempts to cope with severe posttraumatic stress. Rather than attempting to convince either of them to adopt more "rational" beliefs, it was important instead for me to take their reactive thoughts seriously while also articulating and highlighting several key main thoughts that were the foundation for their reactive thoughts. For Monica, this was a belief in her own worth and competence as a parent and that her children had, and would continue to have, success and safety in their lives. For Michael, the foundational main thought that I could discern, reading between the lines, was that he could put the bad memories away and be happy with the people who love him.

- Defining goals: Reactive goals are a synthesis of reactive emotions and thoughts, and thus the reactive goal expressed most clearly by Monica and (albeit indirectly) also Michael was to avoid or escape catastrophic violence or irreparable injury. This survival focus was understandable given the past traumatic violence and the current uncertainty about being subjected to more violence or distressing reminders of the past hurt and helplessness they had experienced. Although I acknowledged this perspective, I also highlighted the seemingly obvious but easily overlooked survival goals that were a source of hope for both Michael and Monica: having a happy and caring family, and having a happy and successful life

- Options: The options that flow from reactive goals tend to be rigid, automatic, and either impulsive or avoidant patterns of behavior that provide a semblance of relief but that exact a high price. For Michael, the reactive options were to go to ground (literally and figuratively) and just attempt to endure whatever violence occurred. For Monica, the reactive options were to demand compliance from her children so that they would avoid any people, places, or activities in which they might be vulnerable and so that she would be able to constantly monitor their safety. Although these reactive options caused, or exacerbated, a state of emotional dysregulation for both Monica and Michael, in that state of dysregulation, it had become virtually impossible for either of them to think clearly enough to realize that the solution was worse than the problem they were attempting to solve. The more they relied on those reactive options, the more unsafe and confused they felt, and this made them less rather than more safe. Rather than highlighting this dilemma of self-defeating behavior, I guided them by modeling and helping each of them to experiment with trying out main options that were more consistent with their main goals. For Monica, this involved being calmly attentive and emotionally available to Michael without anxiously pressuring him. For Michael, this involved doing simple things that helped his body feel calmer and that helped him to know that he and his mother were safe and happy together.

- Making a contribution: By facing the triggers and resultant reactive emotions, thoughts, and goals, Monica was able to see that she could help Michael get through a crisis, and Michael was able to see that he could help his mother to feel happy. These may seem like small "contributions," but for a family in crisis, they are major accomplishments because nothing is more important in a crisis than finding how to handle the stressor(s) so that safety and hope are regained.

The crisis was not just happening to Monica and Michael but also to Trish. Despite her silence and apparent detachment, Trish was watching carefully and feeling the intense distress that was escalating for and between her mother and brother. For Trish, the problem was that her father's violence in the past and her mother's anxiety were threatening to deprive her of the freedom to live a full and meaningful life. Monica clearly did not want her daughter to make the same, or similar, mistakes that she faulted herself for having made as an adolescent and young adult—particularly not to become involved with a boy or man who seemed charismatic at first but then turned out to be a bully and batterer. Monica's guilt for having been seduced and deceived by her ex-husband, and, as a result, exposing her children to his violence, was compounded by her personal sense of loss in having had her youth and young adulthood taken away by entrapment in that controlling, devaluing, and threatening relationship—as well as having lost the chance to have the genuinely happy and healthy family relationships that she had wished for as a wife and mother. Trish knew the general outline of that story, but just as Monica had done with her own mother, Trish was determined (and felt certain) that she would not make her mother's mistakes. However, Trish felt trapped by her mother's anxiety and what she saw as overprotectiveness and being deprived of the freedom to make her own choices and find the right path and relationships to have a fuller and more unequivocally pleasurable and successful life than she viewed her mother's life to be.

So, while Michael was embroiled in intrusive memories or flashbacks and Monica was preoccupied with rescuing him or getting him to pull himself together and act "appropriately," Trish was left as the third wheel, an outsider watching the drama—and with no one in the family reaching out to help her or watching over, and out for, her. The enmeshment experienced by Monica with Michael created an intergenerational coalition that unintentionally excluded Trish. Although in many ways, Trish wanted to be left out and not caught up in the anxiety and panic that her mother and brother were experiencing, she also did not want to be alone or without a family, which would most likely lead her to seek an alternative family in a peer group or (following the exact pattern she did not want to replicate from her mother's life) in an intense romantic relationship with a charismatic partner and an "us against the world" drama. Although this potential future crisis was only briefly alluded to in the current session, it represented just as serious a risk to Trish's ultimate safety and development as did the more immediate and obvious posttraumatic aftereffects that appeared in the form of Michael's dissociative episode.

As the therapist, I knew that it would be upsetting for the son and daughter to learn that their father was being released from prison. I also knew that although I could help them and their mother work through these reactions within the psychotherapy context, my presence as a man whom they did not know might complicate their reactions substantially. Their initial presentation—fairly relaxed but cautious on the part of Michael and mildly annoyed skepticism on the part of Trish—was consistent with how their mother had described them to me. Their first reactions to the news about their father—anxiety on Michael's part and anger and criticism on Trish's part—also were not a surprise. But when Michael abruptly panicked and became dissociated, I felt stunned and confused at first, even though I was well prepared based on advanced knowledge that each member of this family was at high risk of being intensely triggered in the session. I felt far from being able to act with calm confidence and to think clearly with presence of mind.

My first thought was, "What does Michael need to regain a sense of safety?" My immediate second thought was, "What do I need to be calm and confident enough to show Michael that he is safe?" My third thought was, "Monica and Trish are going to need reassurance that I can help Michael because I know that Monica is very protective of Michael." I also thought, "Trish is going to be judging whether she can trust me by how I help her brother recover from freaking out (as she pretends not to freak out)." Those four thoughts became my orienting focal thoughts.

As the session proceeded, I noticed a shift in my internal physical and mental state, feeling a sense of calm and an increasing ability to read and respond to each of the clients' microcommunications with empathic acknowledgment of their distress and the dilemmas as they saw them. I was not primarily concerned with managing or containing the "problem." Instead, I focused on joining with each client in collaboratively negotiating a major turning point in their life. I became aware of not only their distress but also of their courage and their remarkable ability to express their core values and hopes—albeit indirectly and obscured by a flood of fear and grief, In short, I saw the devil of the dilemmas they faced and also the better angels of each of their true selves.

As I reflect on what I did to make that shift in my perspective possible at the moments of crisis when it was most difficult be fully mindfully present and engaged with each of those clients, I believe I moved from an initial state of survival mode—shocked, perplexed, internally agitated and frozen—to an awareness of how my reactions were resonating with each of the clients' sense that the possibility of a recurrence of the past violence posed an existential threat. With that awareness as my focus, I was able to not just observe and react to their distress and confusion but to develop hypotheses attuned to the meaning that this experience was having for each client:

Looking back, I can see how in the midst of the ebb and flow of dissociation, panic, and impulsiveness that occurred as Michael and Monica reacted to the overarching trigger of past violence and current reminders, and to one another's emotion dysregulation, we were able to proceed through the five essential stages of crisis intervention in this session (see Chapter 5):

- Protecting (Step 1): My opening statement was an attempt to explicitly communicate that therapy is a safe place to deal with stressors and to build on and support positive life experiences and relationships. I also was implicitly communicating that the therapist's role is to keep everyone safe while in the session so that they can focus on working together to deal with challenges or problems that they need to face and overcome. Protection was a recurrent theme throughout this session, most obviously in Monica's repeated declarations that all of the family members needed to keep one another safe and that she, as their mother, was determined to protect all of them. On a subtler level, I attempted to help Monica to see that Michael was able to protect himself and needed coregulation and the security of her affirming presence rather than protective instructions or intrusion from her so that he could recover from dissociative panic episode. And Michael (and less obviously, but equally importantly, also Trish) needed protection from their mother's triggering anxiety and intrusiveness, while, as a result, Monica needed protection from inadvertent shame in the form of affirmation of her ability to care for and guide her children as a mother.

- Joining (Step 2): By framing the session as a collaborative decision by Monica and her therapist, and then deferring to her as the family leader until Michael's behavior signaled a crisis, I was joining with Monica in support of her as a mother and then with Michael as a guide to assist him in going through and coming out of the dissociative flashback. Although my explicit focus was on Michael when helping him to coregulate, I also was addressing most of my comments to him as implied statements to his mother (i.e., that her presence, confidence, support, and protection of Michael were helping him solve the problem posed by the intrusive memories) and to Trish (i.e., if it was possible for Michael to face and put away traumatic memories, this represented an alternative to avoidance and denial for her). Once the obvious crisis was resolved and Michael was able to connect with his mother and emotionally self-regulate, I intentionally returned to Trish's goal of greater freedom and independence, and Monica's counterbalancing goal of ensuring safety, to conclude the session by joining with each of them in service of their expressed goals.

- Shifting to present-centered focusing (Step 1): I helped Michael work through the dissociative flashback using a variety of modular tactics for present-centered focusing, including grounding (i.e., bodily self-awareness; repeated statements of my, and his mother's, protective and supportive presence), trigger reduction (i.e., reframing the disturbing internal experience as a memory that could be put away; assisting Monica in disengaging from intrusive escalation of Michael's distress and dissociation); strategic distraction and self-soothing (i.e., helping Michael to use self-touch as a form of self-soothing; reframing dissociative panic as productive work on a solvable problem); resilience building and positive self-talk (i.e., repeatedly emphasizing the "good work" that Michael and Monica were doing in handling the intrusive memories and in making sure they were physically safe from harm); and mindful metacognitive self-awareness (i.e., helping Monica to reflect on her focal goal of protecting her children and also strengthening their autonomous capacities for resilient self-protection and positive development).

- Partnering (Step 2): Throughout the session, I repeatedly affirmed my role as a partner for Monica in her role as her children's caregiver and leader of their family. I deferred to her initially in her dialogue with Trish, and I did not directly interfere with her attempts to physically and psychologically pull Michael out of the dissociative episodes, only stepping in to help when Michael's distress was escalating to a crisis level. When I stepped in, I was focused on not just helping Michael but also helping Monica to coregulate and to recognize the positive impact that her "mere" presence had for Michael to promote a sense of partnership while (paradoxically) interrupting Monica's anxiety-driven intrusion.

- Affirming resilience (Step 3): Most obviously, I focused my intervention with Michael on affirming his resilient capacity to face and "put away" troubling memories, and extended this to affirm his intention and ability to help his mother and sister be safe as well. I also repeatedly affirmed Monica's resilient ability to support and protect her children even when her actions might have seemed to contradict this view. My goal was not to gloss over problematic or triggering behavior by Monica but instead to focus her attention on how she could achieve her goals by focusing on coregulation and guidance of her children rather than instruction, criticism, or panic. In the session's closure period, it was important to reaffirm Trish's resilience by supporting the plan to have a discussion of how her mother could support her achieving her goal of freedom and independence.

- Affirming core values and priorities (Step 3): I attempted to allude to and show support for the core values and priorities of each client in virtually every interchange throughout this session. I also made a point of affirming the shared nature of these goals with all of the family members in agreement in principle about the importance of safety, security, trust, and cooperation as well as having a full and meaningful life, and showing and being shown respect. These are the polar opposites of the antivalues that are expressed by domestic violence (e.g., injury, harm, threat, coercion, dishonesty, betrayal, exploitation).

- Identifying meaningful options (Step 3): The most critical new options for this family in this session were to intentionally face and gain mastery of toxic memories rather than minimize or avoid such memories because of the distress they evoked. An associated new option was to coregulate rather attempt to suppress or vent strong emotions. An additional option that was repeatedly offered and tested was to view oneself and other family members as resilient and capable rather than as dysfunctional and problematic.

- Developing a collaborative action plan (Step 4): The explicit action plan was to continue to meet to fully resolve the emotional and relational difficulties that the family members were experiencing both on an ongoing basis (e.g., the mother–daughter conflict) as well as specifically in relation to the current trigger of the release of the ex-husband/father from prison. In addition, an implicit action plan was of equal or greater importance: This was to intentionally apply the new options to enhancing self-regulation and relationships.

- Accessing resources and ensuring continuity (Step 5): Although the primary overt resource was the therapy, a key implied resource to which the family members were beginning to have increased access was a sense of confidence in themselves and each other, and security in their relationships with one another. The family members were at a relatively early stage of both recognizing and being able to access these crucial implicit resources, so this will be a recurrent theme and goal for the family therapy going forward and for each family member's personal development in or outside of psychotherapy.

CONCLUSION

This session illustrated the value and perils of literally as well as psychologically joining with a client who is panic stricken by moving in physical proximity and using voice, body language, and words to convey a constant protective and nonthreatening presence—and also confidence in a dysregulated client's ability to successfully complete the important internal work they are doing. Thus, this was not a rescue of a helpless client who is unable to cope with distress but rather a partnership with and affirmation of a resilient and highly competent client who is working on solving a crucial problem. This redefinition of the client as courageous, dedicated, and effective, and of the problem as a solvable inner dilemma (in this case, putting bad memories away where they no longer cause unmanageable distress) fundamentally shifted the context from one of panic to one of intense determination and correspondingly intense emotional and physical reactions. The reframe was difficult for the adult to accept, and the teenager was skeptical, but the proof was in the 11-year-old's ability to regain calm and self-regulation. Joining with a client who is in a crisis of panic or dissociation can literally mean going to ground with the client while simultaneously shielding the client from intrusions, so long as this is done with consistent genuine affirmation of the client's resilience and hard work, and careful attention (and modeling and redirection when intrusion is an issue) of safe boundaries and personal space.

QUESTIONS FOR READER SELF-REFLECTION

- What are the potential benefits and the potential adverse consequences when a therapist literally joins a client by moving toward the client to establish proximity in a crisis?

- Why was it important for the therapist to not attempt to physically touch or hold Michael in this situation—and are there any circumstances in which physical touching or holding of a client in crisis could be done safely without violating professional and personal boundaries?

- Should the therapist have intervened earlier to help Michael cope with the anxiety that he clearly was feeling immediately after his mother's announcement about his father's release from prison?

- What were your first thoughts when Michael fell to the floor and appeared to be having a physical and psychological crisis that had the appearance of a panic attack or a seizure?

- Should the therapist have been more assertive or directive to stop Monica from pressuring Michael to stop "freaking out"—or to stop her from trying to make him stop scratching himself?

- What potential countertransference issues should the therapist be aware of? (These might include feeling worried or frustrated that Monica's reactions seem to be escalating Michael's distress, wanting to rescue and protect this family from the previously violent ex-husband/father, or feeling helpless to reach and comfort Michael when he became dissociated.)

12

DEFUSING VIOLENCE AND FACILITATING RECOVERY FROM PROFOUND DISSOCIATION

CASE BACKGROUND[1]

In Chapter 11, we met Monica and her teenage daughter, Trish, and 11-year-old son, Michael. In this vignette, Monica is bringing Trish to meet both with her and her individual psychotherapist as required by child protective services after an incident at their home that a neighbor reported to the police because the neighbor had heard screaming and loud smashing noises. Monica is furious with her daughter for what she considers to be Trish's defiant and irresponsible attitude and behavior, and embarrassed to have had the police called to their home. Trish is equally angry at her mother for "blowing everything out of proportion and trying to take away my freedom."

---

[1]To view the webinar associated with this case, including a video of the psychotherapy session, go online (https://learn.nctsn.org/enrol/index.php?id=512). Alternatively, you can go to the main website (https://learn.nctsn.org), click "Clinical Training" in the menu bar at the top of the page, click "Identifying Critical Moments and Healing Complex Trauma," and then click the webinar associated with this case: "Defusing Violence and Facilitating Recovery From Profound Dissociation." Although you will need to create an account ID and password, there is no fee to access the webinar.

https://doi.org/10.1037/0000225-013
Crises in the Psychotherapy Session: Transforming Critical Moments Into Turning Points, by J. D. Ford

Monica, Trish, and Michael had met with this same therapist earlier in a first family session so that Monica could tell her children that their father, Neil, was being released early from prison. Neil, from whom Monica is divorced, had been incarcerated for 5 years after a violent incident in which he had severely assaulted Monica. Neil had been physically abusive toward Michael and Trish as well as Monica for as long as Michael and Trish could remember. During that session, Trish said that she had never been seriously physically hurt by her father and that she "just puts the bad memories out of my mind, where they can't bother me." Trish had met with a different therapist for a few months after her mother filed domestic battering charges against Neil and had taken the children to a shelter so that they wouldn't have to live with Neil anymore. Trish said that the therapy was "okay— mostly a bunch of drawing and games. I don't remember what we talked about." Describing Trish as a girl growing up, Monica said that she was "really resilient. [Trish just] won't let anything or anyone stop her when she sets a goal, which can be quite a handful." She added, though, that "it's a sign that she's strong and healthy, that the violence by her father hasn't left her with any emotional baggage." At their first family session, Monica was concerned that Trish was having intense nightmares in which she screamed and sounded to Monica like she was fighting some kind of attacker. However, Monica reported that "when [Trish] wakes up she's totally fine, so it seems more like adolescent hormones and brain farts than anything to worry about."

Now it's been several months since that first family session, and things have gotten better for Michael but rockier between Monica and Trish. In that first session, Michael experienced an intense flashback and Monica became terrified, fearing that he was completely "losing it." Monica became progressively more agitated as Michael became more dissociated, and she repeatedly demanded and pleaded with Michael to get up and stop acting strangely. As she did this, Michael became increasingly agitated and detached, and started scratching himself. The therapist was able provide Monica with role modeling for how to nonintrusively connect with Michael and let him know that he was safe without communicating anxiety or criticism. Although Monica was skeptical, she could see that Michael seemed to relax and stopped scratching himself when the therapist gave him explicit permission to do whatever he needed to do to feel safe and told Michael that he was doing a very good job making the bad memories go away—while also calmly emphasizing that it was important to be careful not to hurt his body. As Michael gradually became calmer, the therapist was able to help him to touch his arms and legs in a way that was soothing. Monica also was able to calm herself, and the therapist helped her and Trish to both step back from arguing with one another and think of ways to support one another in achieving shared goals. For Monica, this involved knowing that Trish was not putting herself in danger by hanging out with "the wrong crowd," especially boys who were superficially charming but potentially abusive and controlling like Neil—in other words, to not make the same mistakes that Monica felt she had made in being with Neil. For Trish, this meant being able to be with the friends she chose without her mother criticizing both her and her friends, and forcing her to comply with restrictions that Trish felt confined her, made her look like she was still a child, and made her feel that her mother, rather than she, was controlling her life. By the close of the session, Trish and Monica felt as though they had reached a better understanding. The therapist referred Michael to a therapist colleague with expertise in doing trauma-focused cognitive behavior therapy, and Michael did well with this, enjoying the relaxation and emotion labeling skills, and creating a storybook that encapsulated the trauma memories involving his father's violence.

Things have generally gone well for the family in the months since the family therapy session. Michael feels reassured knowing that his mother and sister are safe, and that he is brave and has done a good job keeping helping them as safe as possible during the scary times—and that now he can get help if his father or anyone else is acting angry and scary. Michael is showing some signs of anxiety at school and occasional nightmares at night, and Monica is remembering to reassure and praise him for how well he's handling things. Michael is responding by being assertive at school and with peers, including going to friends' houses (which he had been avoiding). He also now calms himself and "debriefs" the next morning with his mother rather than needing to go immediately to his mother for reassurance following a nightmare. Monica and Trish almost always catch themselves if they start to argue or when they do things out of frustration—and to call time-out so they can sit down and talk and listen to each other.

A recent argument between Monica and Trish, though, led to visits from the police and then child protective services. This argument occurred when Monica received a phone call from Michael's school because Trish had not picked up her brother and brought him home after school. Monica had to leave work early to get Michael, who was very nervous and more agitated than Monica had seen him be for months. Monica tried to contact Trish on her cell phone several times, but Trish didn't pick up, and Monica went from being angry to feeling terrified that something had happened to Trish. Trish arrived home around midnight and was surprised to find her mother still awake and furious with her. Trish became angry and defensive, accusing her mother of "trying to ruin my life, putting down all my friends, and acting like I'm a dope fiend and a slut." Trish added, "What right do you have to tell me what to do or who to have as friends when you're the one who was the pothead and married a batterer?!"

The argument rapidly escalated into screaming, and Trish smashed dishes on the floor and knocked over a table and lamp, leading Monica to shriek, "You're crazy just like him! I want you out of this house right now before you kill someone!" Trish ran out, and Monica first yelled, "That's right! You better never be like that again in my house!" followed by, "Where do you think you're going? You can't just run away! It's not safe! I don't want you to get hurt! Oh, my god, what's happening?!" After walking around the block several times, Trish returned home to find the police at the house. Their presence somewhat reassured her but also embarrassed her and left her feeling that her mother would never understand or help her. When they had been arguing, Trish had felt a strong impulse to grab and shake mother, to make her see that she (Trish) was really a good person who wasn't going to make the same stupid mistakes she (her mother) had made. Instead, she had smashed the dishes and furniture, and had run out before her mother had come close enough for Trish to lash out at her. Trish was afraid (although she wouldn't admit it to anyone and tried not to think about it herself) that maybe she was just as messed up and had a temper just as violent and out of control as that of her father. Although Trish dreaded having to hear her mother criticize her in front of the therapist, secretly she felt reassured that the therapist would keep her mother in check "so we can get this over with." Monica came to the session feeling terrified that she was losing Trish, yet also enraged that Trish would be so irresponsible as to leave her brother alone and then try to make excuses.

SESSION TRANSCRIPT, ANNOTATIONS, AND COMMENTARY

Monica and Trish are attending this session on the order of child protective services after the loud argument at their home resulted in the police being called to ensure the family's safety.

THERAPIST: You've experienced something that's just like being in an earthquake. I don't know if you've ever been in an earthquake, but when that earthquake happens, you're not sure you're gonna come out of it alive. And then when it stops, it's really, really a moment you never forget, and then there are aftershocks, and I'm thinking that what may have happened here is one of those aftershocks. So, can we talk a little bit about what's happening? What has happened? Did you want to start, Monica?

Therapist's Inner Reflections: I want to put this incident of yelling and violence—which was dangerous but didn't involve either Monica or Trish's physically assaulting the other—in a context of the domestic violence that they had both experienced in the past so that they can think of this as a reaction to that past violence rather than because they fundamentally don't care about or respect each other. That should help me to help them to revive the bond of security that this incident shows has been seriously ruptured and that both of them need to recommit to honoring (for their own sense of security—being loved and safe personally—as well as for their relationship).

MONICA: Yeah. Um. Well (*sniffs*), I've been asking Trish to pick up Mikey after school so they can ride the bus together so he's not alone. It's important that he is not alone, especially on public transportation. We've still got a lotta things to worry about as far as, you know, we don't know where Neil is. I don't know what could happen.

Therapist's Inner Reflections: Monica is understandably vigilant about her children's safety based on their father's (her ex-husband's) past violent behavior, now that he's released from prison. Her reactive emotions and thoughts triggered by the reminders of the past violence and the current uncertainty make sense, but they also probably communicate a mix of weakness and overprotectiveness to a teenage daughter like Trish. I see Trish rolling her eyes in response. I'll validate Monica's legitimate uncertainty and concern before I invite Trish for her perspective.

THERAPIST: There's a restraining order, but you still can't be absolutely sure.

MONICA: Yeah. I mean, there's only so much protection we can have.

THERAPIST: Okay. So, this is very important to you.

MONICA: (*Sighs*) A few weeks ago, she didn't pick him up, and he called from school just very upset, crying, freaking out. I had to leave work early to go get him, which is not good for me, and then she was just gone. All day, she wasn't picking up her phone. She didn't tell me—I—I had no idea where she was. I had no idea what was going on. She walks in at, like, 11:30 at night, and I'm just asking her questions. Like, I need to know where she is. I need to know why she's gone all day, why she would do that to Mikey, why she would do that to me?

Therapist's Inner Reflections: Monica moved very rapidly from expressing her concern and goal of protecting her children to criticizing Trish for negligence and even intentionally hurting her. That puts Trish in a bad spot and certainly could trigger intense defensive reactions of anger and hurt that teenagers tend to express by adopting an attitude of contempt and disgust that is a major trigger for escalating distress by a parent—and potentially violent words or actions.

THERAPIST: So, Trish, your mom, if I'm hearing her correctly, was really scared. I imagine that she might've sounded pretty angry.

TRISH: She was.

THERAPIST: Hmm. Mm-hmm.

TRISH: But it wasn't a big deal. I was just going to hang out with my friends.

MONICA: No, it was a very big deal.

TRISH: No, it wasn't! That was it.

MONICA: You could've told me! You seriously don't understand the situation, do you?

THERAPIST: Hmm.

Therapist's Inner Reflections: I see how volatile this relationship has become. Helping them to see and take seriously each other's perspective is going to be very hard with Monica in survival mode and Trish adamantly asserting her right to freedom as a young adult. The middle path that might be acceptable to both of them is the strong bond they share emotionally. Their intensity is a reflection of that bond but also that the bond has been torn and distorted by the past violence, and could be further damaged by conflict that they're displacing onto one another.

MONICA: Like, we—I need you to be safe! I need you to take care of Mikey when I can't!

TRISH: Why do I need to take of Mikey? It's not my job!

MONICA: But we're all in this together!

Therapist's Inner Reflections: Monica is expressing a sound principle— we need to be together—but she's operationalizing it in the form responsibility that, as a healthy adolescent, Trish doesn't want to be burdened with. Trish wants to not do Monica's job as mother, but Monica interprets this as Trish's being unwilling to be a member of the family and to be a protective older sister. The issue is that Monica can't see Trish's need for autonomy because of her fear for their safety.

THERAPIST: Are you saying that because your ex-husband is out there that you are deeply worried about your children's safety?

MONICA: Yes.

THERAPIST: That's the situation.

MONICA: Yes.

TRISH: He's not gonna do anything!

MONICA: Oh. Ha!

TRISH: What is he gonna do?

MONICA: Take you.

THERAPIST: You don't think that's gonna happen.

TRISH: No!

THERAPIST: Hmm.

TRISH: If I'm with my friends, I'm with people. It's not like I'm by myself.

> *Therapist's Inner Reflections:* Trish is expressing a teenager's naive sense of invulnerability and the shift she's making from seeking security in her family to finding security in her peer group. She may be right that her father is unlikely to abduct or harm her, but Monica's concern about that shouldn't be dismissed because of the past history of violence and the current uncertainty with the family's equilibrium disrupted by the ex-husband/father's return to the community. I'm again going to try to find a middle path by not privileging either's view over the other's but instead focusing on helping each of them to have a better understanding of what's important to the other person that they can support so that they can actually partner rather than fight. I'm guessing that something was happening on the day of the incident that had a special meaning for Trish and was significant enough to her to justify not doing her "job" of watching over her brother.

THERAPIST: So, what happened this particular time, Trish? How come if you've been picking up your brother, is this different? Was there something different about this particular day?

TRISH: Yes!

THERAPIST: What was different?

TRISH: Someone asked me to go hang out.

THERAPIST: Oh. Is that not something that happens all the time?

TRISH: No, because I always have to pick up Mikey!

THERAPIST: Oh.

TRISH: That's my job.

THERAPIST: Hmm.

MONICA: You can go out afterwards, but you just need to let me know where you are. That is all I'm asking.

TRISH: You never let me!

MONICA: You stopped telling me what's going on! We had an agreement. An agreement!

TRISH: Well, I wonder why . . .

MONICA: You can go out . . .

TRISH: . . . you always freak out on me!

MONICA: I think I have a right to freak out.

> *Therapist's Inner Reflections:* I thought I was following them despite the ambiguity and surface contradictions—Trish says I want my freedom, Monica says fine but invokes her prerogative as a parent to put some restrictions on Trish with a bottom line of not being kept in the dark and having to worry about Trish—which Trish interprets as "you never let me" and protests the she shouldn't be controlled by her mother as an emerging adult. But I'm confused: What does it mean that Monica "freaks out," and why does Monica feel entitled to do so? There's clearly something more that they're talking around but not saying directly. Is Trish getting into an intense relationship that scares Monica? Or does Monica just want Trish to not grow up, and this relationship with a boy is taking her "little girl" away from her? I need to clarify, not to assume.

THERAPIST: Is there something about this someone that's of concern to both of you? This sounds like this is not just the average situation. Sounds like it's been working out, and yet here we have a time where it just didn't happen at all. Is there something about this particular someone, Trish?

TRISH: (*Shrugs shoulders*)

THERAPIST: Maybe.

TRISH: I guess.

THERAPIST: Okay. Is that a secret? You're talkin' about it like you both know, and I'm the only one who doesn't know, and I don't need to . . .

MONICA: She has a boyfriend.

THERAPIST: Oh! Okay.

MONICA: Yeah.

THERAPIST: Well, that sounds like something that could be a good thing, but it could also . . .

MONICA: Not in this case.

THERAPIST: . . . be a worry.

TRISH: Not to her it's not.

MONICA: Not in this case.

> *Therapist's Inner Reflections:* Monica has shifted from being worried, angry, and disappointed to having a look of steely determination. Although I need to be cautious and not simply join with her in a way that will feel to Trish like being ganged up on, Monica's demeanor signals to me that she's not just worried based on past bad experiences but that she may be seeing danger signs that are real and that her experience as a survivor of intimate partner violence may make her able to more acutely and accurately detect than someone without that adverse history. I could write off Monica as an overprotective mother who is overcompensating based on her own past victimization, but that would be a serious disservice to her and to Trish as well. There is ample evidence of intergenerational vulnerability to victimization, and Trish is especially at risk for that if I undermine her mother's credibility by discounting her concerns. That could inadvertently signal to Trish that I take her side and minimize the potential danger in this relationship because I think that Trish is stronger and wiser than her mother. I really don't want to make that mistake.

THERAPIST: What are you worried about, Monica? What's your concern?

TRISH: Yeah, what are you worried about?

MONICA: I'm worried about how you're changing.

TRISH: Me?

MONICA: Yes.

TRISH: How I'm changing.

MONICA: Yes.

TRISH: Okay.

MONICA: And I think I know exactly why you're making some of those changes. I see you leave home wearing something that changes in the middle of the day.

TRISH: (*Expression is incredulous.*) *What*?!

MONICA: Yeah. Yeah. And I don't know . . .

TRISH: *What* are you even talking about?

MONICA: Um.

TRISH: (*Speaks shrilly*) Do you hear her?

> *Therapist's Inner Reflections:* Monica's really touched on a raw nerve for Trish, apparently saying that Trish is trying to appeal to her boyfriend by changing how she dresses when she's going to be with him. That could be innocuous—just a teenager's attempt to be pretty in the eyes of a flame and with her peers. But it could be one of the red flags for intimate partner coercion if Trish feels she has to dress or act in certain ways to be approved of by a controlling boyfriend. I need to understand how much of Trish's outrage is because Monica is reading too much into her behavior and how much is because Trish doesn't want to see that her mother has a valid concern.

THERAPIST: I hear it.

TRISH: (*Looks outraged*) She's so crazy.

MONICA: (*Escalates*) You—you leave . . .

TRISH: (*Further escalates*) Are you kidding me?

MONICA: (*Looks outraged*) No. No, don't do that. You do not get to do that to me.

TRISH: (*Expression is defiant.*) No.

> *Therapist's Inner Reflections:* I worried that they were losing control and escalating into the kind of incident that is the reason we're meeting. I couldn't stand by and let that happen. I almost stepped in to be the voice of calm and reason, but I'm glad I didn't because that would have been more for my own benefit than theirs. Yes, my concern is genuine but also (I must admit) is driven by a fear that I'm failing to do my job and not wanting to seem neglectful. What I learned by waiting watchfully instead was that they are able to catch themselves and de-escalate. I'll look for opportunities to point that strength out to

them, but at the moment, it's best that they continue to carry on with this difficult discussion without my interrupting.

MONICA: You know exactly what I'm talking about.

TRISH: (*Expression is defiant.*) No, I don't.

MONICA: (*Voice is angry but contained.*) Yes, you do.

TRISH: (*Expression is defiant.*) So, why don't you explain it to me.

MONICA: You leave home in sensible clothes and then, you know, you go to pick up Mikey, you're wearing, like, crop tops and all sorts of crazy shit. Like, who's telling you to do that?

TRISH: I wear what I want.

MONICA: (*Tone is skeptical.*) Do you?

TRISH: Yes. Yes, I do.

MONICA: You do? 'Cause you've never worn that stuff before.

TRISH: Maybe I didn't feel comfortable wearing it around you because you'll judge me all the time.

MONICA: You know what? I wouldn't have a prob—why, why are you hiding it though? You don't need to hide that from me.

TRISH: (*Expression is defiant.*) I'm not hiding anything!

MONICA: (*Escalates*) Yes, you are!

TRISH: (*Further escalates*) No, I'm not!

MONICA: (*Further escalates*) Yes, you are!

TRISH: (*Further escalates*) No, I'm not!

Therapist's Inner Reflections: I'm uncertain if this is the right time, but I'm going to step in so that the key question that Monica is asking—about Trish hiding a secret—doesn't get lost in the repetitive contest of accusation and denial ("Yes, you are"–"No, I'm not"). This is not because I'm worried that their escalating conflict will become a crisis. It's to help them find shared ground based on recognizing what they actually agree on instead of seeing each other as the enemy.

THERAPIST: Monica, what are you worried about? What, what does the clothing mean? From your experience. It may not be true for Trish, but what's it mean from your experience?

TRISH:	And it's not true.
THERAPIST:	What's it mean from your experience?
MONICA:	It's just not a good sign if . . .
THERAPIST:	Of what?
MONICA:	Of—it's—it's a controlling guy.
THERAPIST:	Oh. So, you think Trish's boyfriend is telling her how to dress and telling her to dress in a way that is kind of sexy.
MONICA:	Yes, among other things.
THERAPIST:	Have you had experiences in your life where that happened to you?
MONICA:	Yes.
THERAPIST:	And did it turn out badly?
MONICA:	Yes!
THERAPIST:	(*Speaks to Monica*) Okay, you're concerned. You're deeply concerned. (*Turns to Trish*) But you don't wanna be put into a box because something's happened to your mom.
MONICA:	(*Speaks plaintively*) No, you don't—you're not understanding the situation.

Therapist's Inner Reflections: Monica's signaling she's feeling abandoned and let down by me. I intended to provide a balanced view, summarizing both her and Trish's perspectives as valid. But I made a mistake by implying that Monica's concern was just based on her own past experience and not on a genuine problem in the present. I'm frustrated with myself and feeling flustered.

THERAPIST:	What's—what's the deal?
MONICA:	You're not understanding this. You're not understanding this. No . . .
TRISH:	(*Escalates*) No!
MONICA:	. . . you need to listen for a second.
THERAPIST:	I might not be understanding.

Therapist's Inner Reflections: Now I sound really pathetic. I'm trying to think how to throw a lifeline to Monica and restore her confidence in me, but I feel like a pinball in the arcade with Monica and Trish pulling the levers and me just bouncing around and at a loss for what to say.

MONICA: (*Pleads*) Okay?

TRISH: He *is* listening to you.

MONICA: (*Looks despondent and is almost wailing*) No. No. No.

TRISH: You're the one that's being a lunatic.

MONICA: Stop it. She got her hair cut . . .

Therapist's Inner Reflections: I think I need to stop trying to find the right thing to say and just listen and focus entirely on understanding what Monica needs me—and Trish—to understand. They need a calm, empathic presence now, not any "brilliant" therapeutic words or strategy.

THERAPIST: Okay.

MONICA: . . . a few weeks ago.

THERAPIST: Fill me in. Mm-hmm.

TRISH: So?

MONICA: Okay? It looked fantastic. You were very happy. You were so psyched about this beautiful, new haircut. Then you come back 2 days later crying about your hair.

THERAPIST: Hmm.

TRISH: Well, maybe because I didn't like it anymore.

MONICA: What made you change your mind?

TRISH: I just didn't like it anymore. Why can't that be enough for you?

Therapist's Inner Reflections: Monica's being quite the prosecuting attorney, drawing out the defendant to prove her case. Monica's feeling stronger and not desperate, which is good. But Trish is deflating rather than calming and working hard to resist despite apparently recognizing that her mother is voicing a valid concern. The problem is getting clearer, but the relationship is still very unsteady, leaving them both feeling more, not less, insecure. I'm looking for a chance to help them find a middle ground where they can work on this together rather than as adversaries.

MONICA: He doesn't like your hair, does he?

TRISH: I don't know.

THERAPIST: And what does that mean?

MONICA: See?

THERAPIST: To you, what does that mean?

MONICA: That means he is not a good guy.

TRISH: Just because he doesn't like my hair?

MONICA: Yes.

TRISH: (*Looks outraged*) What? Are you kidding me? Are you serious?

THERAPIST: I think—I think your mother is talking about her past experience, and you're telling her it's not the same, right?

MONICA: It's a sign of abuse.

TRISH: (*Responds emphatically*) No, it's not!

MONICA: It's a sign of abuse.

TRISH: (*Escalates*) No, it's not! You don't know him!

MONICA: Yes, it's the beginning of it.

TRISH: (*Escalates*) Are you kidding me?

MONICA: First of all, he's a teenage boy, okay?

TRISH: And what does that mean?

MONICA: They suck.

TRISH: There—there's a lotta teenage boys.

MONICA: Yeah, there are.

TRISH: There's a lot of them.

MONICA: And there are a lot of really nice boys that would . . .

TRISH: Like him!

MONICA: (*Responds emphatically*) No. No. Oh, no.

TRISH: But you wouldn't know that because you've never gotten to know him.

MONICA: (*Responds emphatically*) No. No. You should not be with somebody that's gonna make you cry over your haircut. You should not be with somebody who's gonna try and tell you that the way you dress is not acceptable. You should not be with somebody who's trying to change you.

TRISH: (*Responds emphatically*) He doesn't!

MONICA: What do you mean? So, you're making all of these decisions on your own?

TRISH: Yes.

MONICA: See, 'cause your haircut was your decision. Was your decision.

TRISH: And I decided I didn't like it anymore. Why is that not okay for you? Why do you have to make it . . .

MONICA: Why are you lying to yourself?

TRISH: . . . all about you and your own . . .

MONICA: No, you're lying to yourself.

TRISH: . . . experiences because it's not mine!

MONICA: I'm not (*Sighs*) s—okay. I'm just trying . . .

TRISH: (*Responds emphatically*) No. Uh-uh.

MONICA: . . . to look out for you, okay? I do not wanna see you make the same mistakes that I did. I don't want you to be—I don't (*speaks tearfully*)—I just really, really don't want you to be with somebody that's going to hurt you. There are signs. There are big, fucking, red flags.

Therapist's Inner Reflections: I appreciate how hard Monica is trying to show Trish that this is coming from a place of caring for her and wanting to protect her. I think Trish is having a hard time with this because she's felt she has had to put up a wall to defend against her mother's intensity, and she's not getting the message that Monica supports her in living her own life.

TRISH: Why is this always about you?

MONICA: It's not about me.

TRISH: It always comes back to you.

MONICA: What are you talking about?

TRISH: You and your relationship.

MONICA: (*Speaks plaintively*) It's about you. No, this is about you and this is about me protecting you. This is about me protecting all of us.

> *Therapist's Inner Reflections:* The shift in power balance is really striking: One moment Monica seems very much in control and authoritative while Trish is back on her heels trying to resist, but now Monica is pleading, and Trish feels she must take the opportunity to get the upper hand. This is eerily similar to an abusive intimate partner relationship, so I think that pathological context that the domestic violence created for this family in the past is flooding into this mother–daughter relationship now. They're both feeling unsafe and viewing each other as the threat rather than as an ally, and now Monica seems to be backing down rather than finding a way they both can win.

TRISH: (*Speaks defiantly*) You let this happen. I wouldn't be in this position if it weren't for you!

MONICA: Okay. I'm sorry. I'm sorry that you don't get to be a normal teenager. I'm sorry that you have to do these extra things so that we can all stay safe. Okay? I am sorry. I didn't know. I didn't know. Now I know, which is why I don't think it's okay for you to be doing this stuff. I see it. I see it. I see it. It is not okay. Do not do this. (*Speaks plaintively*) Please don't do this.

THERAPIST: So, the questions is how do you as a mother stop your daughter from doing something that might be dangerous?

> *Therapist's Inner Reflections:* I should have said "help your daughter be safe," not "stop her"—I need to make a course correction so I don't escalate Trish's sense of being coerced by Monica.

MONICA: I just . . .

THERAPIST: That's—that's a tough one because I don't think that giving orders is probably going to cut it, and, yet, I don't think that's what you're intending to do.

MONICA: So, how would you deal with this? Do you have any daughters?

> *Therapist's Inner Reflections:* Sounds like I overcorrected. Monica's feeling criticized by me. I'll have to walk a fine line by being open but not letting this become about me as a parent.

THERAPIST: I do.

MONICA: Okay. How old are they?

TRISH: Why does it matter?

MONICA: It matters. How old are they?

THERAPIST: For right now, I think we need to talk about the two of you.

MONICA: No. Tell me. Tell me. You have taught—you have daughters.

TRISH: No, you're being insane.

MONICA: How many daughters?

TRISH: You're being crazy.

MONICA: How many daughters?

> *Therapist's Inner Reflections:* I get Monica's point that a parent is protective of their teenage daughter especially when it comes to the possibility of her being victimized. Her interrogation feels really intrusive, which is very uncomfortable, but I think it gives me a sense of what it may be like for Trish when Monica is pressing her to agree or comply with her. I can model how to maintain my privacy and the boundaries of our relationship, but I also need to let Monica know that I'm aware of why this is so important for her, including not feeling powerless to prevent harm from coming to her daughter. I'll have to be careful not to appear to align with her against Trish and to communicate to Trish that the pressure she feels from her mother is understandably triggering for her—and that that is equally as important as Monica's concern about safety.

THERAPIST: I think it's important that we talk about the two of you.

MONICA: Teenage daughters?

THERAPIST: I hear you, Monica.

MONICA: Did you have any teenage daughters that went through severe trauma . . .

THERAPIST: At this point in time . . .

MONICA: What are d—do you have—you don't seem to understand, do you? I—I don't understand how you're doing this right now. You know how incredibly dangerous the situation is. You know what we've gone through.

THERAPIST: I certainly know what you've gone through. I absolutely do.

MONICA: Excuse me?

THERAPIST: I certainly know what you've . . .

TRISH: Ha!

THERAPIST: . . . gone through, and I also know what you're trying to protect your daughter from going through. Absolutely. You make
complete sense about that. But I . . .

MONICA: This is not okay.

THERAPIST: . . . but I also think that we're at a difficult position here
because you're fighting to protect your daughter and (*turns to
Trish*) you're fighting to preserve your life, your freedom, but
you're fighting each other.

> *Therapist's Inner Reflections:* I'm finding it really difficult to help
> Monica and Trish slow this down just enough to remember that they
> can trust and support one another. The reactive feelings of fear and
> anger are just exploding, and I don't know how to help them out of
> this black hole.

MONICA: I'm trying to preserve her life and her freedom. She's about to,
like, get locked in to—god, god I can't—I just can't do it, okay?
'Cause I . . .

THERAPIST: It's asking a lot to even consider that Trish might be okay with
this boyfriend, but, Trish, I really think your mom is making
an important point here. She—it's not about this particular
young man. I don't know him.

TRISH: Yes, it is.

MONICA: No, it is about this particular young man.

THERAPIST: It's not . . .

TRISH: It is about this young man.

MONICA: No, it is.

THERAPIST: . . . just about this particular young man.

TRISH: It is . . .

MONICA: No, it is.

TRISH: . . . about this guy. It's all about this guy.

MONICA: It is!

TRISH: It's always been about this . . .

MONICA: Because he's a piece of shit!

TRISH: How do you know?

MONICA: I don't need to know that much. All I need to know are those two things. You can hate me. You can do whatever you want. But I do not want you throwing your life away getting into a situation that's . . .

TRISH: I'm not!

MONICA: . . . potentially dangerous among all this other shit that's going on.

Therapist's Inner Reflections: Well, that was a not helpful intervention on my part. Now instead of looking past the specific boyfriend and seeing that they need to find common ground, they're locked even more tightly into this "I'm right—no, I'm right" battle of the wills. It's getting ugly.

THERAPIST: I think what's happening right now might not be entirely okay either.

MONICA: Excuse me?

THERAPIST: I think what's happening right now might not be entirely okay for you two.

MONICA: What is that?

THERAPIST: The fact that this has become a fight between the two of you when it's really about something and someone else.

MONICA: That doesn't make any sense.

THERAPIST: I know it probably doesn't seem like it makes any sense, but I hear you fighting to protect each other, to preserve your life.

TRISH: Is this guy helping you? Is this gonna fix all your problems? Is this really what you want?

Therapist's Inner Reflections: That came out of left field and caught me off guard! But it makes sense: Monica is angry with me; she feels abandoned and betrayed—that I let her down. Trish recognizes that and sees it as a way out of this therapy: If I'm useless, then they can make me and therapy the focus of shared anger. Then they're on the same side again, and Trish can avoid further conflicts with her mother in which she is put on the hot seat by Monica.

MONICA: I just want you to be safe, okay? I've seen a lot of shit. I've gone through a lot of shit. I am so sorry that you have gone through all of this.

TRISH: But that doesn't mean that it's my life. It's your life, but it's not mine.

MONICA: No—okay. You can have a life. I want you to have a life. I want you to have a wonderful life and as—as safe . . .

Therapist's Inner Reflections: Monica did a great job of refocusing on Trish's well-being and safety, and then supporting Trish's desire for autonomy. But Trish doesn't trust that to last.

TRISH: Then act like it.

MONICA: Because—this is not what you need! This is not what you need right now!

TRISH: How do you know what I need?

MONICA: I know you need to be safe, and I know you need to be with somebody that loves you and cares about you and supports you.

TRISH: I am safe and with someone that loves me . . .

MONICA: No, you are not. No, you are not.

TRISH: . . . unlike you.

MONICA: No, it's your job to not do what I did.

TRISH: If we're over it, then why do you keep bringing it up?

MONICA: Because you're doing what I did!

TRISH: (*Turns and leans pointedly toward her mother*) No, I'm not!

Therapist's Inner Reflections: This is not good. They're stuck in the power struggle again. I don't want to intrude after they've both told me to stay out of their conversation because I don't understand and I'm not helpful. But this is escalating even more rapidly, and I'm concerned.

MONICA: (*Sits up defensively*) Yes, you are!

TRISH: (*Gets up, starts to walk out of the office*) No. I'm not doing this anymore.

MONICA: (*Gets up, reaches to hold her daughter from behind by both shoulders*) Yes, you are. You can't—you can do the–don't you dare walk away from me.

TRISH: (*Turns to face her mother, arches her back, lunges, and pushes her mother forcefully back onto the couch*) Are you kidding me?

MONICA: (*Falls backward onto the couch, gasps*)

Therapist's Inner Reflections: This is really bad! I don't want the physical aggression to go any further, I have to step in.

THERAPIST: (*Stands up, puts his hand lightly on Trish's shoulder*) Trish. Trish.

TRISH: (*Turns away from the therapist and her mother, steps back, walks forcefully toward the office door*) No. Get off'a me.

Therapist's Inner Reflections: Trish's assertive reaction was right on. My physical contact with her was a mistake, even as a gentle reminder to her to calm down. Now I need to use words and my voice to help all three of us stay (or, for Monica, return to being) present. I want to restore a sense of calm by slowing things down and reminding them that we're still here together, and we're going to find a way through the hurt and anger that brings them together to a safer place.

THERAPIST: (*Remains standing in place; turns to partially face both Monica and Trish; speaks in a soft, hypnotic voice*) Okay. Just slow it down. Slow it down. Slow it down. Monica? I'm right here. Trish? We're right here just for a moment. That was a big, big explosion, but you're both okay. We're all here together. We're gonna find a way through this. I know it sounds like I don't understand, and I probably don't, but I see two women who care very deeply about each other and are also very, very hurt by violence, and I see how important it is that there be no more violence and no more hurt. I don't think that either of you intends to hurt the other at all. (*Turns to Monica*) You're trying so hard to protect your daughter and your family to make sure that you (*turns to Trish*) can make the choices that are right for you, Trish.

Therapist's Inner Reflections: I'm tracking Trish with brief moments of eye contact to signal that I'm staying with her but not being intrusive. I'm also speaking to Trish indirectly while I speak directly to Monica to help her gradually come back from the dissociated state she fell into when she literally fell back onto the couch after Trish lunged at her. I'm starting with a reframe: that what happened was scary for both of them, but it was not based on an intent to hurt one another, and the hurt they're both feeling can be repaired. I want to emphasize that they're both resilient survivors of violence, and this is a chance to join together in supporting each other in recovery from that.

THERAPIST: Right now, we just need to regroup for a moment. I know it's really scary, but I'm here and your daughter's here. It's going to be alright. I know it's a scary place where you're going now, but you can come back. Trish is right here and I'm here.

There's not gonna be any more violence. No more. No more. You've worked so hard to make that true, and you've made it true. It's truer than you realize, but right now, you just need to be here in the room. Your daughter's still right here. I know you can't see her, but she's right here. She hasn't left. She's not gone. She's doing a really good thing. Thank you for staying with us, Trish. I know this is very hard. You don't wanna give up what's important to you, but staying here is really important, so thank you.

Therapist's Inner Reflections: Now I want to help Monica come out of the dissociative state, and I think helping her feel more connected to Trish right in the moment is the best way to do that.

THERAPIST: Monica, Trish is here because she really is listening to you, but she's got to speak her piece, too. We'll figure that out—not right now, but we'll figure that out. She's hearing you, and she's here for you, and she knows that you're here for her. Just keep breathing. Just remember we're here together. We're gonna figure this out.

Therapist's Inner Reflections: Monica's still dissociated but seems calmer and gradually more oriented. I can reach out to Trish, let her know I appreciate her staying with us and that she needs to keep her distance. Then I can shift back to helping Monica reorient to the present.

THERAPIST: Trish, if, if you'd like to come back in at any point over—over here, you're more than welcome. You don't have to. I understand. You needed some space. You got it. I'm s—I'm sorry if I did anything that felt wrong to you. I really do wanna be careful for both of you. (*Trish slowly walks back toward the couch and tentatively stands aside her mother. The therapist looks at Monica, then at Trish.*) Just breathe. Just feel. You know where you are. Your daughter's right here. Great to have you back, Trish. Thank you. We'll just sit together for a moment— kind of breathe and just regroup.

Therapist's Inner Reflections: Trish is coming back, so I can affirm their bond with each other and again that they're both survivors who are working hard to make a good life, not perpetrators. And to do that, they need to face the past together when it intrudes on their current lives in the form of the kind of angry emotional confrontations that just led to a physical confrontation—and commit to not letting that violence come between them and cause hurt, emotional or physical.

THERAPIST: I see so much caring between the two of you. So much hurt and so much anger, but I don't think that that's what you've done to each other. It's what's happened to both of you, and you're both working so hard to have the right kinda life with the right kind of young man and the right kind of family. I think there's a way to do that, but we've gotta figure out a way to just close the chapter and the book on the past. You're doing that Monica. You're workin' really hard, and I'm sorry.

Therapist's Inner Reflections: I think they're both feeling sorry to have said and done hurtful things to each other. That can be painful to realize, when the inner alarm turns down and calmer reflective thought kicks back in. If I model a way to apologize while not taking on blame or shame—which is genuinely what I am feeling because I know I made mistakes as the anger escalated—that can help each of them see that taking responsibility does not involve blame or shame.

THERAPIST: I know it seemed like I didn't understand, and we can talk about what I know and what I don't know, but what's most important now is you're here. Trish, are you—I can see you're just kinda not sure which way to go. Are you worried that your mom is gonna be really upset 'cause you pushed her?

Therapist's Inner Reflections: I don't expect that Trish will answer that directly, nor does she have to, but my saying it takes that burden off of her and signals to Monica that Trish needs her reassurance—which is what Trish has been asking for, without saying it directly, this whole time.

TRISH: (*Walks slowly, unsurely, back to the edge of the couch on which her mother is sitting, looks at her mother questioningly, then looks away, then leans gradually toward her mother, and walks closer until she is within arm's length of her mother and is tearful*)

MONICA: (*Reaches out, gently pulls Trish toward her, and embraces and enfolds Trish as they sit together, tearfully*) Come here.

THERAPIST: Okay.

MONICA: It's okay. Come here. It's okay. It's okay.

Therapist's Inner Reflections: Monica is back now, too. I'll just confirm that for them with a few brief words and not interrupt their private experience of coming back together.

THERAPIST: That's what we're talking about.

MONICA: I love you so much. It's gonna be okay. Okay.

THERAPIST: She's here, Monica. She's right here. So are you.

MONICA: You're a good girl, okay? I just want you to be safe. Okay? I love you so much.

> *Therapist's Inner Reflections:* Monica's remembering what's really most important to her: that she hasn't lost Trish, that she's been able to protect Trish even though they've been through the hell of domestic violence, and they're on the roller coaster of a daughter becoming a woman.

THERAPIST: You haven't lost her. You've held real tight, and you haven't lost her, and that's where we could start from.

MONICA: Okay. I'm sorry. I'm sorry. I love you. It's gonna be okay. Okay.

THERAPIST: It's great to see you both back.

MONICA: Okay. Don't be scared, okay?

TRISH: It's okay.

MONICA: I need you to work with me, okay? Okay. I hope I didn't scare you. I love you. Okay?

> *Therapist's Inner Reflections:* This is a good rapprochement, and it can be the beginning of a new way for them of handling conflict. For now, I just want to support them in imprinting the memory of how it feels to be truly together so that can be a lasting shared orienting thought.

Monica's and Trish's Observations

Monica described her hopes for the session and reflections on what actually happened in the session as follows:

> During this session, I was hoping to get help in talking to Trish—in getting her to understand where I'm coming from and understand the situation. I wanted her to see that I'm not trying to be the bad guy. The most challenging part of the session was my struggle with some of the therapist's responses. I have felt supported in previous sessions with him but wasn't feeling supported in this session. It felt like he was taking her [Trish's] side, like I wasn't being listened to, and the situation was being minimized.

Monica continued by saying,

> I was really shocked and surprised that Trish pushed me, especially because there had never been any physical aggression in our relationship. I'm worried that this was another blowup like she did when she was smashing things and

screaming at me on that night when the police were called, and I don't understand where all that anger comes from and why she can't control herself—it reminds me of my abusive ex—but I can't believe Trish would be like him in that way. When she blew up this time and pushed me down, what helped in the moment was the therapist reminding me where I was: that we were in a safe space and that Trish was right there with me. I realized that I had been so angry and scared about her getting trapped in abusive relationship with that boyfriend that I was doing exactly the opposite of what I intended: criticizing and lecturing her instead of showing her how much I value our relationship, letting her know that I love and appreciate her.

Trish described her hopes for the session and reflections on what actually happened in the session as follows:

In this session, I was hoping to get my mom to understand where I'm coming from and to not pin everything on a boy or my dad. When things get heated between my mom and me, I feel like my mom shuts down and doesn't think or process what I'm saying. She wasn't listening to me, and I kept trying to force her to understand where I'm coming from. When I moved away from the sofa, I just needed to get away from everything that was going on—away from the anger and tension, and to take a break from everything. I could feel my mom breaking down, like she wasn't her normal self. It felt like she was disappearing.

Trish continued by saying,

When I got up to leave and she grabbed me, I pushed back harder than I should have. I was so angry that I just lost it like I did when I smashed the dishes the night the police were called. I was thinking,

> It's always all about you. You say you care and you trust me, but you really think I'm going to make you look bad, and you act like I'm just rotten and evil to the core like my father. I know that's what you think, and I hate you. You have to stop treating me like that. You're making me be like him just like you made him be so horrible and mean. It's all because you make people feel like they're nothing. . . .

I don't really think my mom treats people that way or that she is to blame for my father's anger, but at that moment, I felt so overwhelmed and confused that those thoughts just sort of took over and I wanted to run away and lash out at the same time. Really, I'm worried that I'm too much like my mom and my dad, making stupid choices about who to be with because I put myself down and feel like nobody would want to be with me, and then getting so angry that I say mean things or get out of control and smash things so people do think I am crazy or just trouble.

Trish added that,

In the session, when I lost it, I was just about to run out the door, when I looked back, and the calm aura of the therapist helped to de-escalate the situation. He helped us—me and my mom both—get on the same level so we could understand each other and listen. Then I felt like I was back to my real self again, and my mom was, too, so I could reach out to her and trust her, which was all I wanted to begin with. I know we have a lot of work to do to make things right again, and I feel guilty that I was so mean, but I need her to understand that I have my own life, and she can't keep treating me like a child or get in my business, when she should just trust me and let me handle it.

Commentary

As the therapist in this dramatized therapy session, I found myself almost constantly confronted by dilemmas for which there didn't seem to be any right answer. I tried to act as if I always knew what I was doing and to project a sense of calm confidence that I hoped would help both Monica and Trish to coregulate with me when they were going from the peaks to the valleys of feeling hurt and hurtful, angry and attacked, guilty and blaming, and enmeshed and abandoned. I'm not sure that anything I did until I was bringing both of them back after the sudden physical altercation was getting through to either of them or was helping. But, looking back at the session, I can see a progression that may have laid the groundwork for that rapprochement, even though I wasn't able to prevent the escalation of their mutually triggering dysregulation from becoming a crisis.

The session began with my providing a context that I hoped helped both Monica and Trish to view the recent crisis incident at their home as an aftershock from which they could recover and that we could find ways to prevent from recurring. Monica seemed to feel safe enough with that protective context and with me as a guide to join with me by describing the beginning of the crisis incident clearly from her perspective. When Trish minimized the seriousness of her mother's concern about safety, Monica became dysregulated, and I was able to help her to refocus on the immediate issue (and to get some distance, temporarily, from the larger issues and fears in which she was beginning to become lost) by engaging Trish in describing the specific incident from her point of view. Fairly quickly, Trish identified the issue as her feeling that her mother was not letting her have the freedom to be with her friends, and both Trish and Monica became intense and then dysregulated, debating the issue in generalities that were vague and extreme, and that seemed to imply a disagreement about Trish's choice of a particular friend. I asked for clarification, and Monica launched into an extended critical analysis, implying that Trish's new boyfriend was controlling and abusive, for which she provided some telling but not definitive circumstantial evidence.

I commented on the parallel to Monica's own experience with her ex-husband to suggest that Monica's experience made her concerns worth considering but that they also needed to be taken with caution because she might be projecting characteristics of her ex onto the boyfriend (although I didn't use that technical and potentially pejorative term to describe the caution). I said to Monica, "Okay, you're concerned. You're deeply concerned." I then turned to Trish and said, "But you don't wanna be put into a box because something's happened to your mom." Monica reacted to my statement as showing a lack of understanding on my part and began to become more dysregulated. I (with Trish also contributing, albeit in an oppositional tone) was able to acknowledge that I might not be understanding and to encourage Monica to "fill me in." She became calmer temporarily, but then both she and Trish escalated into dysregulation and debated whether the signs of a controlling/abusive relationship were present. As Monica asserted this view, Trish responded with disbelief that her mother was being unfairly judgmental and trying to interfere in her life in a way that Trish felt was demeaning and controlling—saying that Monica was imposing her (Monica's) own issues and mistakes onto her (Trish). At this point, it seemed to me that both Monica and Trish had valid points, but they were communicating their views in the form of criticisms of the other (and feeling both assaulted and invalidated by the other) rather than as perceptions or goals that they could join together to deal with. So, my focus shifted to helping them to step back, refocus on the value and importance of their relationship with each other, and redefine the problem as finding a way to restore their mutual trust and the potential solution as talking together about how to support one another by drawing on their strengths as people and as a team to achieve both of their priorities. To not overcomplicate this idea, I framed the message as the need to disengage from fighting each other to "protect each other."

Before I got there, however, I made what I still think was a mistake: I described what Monica was doing as "giving orders" to Trish. Although I caught myself immediately and tried to soften the blow by asserting that this was not Monica's intent, she clearly heard the thinly veiled criticism. This is a clear example of a countertransference enactment on my part, which shows that such enactments can seep into what seems like an innocuous choice of a single phrase. Her response was to insist that I disclose whether I'd had any similar experiences as a father with the implication (that she ultimately made explicit) that I didn't understand the situation and that I should not be challenging her when she was trying to get Trish to recognize the danger she faced. This probably undermined Trish's confidence in me, which was not great to begin with, leaving her feeling more alone in defending herself against her mother's criticisms and in resisting her mother's attempts to control her choices. From that point until the physical altercation, I tried to reframe the problem so that it was not whether the boyfriend was a good or bad person. Instead, I tried to focus on the importance of Trish's being able to be safe and respected in her relationship with her boyfriend while also having a mutually supportive relationship with her mother. However, I was not a credible voice for either client. However, it is possible that some of my attempts to help Monica and Trish refocus from fighting each other to recalling their bond and finding common ground did get through to them, and that may have helped them to be receptive to my help after the altercation.

When Trish said she was finished and jumped up, I believe she was making a good choice to disengage from the escalating conflict, and physical separation may have been the only way that she could reduce the intense input and cognitive/affective load of processing her own internal experience. Monica further triggered Trish by physically grabbing and holding her back. This literally was a replication of the aggressive physical domination that Trish had witnessed and directly experienced when her father was abusive in the past as well as a metaphorical enactment of the psychological/emotional restraint that Trish felt Monica was exerting to hold her back from having her own life and trapping her in Monica's dysfunctional (from Trish's perspective) life. Trish's reaction of pushing back was self-defensive but also was a further replication of the past violence she had witnessed—and Monica had experienced—from the battering ex-husband/father. At that point, Monica clearly had a dissociative reaction, fortunately physically uninjured but stunned and probably experiencing a flashback of the past violence. My immediate concern was that Trish not feel that she had to lash out further to defend herself, hence I rose and put my hand on her shoulder firmly but as gently as possible to signal that she could pull back and safely disengage (without actually trying to pull her back as her mother had done). This was an inevitable further replication for Trish of experiencing both the past physical aggression and the current physical and psychological restraint, and she understandably reacted by pulling away from me, batting my hand away, and telling me to back off—all of which seemed like very legitimate self-protection and self-assertion on her part. When Trish then rushed off toward the office door, I feared that I had frightened and further alienated her, and I was afraid that Monica also had been sufficiently injured psychologically by my failure to protect her that she would have difficulty recovering.

As a result, the peak moment of crisis was extremely complicated for both of the clients and also for me. My response to the vicarious intensity and to my own intense countertransference reactions was to draw on the therapeutic process from the TARGET (Trauma Affect Regulation: Guide for Education and Therapy; Ford, 2020c) model. Without consciously recalling the FREEDOM steps (i.e., focusing, recognizing triggers, emotion awareness, evaluating thoughts, defining goals and options, making a contribution; see the Introduction to this volume), I followed them while I attempted to regroup and help Monica to reorient from the flashback to being safely in the present moment and place, and to help Trish to feel sufficiently secure to stay within contact and then return to be with her mother. My focal point initially was the orienting thought that nothing was more important than helping both Monica and Trish to know that they were safe to stay here together and with me, and that we, together, would find our way out of the memories of violence and on to the life they both were working so hard to achieve: one in which violence has no place and relationships are based on honesty, trust, and caring. Although my emphasis was on affirming their resilience and their core values and goals, I added the caveat about past and future violence to signal that this was the primary trigger that we all were working on understanding and eliminating from their lives, to shift the focus from any specific external person (e.g., the ex-husband/father, the boyfriend)—and related anxieties and frustrations with themselves and one another—to their shared goal of forever stopping violence.

I was aware that much was unresolved and required therapeutic reflection and discussion in relation to those specific people, and to how Monica and Trish viewed and treated one another, but my goal was to identify a starting point for that specific moment that addressed the trigger but focused on the path we could take to neutralize or eliminate that trigger. That path led next to their emotions, which I attempted to describe as intense feelings of determination and mutual caring. I characterized their essential thoughts as a belief that honoring those emotions provided a basis for hope and would actually achieve the life, together and as individuals, that they had courageously been pursuing as well as their core goals as honoring their bond and creating the life they each deserved and wanted for one another. Based on those goals, I described our best immediate option as focusing our minds on the fact that we were keeping one another safe by staying with one another and mentally tuning into the signs from our bodies of the safety and caring we each were feeling. In thus reviewing emotions, evaluating thoughts, defining goals, and identifying options (the "EEDO" components of the FREEDOM template), I drew on a combination of techniques from therapeutic modules for grounding, mindful present-centered bodily and contextual awareness, metacognitive observation of emotions and thoughts, self-soothing, and positive self-talk focused on resilience and signs of achieving core goals. My ultimate goal was to engage Monica and Trish simultaneously in coregulating with me as the conductor/guide/role model.

As I spoke with them, I observed Monica gradually showing nonverbal signs of reduced dissociation and distress, and increased present-centered orientation, and Trish gradually returning to the room both physically and psychologically (i.e., nonverbally expressing interest, relaxation, and warmth instead of detachment, tension, and anger). My focal goal was to help both Monica and Trish become aware that they each were making a crucial combination to one another's lives by being willing to return to the room and reaffirming their caring and respect for each other (i.e., the final "Making a contribution" step in the FREEDOM template). My practical goal was to restore Monica and Trish's confidence in the therapy and in me as a therapist so that they would feel motivated to continue to work together to (a) collaboratively redefine the problem(s) they were facing; (b) establish shared or mutually supported goals; and (c) develop, implement, and test new options that could enhance current or past successful solutions and replace or modify attempted solutions that have proven unsuccessful.

Perhaps the strongest trigger for countertransference for me in this session was not the altercation, as disturbing and stressful as that was for me personally as well as for the clients. Instead, it was when Monica repeatedly expressed frustration that I did not understand—both her and the problem that she was raising—and insisted that I self-disclose about my own daughters. This seemed very intrusive and unappreciative to me, which gave me a window into how Trish might have been feeling—and also into how vulnerable and unappreciated Monica might feel in relation to Trish (and possibly other formative relationships). In addition, this eventually led Trish as well as Monica to question my ability to help them, which intensified my own self-doubt and my fear that I was failing them and failing to meet the professional standards to which I aspire (and that my peers and role models might judge me by). I also felt somewhat guilty by choosing not to answer more than Monica's first question, as if I were falling back on a formulaic response of answering her question with another question instead of being authentic and as transparent as I was asking Monica to be in her own self-reflection and self-disclosures.

While I believe that I was able to remain outwardly steady and client centered in responding to Monica, I cannot rule out the possibility that I withdrew somewhat and assumed a more passive stance than might have been most therapeutic as she and Trish escalated their dysregulation and ultimately had an altercation. Although there is no definitive evidence-based answer to this question, it is something that I would plan on raising in future sessions with Monica and Trish (and in one-to-one sessions with Monica)—not to get their reassurance and not to determine exactly how I should handle this or similar countertransference challenges in the future but to engage them as collaborative partners in the self-reflective process that is the essence of psychotherapy. If we can talk about what happened in this crisis session from the observing ego position of participant observers, then they are active contributors to both understanding and shaping the process of their own psychotherapy—and that also prepares all of us to step back and reflect should similar dynamics develop in another session.

At the start of the session and in places throughout, I made a point to explicitly establish and emphasize (yet without revealing my intentions in doing so) the separate, yet not wholly incompatible, goals of Monica and Trish. Both Monica and Trish appeared to have conceptualized the other's goals in a way that made them defensive and emotionally reactive. Although not explicit, Monica appeared to be locked into believing that her daughter was willfully defying her desperate attempt to keep the family safe—perhaps she even felt her daughter was trying to sabotage the family's safety. Trish, on the other hand, appeared to hold onto the perception that her mother was trying to keep her from gaining her independence and perhaps even felt her mother was punishing her for being interested in dating and peer relationships. Monica's goal, though, was to keep her daughter and son safe from her abusive ex-husband and anyone else like him, and Trish's goal was to be what she considered a "normal teenager" and to explore healthy adolescent relationships. Revising how mother and daughter saw each other's goals would possibly enable them to let go of some of their defensiveness and start to listen and communicate in healthier ways.

It was clear at various points throughout the session that Monica's relationship with the therapist was being challenged. When the therapist attempted to clarify a point that Trish was making or to reframe how Monica might have been thinking about her daughter's intentions, Monica said, "You're not understanding." Ultimately, she became angry and pressed the therapist as to whether he had teenage daughters and daughters who had suffered trauma; she felt offended and that the therapist had taken sides with her daughter, Trish. Challenging his competency to understand and provide insight on what is going on with her daughter was a desperate attempt to regain control of the session. She perhaps felt threatened and a little betrayed. I was conscious of being careful to follow my challenge to Monica's perception by validating her feelings and emphasizing her ultimate goal: to keep her daughter and family safe. This prevented Monica from fully giving up on the conversation and retreating. What happened during this session was a good example of how ruptures in the therapeutic alliance are sometimes necessary consequences of the therapeutic process and how therapists can navigate that process.

I was very aware throughout the session that as a White man in a position of ostensible authority, I had to be particularly mindful of the possible triggering that my presence and my behavior could have for both mother and daughter. Also, because Monica is African American and my observations of the family suggested the ex-husband and batterer might be White, I attempted to clearly show deference to Monica as the expert and decision maker—and to not inadvertently usurp that role and authority from her. I was glad to hear Monica refer to me by my first name in the after-session commentary; although her doing so could have many possible meanings, I thought it suggested that she saw me as a person and a peer, albeit with a special role and some potentially helpful expertise, and not as a detached or disempowering voice of the White male establishment. Whether that was indeed true would be an important question to explore with her in her individual therapy when there was no longer an immediate crisis.

The use of touch in session also was complicated. It was clear (after the fact) that when I touched Trish on the shoulder, she experienced that touch as intrusive, swatting my hand away and saying, "Get off'a me!" However, it also was possible that she may have found this to have been a helpful example of an alternative way to experience a male in a position of authority who responds to conflict with self-control and respect for her privacy, and with a nonverbal and nonjudgmental reminder of the importance of maintaining everyone's safety from physical (or emotional) harm. My intent, by standing in the manner in which I did, was to communicate that "you're not alone" and "let's all calm down—no one is going to get hurt here." Rather than jumping up and into the fray, I tried to communicate active involvement and calm self-control, something that was both new and reassuring to Monica and Trish. However, the possibility that Trish or Monica interpreted my having physically intervened by touching Trish as an assault or violation also would be important to discuss with them.

In the aftermath of the altercation, I purposefully raised this concern with Trish and apologized if I had done anything to hurt her. Earlier, I had apologized to Monica for seeming not to understand her perspective leading up to the altercation. My hope was that those apologies conveyed to Monica and Trish that a person's taking responsibility for actions that cause hurt or distress does not have to be humiliating or a burdensome acceptance of fault or blame. The message I conveyed was that I care about both of their feelings and respect their personal views, integrity, and boundaries. This may have helped them to be open to receiving my guidance in the aftermath of the altercation by reducing the likelihood that either of them would shut down or become aggressively defensive to dispel a sense of guilt or because they feared I would judge them harshly for their actions.

Monica noted that what really helped her in the most difficult moments was simply being reminded of where she was and that she was not alone. That is why, when talking to them in the aftermath of the altercation, I repeatedly said that I am here, that Trish is here, and that "we" are present in the room together. This approach seems so simple, but it is crucial to reduce the sense of (and fear of) abandonment that was a central issue both for Monica (who had gone "somewhere else" in a dissociative state—very possibly a flashback) and for Trish (who was unsure whether she should stay or go, literally as well as figuratively). Sometimes simple reassurances are critical ways to evoke a sense of security and hope during and in proceeding beyond pivotal moments in therapy, which might otherwise either result in termination of progress or of therapeutic growth.

In reflection, Trish noted her mother's reaction following the physical altercation and how she was not her "normal" self. Trish may or may not have witnessed her mother in a dissociative state, and I think witnessing this may have been an opportunity for Trish to empathize with her mother and better understand where she was coming from. Monica may not have previously revealed her pain and vulnerability to Trish, perhaps wanting to convey strength and protection and but being fearful that opening up to Trish would compromise her role as a parent. However, seeing this side of her mother provided Trish with an opportunity to identify with Monica, to validate her own feelings of vulnerability, and to further develop a sense of her own identity.

CONCLUSION

As the crisis of mutually escalating dysregulation between a mother and her teenage daughter emerged in this psychotherapy session, my overarching goal was to help them bridge the separation that had grown between them and to heal the emotional wounds that the conflict in their relationship was reopening. To do this, my strategy was to unobtrusively facilitate the (a) expression and clarification of deeply felt concerns, (b) clarification of the specific events and circumstances that were causing those concerns, (c) understanding and nonjudgmental acceptance of the other person's feelings and views (i.e., empathy), (d) sense of control and freedom in their lives that had been diminished by past domestic violence, (e) repair of the emotional wounds that each felt as a result of the other's anger and anxiety, and (f) maintenance of a tolerable and manageable window of arousal so as to prevent hyperarousal or dissociation. These objectives were important because, throughout the session, both Monica and Trish continuously expressed the need to feel heard and understood. Monica told me that she just needed Trish "to understand where I'm coming from . . .," and Trish implied that her mother didn't understand her perspective, angrily telling her mother, "This is about you!" (i.e., "and your needs, not mine").

As is typical in family therapy sessions, the therapist's task is to align, validate, and empathize with both clients separately despite seemingly disparate/opposing perspectives while simultaneously forming and maintaining an "alliance" with a third entity—the "family unit," which, in this case, was the mother–daughter relationship. This is a difficult task to balance, and, at times, it was clear that Monica did not feel understood by the therapist or by her daughter. By alternating my attention between Monica and Trish throughout the session in an attempt to have each of them understand the other, I tried to communicate the importance not only of each of their needs and perspectives individually but also of the importance of the relationship as a whole—and that I was not on one person's side over the other but rather was "on the side" of the relationship. This proved to be particularly important as a theme to help Monica and Trish recover at the most critical point in the session, when both experienced extreme dysregulation during and after the physical altercation.

QUESTIONS FOR READER SELF-REFLECTION

- Would you have intervened earlier or differently than the therapist did in this session?

- What were the moments in this session when Monica's inner alarm was most reactive, and what behaviors by Trish, and by the therapist, appeared to trigger her escalating reactions?

- Similarly, at what moments in this session was Trish's inner alarm was most reactive, and what behaviors by Monica, and by the therapist, appeared to trigger her escalating reactions?

- What were Monica's most evident alarm-based reactive emotions?

- What underlying main (i.e., fundamental) emotions did Monica express indirectly (e.g., love for her daughter and son, hope for her daughter to enjoy success in her life)?

- Similarly, what were Trish's most evident alarm-based reactive emotions?

- What underlying main (i.e., fundamental) emotions did Trish express indirectly (e.g., determination in relation to being able make her own choices, hope and happiness in relation to her relationship with her new boyfriend)?

- What were Monica's most evident alarm-based reactive thoughts and goals? What underlying main (i.e., fundamental) goals did Monica express indirectly?

- Similarly, what were Trish's most evident alarm-based reactive thoughts and goals? What underlying main (i.e., fundamental) goals did Trish express indirectly?

- What orienting thoughts did the therapist use to maintain, or regain, his sense of calm and to focus on listening carefully and responding helpfully to Monica and Trish—both before and after the brief physical altercation between Trish and Monica?

- What orienting thoughts did the therapist use to help Monica recover from the state of shock and dissociation that she experienced after the physical altercation, and how were those main thoughts consistent with the main (i.e., fundamental) goals that Monica was expressing?

- What potential countertransference issues should the therapist be aware of? (These might include feeling worried or frustrated that Monica's commands and criticisms seem to be escalating Trish's anger, wanting to rescue and protect this family from the previously violent ex-husband/father, or feeling helpless to prevent Trish from physically assaulting her mother.)

Epilogue

Despite the almost infinite variability in the crises that can occur in the psychotherapy session, one common denominator can guide therapists in preventing and resolving those critical incidents: Clients in crisis are experiencing emotional dysregulation that has become sufficiently extreme to lead them to shift into a state of mind (and body) that is essentially survival mode. Severe emotional dysregulation and survival mode are an extreme case of the classic defensive stress reaction: freeze, fight, flight, and immobilization. To help a client replace those stress reactions with self-regulation, the therapist's challenge is to engage in their own self-regulation while simultaneously reinstating the client's sense of being understood, nonjudgmentally accepted, and genuinely supported in achieving reachable goals, and of feeling secure in being protected by and collaboratively partnered with a calm and confident helper.

This is a tall order indeed. Yet it is attainable, as illustrated by each of the case vignettes. The specific sequence in which a therapist deploys the tools—both attitudinal as well as overt behavioral practices—that communicate these vital messages to the client in crisis also varies. However, the fundamental process of engaging in coregulation to assist the client in crisis to

https://doi.org/10.1037/0000225-014
Crises in the Psychotherapy Session: Transforming Critical Moments Into Turning Points, by J. D. Ford

regain and strengthen self-regulation is a constant that follows the progression described by the FREEDOM acronym (see the Introduction):

- **F**ocus on self-reflection and on modeling and helping the client to access self-regulation by unconditionally communicating support for the main goals that the client holds.

- **R**ecognize and help the client nonjudgmentally understand triggers for survival mode.

- Identify and help the client to nonjudgmentally accept dysphoric and core **e**motions.

- Help the client to nonjudgmentally **e**valuate and accept core values and priorities.

- Help the client to nonjudgmentally **d**efine core personal and relational goals.

- Help the client to identify **o**ptions consistent with their core emotions, values, priorities, and goals.

- Recognize and help the client to take credit for **m**aking a contribution by being willing to engage in this rigorous self-reflection and basing their actions on their core values, priorities, and goals.

In each case vignette, the therapist struggled with their triggered reactions to the client's crisis, challenging behavior, or both, but quickly focused on the client's core priorities and values that had been compromised as the triggers for the current crisis (e.g., safety violated by violence and exploitation, trust violated by betrayal, security denied by abandonment, self-respect compromised by abuse and invalidation, love and caring violated by domination). They proceeded to listen and observe carefully to identify and understand both the client's and their own emotions, articulating in down-to-earth terms the spoken and the deeper unspoken or implied emotions the client was indirectly expressing as well as obviously feeling. They then affirmed the core beliefs or cognitive evaluations (i.e., values and priorities) the client was expressing through their statements and actions (past as well as present), as well as the strengths and sources of resilience (internal and external) that the client was drawing on (or had in the past drawn on) to regain a sense of hope and confidence. This provided a natural basis for helping the client to clarify the core goals that seemed to be thwarted or undermined in the crisis and for the therapist to affirm support and willingness to partner with the client in achieving those goals based on feasible steps (i.e., options) that embodied the client's past successes or potentially viable adaptations of those past successful solutions.

Without artificially praising or complimenting the client, in an understated but authentic manner, each therapist was able to affirm the client's achievement in having navigated the crisis and having regained self-regulation—most often by simply nonverbally joining with the client as they experienced a renewed sense of hope and confidence. Each therapist also developed plans for reviewing in future sessions the process that the client went through in this session to highlight for the client the value and accomplishment represented by their successful efforts in restoring self-regulation.

Although there are valuable nuances in each vignette that this summary does not adequately address, the cross-cutting themes that I am highlighting are much easier to recall and implement in the moments of crisis than the much longer list of techniques and strategies that are described in Chapters 3, 4, and 5. That longer list is valuable as a set of possible specific foci for understanding the client's core goals and setting a course to intervene in crises or as the full set of tools in the therapist's memory storehouse. Rapid selection of the most appropriate tool or tools hinges on having a much more concise map for traversing the crisis, which the FREEDOM framework can provide.

So, in closing, I hope you'll find the following seven key take-home points useful:

- Crises in therapy result when clients experience extreme emotional dysregulation that exceeds, at least temporarily, their capacity for emotion regulation and they shift automatically into survival mode and extreme stress reactions.

- The restoration of emotion regulation involves more than simply performing "adaptive" emotion regulation skills to reduce the intensity of emotional dysregulation. It requires restoring the fundamental prerequisites for emotion regulation, as well as security and control.

- Crises occur when people are blocked or frustrated in their attempts to achieve a goal of central personal relevance, so crisis resolution always requires identifying and developing feasible steps toward achieving the client's thwarted goal.

- Psychotherapy provides a framework for the psychotherapist and client to understand how the client's personality and learning history have led to formative experiences in which their sense of security and control has been damaged or underdeveloped—thus causing or contributing to problems with emotional dysregulation—but also to understand how other experiences have affirmed and strengthened the client's sense of security or control (and resilience) that they can and must draw on to restore self-regulation.

- Emotional dysregulation is contagious: Empathically attuned therapists experience a vicarious state of emotional dysregulation when clients are in crisis, which tends to manifest in countertransference reactions that can trigger enactments and worsen a crisis—or that also can point toward a path to resolve the crisis.

- Simultaneous restoration of self-regulation—and active intentional engagement in coregulation—by the therapist and client, therefore, is the key to resolving as well as anticipating and preventing crises in psychotherapy.

- The alpha-and-omega for psychotherapists when clients are in crisis is to demonstrate through actions as well as words a commitment to be sufficiently self-regulated to effectively partner with the client in service of the client's core values, priorities, goals, and sense of self efficacy, self-worth, and relational security.

This is a lot to ask of any professional or other helper—or human being. Yet, as the case vignettes illustrated, it is possible, albeit with many bumps on the road and even clear missteps (from which a strong focus and presence of mind are essential for the therapist to recover their balance and restore the therapeutic alliance). Fortunately, when crises are prevented or resolved, the rewards for both client and therapist are profound.

References

Abblett, M. (2013). *The heat of the moment in treatment: Mindful management of difficult clients*. W. W. Norton.

Aldao, A., Nolen-Hoeksema, S., & Schweizer, S. (2010). Emotion-regulation strategies across psychopathology: A meta-analytic review. *Clinical Psychology Review, 30*(2), 217–237. https://doi.org/10.1016/j.cpr.2009.11.004

Alexander, F., & French, T. M. (1946). The principle of corrective emotional experience. In F. Alexander & T. M. French (Eds.), *Psychoanalytic therapy: Principles and application* (pp. 66–70). Roland Press.

Allen, V. C., & Windsor, T. D. (2019). Age differences in the use of emotion regulation strategies derived from the process model of emotion regulation: A systematic review. *Aging & Mental Health, 23*(1), 1–14. https://doi.org/10.1080/13607863.2017.1396575

Anderson, K. N., Bautista, C. L., & Hope, D. A. (2019). Therapeutic alliance, cultural competence and minority status in premature termination of psychotherapy. *American Journal of Orthopsychiatry, 89*(1), 104–114. https://doi.org/10.1037/ort0000342

Andreotti, C., Thigpen, J. E., Dunn, M. J., Watson, K., Potts, J., Reising, M. M., Robinson, K. E., Rodriguez, E. M., Roubinov, D., Luecken, L., & Compas, B. E. (2013). Cognitive reappraisal and secondary control coping: Associations with working memory, positive and negative affect, and symptoms of anxiety/depression. *Anxiety, Stress, and Coping, 26*(1), 20–35. https://doi.org/10.1080/10615806.2011.631526

Arkowitz, H. (2008). *Motivational interviewing in the treatment of psychological problems*. Guilford Press.

A-Tjak, J. G., Davis, M. L., Morina, N., Powers, M. B., Smits, J. A., & Emmelkamp, P. M. (2015). A meta-analysis of the efficacy of acceptance and commitment therapy for clinically relevant mental and physical health problems. *Psychotherapy and Psychosomatics, 84*(1), 30–36. https://doi.org/10.1159/000365764

Atwood, G. E., & Stolorow, R. D. (1984). *Structures of subjectivity: Explorations in psychoanalytic phenomenology.* The Analytic Press.

Auerbach, S. M., & Kilmann, P. R. (1977). Crisis intervention: A review of outcome research. *Psychological Bulletin, 84*(6), 1189–1217. https://doi.org/10.1037/0033-2909.84.6.1189

Bailey, T., Shahabi, L., Tarvainen, M., Shapiro, D., & Ottaviani, C. (2019). Moderating effects of the valence of social interaction on the dysfunctional consequences of perseverative cognition: An ecological study in major depression and social anxiety disorder. *Anxiety, Stress, and Coping, 32*(2), 179–195. https://doi.org/10.1080/10615806.2019.1570821

Balint, E. (1963). On being empty of oneself. *The International Journal of Psycho-Analysis, 44,* 470–480.

Bandler, R., & Grinder, J. (1975). *The structure of magic I: A book about language and therapy.* Science & Behavior Books.

Bandler, R., Grinder, J., & Satir, V. (1976). *Changing with families: A book about further education for being human.* Science & Behavior Books.

Banks, S. A. (1965). Psychotherapy: Values in action. *International Psychiatry Clinics, 2*(2), 497–514.

Barber, J. G. (1995). Working with resistant drug abusers. *Social Work, 40*(1), 17–23. http://www.ncbi.nlm.nih.gov/pubmed/7863369

Beck, J. S. (2005). *Cognitive therapy for challenging problems: What to do when the basics don't work.* Guilford Press.

Bendezú, J. J., Cole, P. M., Tan, P. Z., Armstrong, L. M., Reitz, E. B., & Wolf, R. M. (2018). Child language and parenting antecedents and externalizing outcomes of emotion regulation pathways across early childhood: A person-centered approach. *Development and Psychopathology, 30*(4), 1253–1268. https://doi.org/10.1017/S0954579417001675

Benjamin, L. S. (2003). *Interpersonal reconstructive therapy: Promoting change in nonresponders.* Guilford Press.

Berg, I. K. (1994). *Family based services: A solution-focused approach.* W. W. Norton.

Berrino, A., Ohlendorf, P., Duriaux, S., Burnand, Y., Lorillard, S., & Andreoli, A. (2011). Crisis intervention at the general hospital: An appropriate treatment choice for acutely suicidal borderline patients. *Psychiatry Research, 186*(2–3), 287–292. https://doi.org/10.1016/j.psychres.2010.06.018

Berthelsen, D., Hayes, N., White, S. L. J., & Williams, K. E. (2017). Executive function in adolescence: Associations with child and family risk factors and self-regulation in early childhood. *Frontiers in Psychology, 8,* Article 903. https://doi.org/10.3389/fpsyg.2017.00903

Bion, W. (1963). *Elements of psychoanalysis.* William Heinemann.

Birk, J. L., Cornelius, T., Edmondson, D., & Schwartz, J. E. (2019). Duration of perseverative thinking as related to perceived stress and blood pressure: An ambulatory monitoring study. *Psychosomatic Medicine, 81*(7), 603–611. Advance online publication. https://doi.org/10.1097/PSY.0000000000000727

Bisson, J. I., Roberts, N. P., Andrew, M., Cooper, R., & Lewis, C. (2013). Psychological therapies for chronic post-traumatic stress disorder (PTSD) in adults. *Cochrane Database of Systematic Reviews.* https://doi.org/10.1002/14651858.CD003388.pub4

Blair, C., & Raver, C. C. (2015). School readiness and self-regulation: A developmental psychobiological approach. *Annual Review of Psychology, 66*(1), 711–731. https://doi.org/10.1146/annurev-psych-010814-015221

Boesky, D. (2005). Psychoanalytic controversies contextualized. *Journal of the American Psychoanalytic Association, 53*(3), 835–863. https://doi.org/10.1177/00030651050530030301

Bosmans, G., De Raedt, R., & Braet, C. (2007). The invisible bonds: Does the secure base script of attachment influence children's attention toward their mother? *Journal of Clinical Child & Adolescent Psychology, 36*(4), 557–567. https://doi.org/10.1080/15374410701662717

Boumparis, N., Karyotaki, E., Kleiboer, A., Hofmann, S. G., & Cuijpers, P. (2016). The effect of psychotherapeutic interventions on positive and negative affect in depression: A systematic review and meta-analysis. *Journal of Affective Disorders, 202,* 153–162. https://doi.org/10.1016/j.jad.2016.05.019

Bowlby, J. (1969). *Attachment and loss: Vol. 1. Attachment.* Basic Books.

Bowlby, J. (1982). Attachment and loss: Retrospect and prospect. *American Journal of Orthopsychiatry, 52*(4), 664–678. https://doi.org/10.1111/j.1939-0025.1982.tb01456.x

Bracha, H. S. (2004). Freeze, flight, fight, fright, faint: Adaptationist perspectives on the acute stress response spectrum. *CNS Spectrums, 9*(9), 679–685. https://doi.org/10.1017/S1092852900001954

Brereton, A., & McGlinchey, E. (2020). Self-harm, emotion regulation, and experiential avoidance: A systematic review. *Archives of Suicide Research, 24*(Suppl. 1), 1–24. https://doi.org/10.1080/13811118.2018.1563575

Briere, J. (2019). *Treating risky and compulsive behavior in trauma survivors.* Guilford Press.

Briggs-Gowan, M. J., Carter, A. S., & Ford, J. D. (2012). Parsing the effects violence exposure in early childhood: Modeling developmental pathways. *Journal of Pediatric Psychology, 37*(1), 11–22. https://doi.org/10.1093/jpepsy/jsr063

Brodsky, S. L. (2011). *Therapy with coerced and reluctant clients.* American Psychological Association. https://doi.org/10.1037/12305-000

Bryan, C. J., Rozek, D. C., Burch, T. S., Leeson, B., & Clemans, T. A. (2019). Therapeutic alliance and intervention approach among acutely suicidal patients. *Psychiatry, 82*(1), 80–82. https://doi.org/10.1080/00332747.2018.1485371

Brymer, M., Jacobs, A., Layne, C., Pynoos, R., Ruzek, J., Steinberg, A., Vernberg, E., & Watson, P. (2006, July). *Psychological first aid: Field operations guide* (2nd ed.). The National Child Traumatic Stress Network and National

Center for PTSD. https://www.ptsd.va.gov/professional/treat/type/PFA/PFA_2ndEditionwithappendices.pdf

Butcher, J. N., Stelmachers, Z. T., & Maudal, G. R. (1983). Crisis intervention and emergency psychotherapy. In I. B. Weiner (Ed.), *Clinical methods in psychology* (2nd ed., pp. 572–633). John Wiley & Sons.

Calcott, R. D., & Berkman, E. T. (2014). Attentional flexibility during approach and avoidance motivational states: The role of context in shifts of attentional breadth. *Journal of Experimental Psychology: General, 143*(3), 1393–1408. https://doi.org/10.1037/a0035060

Calcott, R. D., & Berkman, E. T. (2015). Neural correlates of attentional flexibility during approach and avoidance motivation. *PLOS ONE, 10*(5), Article e0127203. https://doi.org/10.1371/journal.pone.0127203

Canada, E. (2017, July 7). *One day at a time: A slogan bonded in recovery principles*. Retrieved June 18, 2020, from https://www.edgewoodhealthnetwork.com/blog/one-day-time-slogan-bonded-recovery-principles/

Caplan, G. (1964). *Principles of preventive psychiatry*. Basic Books.

Caplan, G. (1989). Recent developments in crisis intervention and the promotion of support service. *The Journal of Primary Prevention, 10*(1), 3–25. https://doi.org/10.1007/BF01324646

Carcione, A., Nicolò, G., Pedone, R., Popolo, R., Conti, L., Fiore, D., Procacci, M., Semerari, A., & Dimaggio, G. (2011). Metacognitive mastery dysfunctions in personality disorder psychotherapy. *Psychiatry Research, 190*(1), 60–71. https://doi.org/10.1016/j.psychres.2010.12.032

Cardoso, C., Ellenbogen, M. A., Serravalle, L., & Linnen, A. M. (2013). Stress-induced negative mood moderates the relation between oxytocin administration and trust: Evidence for the tend-and-befriend response to stress? *Psychoneuroendocrinology, 38*(11), 2800–2804. https://doi.org/10.1016/j.psyneuen.2013.05.006

Casey, B. J., Getz, S., & Galvan, A. (2008). The adolescent brain. *Developmental Review, 28*(1), 62–77. https://doi.org/10.1016/j.dr.2007.08.003

Cassidy, J., Jones, J. D., & Shaver, P. R. (2013). Contributions of attachment theory and research: A framework for future research, translation, and policy. *Development and Psychopathology, 25*(4, Part 2), 1415–1434. https://doi.org/10.1017/S0954579413000692

Cassotti, M., Agogué, M., Camarda, A., Houdé, O., & Borst, G. (2016). Inhibitory control as a core process of creative problem solving and idea generation from childhood to adulthood. *New Directions for Child and Adolescent Development, 2016*(151), 61–72. https://doi.org/10.1002/cad.20153

Chadwick, R. A., Bromgard, G., Bromgard, I., & Trafimow, D. (2006). An index of specific behaviors in the moral domain. *Behavior Research Methods, 38*(4), 692–697. https://doi.org/10.3758/BF03193902

Chakhssi, F., Kraiss, J. T., Sommers-Spijkerman, M., & Bohlmeijer, E. T. (2018). The effect of positive psychology interventions on well-being and distress in clinical samples with psychiatric or somatic disorders: A systematic review and meta-analysis. *BMC Psychiatry, 18*(1), 211. https://doi.org/10.1186/ s12888-018-1739-2

Chefetz, R. A. (2017). Issues in consultation for treatments with distressed activated abuser/protector self-states in dissociative identity disorder. *Journal of Trauma & Dissociation, 18*(3), 465–475. https://doi.org/10.1080/ 15299732.2017.1295428

Cicchetti, D. (2010). Resilience under conditions of extreme stress: A multilevel perspective. *World Psychiatry, 9*(3), 145–154. https://doi.org/10.1002/ j.2051-5545.2010.tb00297.x

Clancy, F., Prestwich, A., Caperon, L., & O'Connor, D. B. (2016). Perseverative cognition and health behaviors: A systematic review and meta-analysis. *Frontiers in Human Neuroscience, 10*, Article 534. https://doi.org/10.3389/ fnhum.2016.00534

Cohen, S., Hamrick, N., Rodriguez, M. S., Feldman, P. J., Rabin, B. S., & Manuck, S. B. (2002). Reactivity and vulnerability to stress-associated risk for upper respiratory illness. *Psychosomatic Medicine, 64*(2), 302–310. https://doi.org/10.1097/00006842-200203000-00014

Cohen, S., Janicki-Deverts, D., & Miller, G. E. (2007). Psychological stress and disease. *JAMA, 298*(14), 1685–1687. https://doi.org/10.1001/jama. 298.14.1685

Cohen, S., Tyrrell, D. A., & Smith, A. P. (1991). Psychological stress and susceptibility to the common cold. *The New England Journal of Medicine, 325*(9), 606–612. https://doi.org/10.1056/NEJM199108293250903

Cole, P. M., Bendezú, J. J., Ram, N., & Chow, S. M. (2017). Dynamical systems modeling of early childhood self-regulation. *Emotion, 17*(4), 684–699. https://doi.org/10.1037/emo0000268

Compas, B. E., Jaser, S. S., Bettis, A. H., Watson, K. H., Gruhn, M. A., Dunbar, J. P., Williams, E., & Thigpen, J. C. (2017). Coping, emotion regulation, and psychopathology in childhood and adolescence: A meta-analysis and narrative review. *Psychological Bulletin, 143*(9), 939–991. https://doi.org/10.1037/ bul0000110

Compton, M. T., Bahora, M., Watson, A. C., & Oliva, J. R. (2008). A comprehensive review of extant research on crisis intervention team (CIT) programs. *The Journal of the American Academy of Psychiatry and the Law, 36*(1), 47–55.

Cona, G., Scarpazza, C., Sartori, G., Moscovitch, M., & Bisiacchi, P. S. (2015). Neural bases of prospective memory: A meta-analysis and the "attention to delayed intention" (AtoDI) model. *Neuroscience & Biobehavioral Reviews, 52*, 21–37. https://doi.org/10.1016/j.neubiorev.2015.02.007

Conte, H. R. (1994). Review of research in supportive psychotherapy: An update. *American Journal of Psychotherapy, 48*(4), 494–504. https://doi.org/10.1176/ appi.psychotherapy.1994.48.4.494

Contreras, A., Nieto, I., Valiente, C., Espinosa, R., & Vazquez, C. (2019). The study of psychopathology from the network analysis perspective: A systematic review. *Psychotherapy and Psychosomatics, 88*(2), 71–83. https://doi.org/10.1159/000497425

Cooke, J. E., Kochendorfer, L. B., Stuart-Parrigon, K. L., Koehn, A. J., & Kerns, K. A. (2019). Parent–child attachment and children's experience and regulation of emotion: A meta-analytic review. *Emotion, 19*(6), 1103–1126. https://doi.org/10.1037/emo0000504

Copeland, W. E., Keeler, G., Angold, A., & Costello, E. J. (2007). Traumatic events and posttraumatic stress in childhood. *Archives of General Psychiatry, 64*(5), 577–584. https://doi.org/10.1001/archpsyc.64.5.577

Coubard, O. A. (2015). Attention is complex: Causes and effects. *Frontiers in Psychology, 6*, Article 246. https://doi.org/10.3389/fpsyg.2015.00246

Courtois, C. A. (2020). Therapeutic alliance and risk management. In J. D. Ford & C. A. Courtois (Eds.), *Treating complex traumatic stress disorders in adults: Scientific foundations and therapeutic models* (2nd ed., pp. 99–130). Guilford Press.

Courtois, C. A., & Ford, J. D. (2013). *Treating complex trauma: A sequenced relationship-based approach*. Guilford Press.

Critchfield, K. L., Levy, K. N., Clarkin, J. F., & Kernberg, O. F. (2008). The relational context of aggression in borderline personality disorder: Using adult attachment style to predict forms of hostility. *Journal of Clinical Psychology, 64*(1), 67–82. https://doi.org/10.1002/jclp.20434

Crone, D. L., Bode, S., Murawski, C., & Laham, S. M. (2018). The Socio-Moral Image Database (SMID): A novel stimulus set for the study of social, moral and affective processes. *PLOS ONE, 13*(1), Article e0190954. https://doi.org/10.1371/journal.pone.0190954

Cross, A. B., Mulvey, E. P., Schubert, C. A., Griffin, P. A., Filone, S., Winckworth-Prejsnar, K., DeMatteo, D., & Heilbrun, K. (2014). An agenda for advancing research on crisis intervention teams for mental health emergencies. *Psychiatric Services, 65*(4), 530–536. https://doi.org/10.1176/appi.ps.201200566

Dales, S., & Jerry, P. (2008). Attachment, affect regulation and mutual synchrony in adult psychotherapy. *American Journal of Psychotherapy, 62*(3), 283–312. https://doi.org/10.1176/appi.psychotherapy.2008.62.3.283

Daniel, S. I. F., Poulsen, S., & Lunn, S. (2016). Client attachment in a randomized clinical trial of psychoanalytic and cognitive-behavioral psychotherapy for bulimia nervosa: Outcome moderation and change. *Psychotherapy, 53*(2), 174–184. https://doi.org/10.1037/pst0000046

Daros, A. R., & Williams, G. E. (2019). A meta-analysis and systematic review of emotion-regulation strategies in borderline personality disorder. *Harvard Review of Psychiatry, 27*(4), 217–232. https://doi.org/10.1097/HRP.0000000000000212

Dash, S. R., Meeten, F., & Davey, G. C. (2013). Systematic information processing style and perseverative worry. *Clinical Psychology Review, 33*(8), 1041–1056. https://doi.org/10.1016/j.cpr.2013.08.007

Davey, G. C., & Meeten, F. (2016). The perseverative worry bout: A review of cognitive, affective and motivational factors that contribute to worry perseveration. *Biological Psychology, 121*(Part B), 233–243. https://doi.org/10.1016/j.biopsycho.2016.04.003

David, D. H., & Lyons-Ruth, K. (2005). Differential attachment responses of male and female infants to frightening maternal behavior: Tend or befriend Versus fight or flight? *Infant Mental Health Journal, 26*(1), 1–18. https://doi.org/10.1002/imhj.20033

Davis, D. R. (1961). The family triangle in schizophrenia. *British Journal of Medical Psychology, 34*(1), 53–63. https://doi.org/10.1111/j.2044-8341.1961.tb00930.x

de Kleine, R. A., Hagenaars, M. A., & van Minnen, A. (2018). Tonic immobility during re-experiencing the traumatic event in posttraumatic stress disorder. *Psychiatry Research, 270*, 1105–1109. https://doi.org/10.1016/j.psychres.2018.06.051

de Shazer, S. (1988). *Clues: Investigating solutions in brief therapy.* W. W. Norton.

Dingemans, A., Danner, U., & Parks, M. (2017). Emotion regulation in binge eating disorder: A review. *Nutrients, 9*(11), Article 1274. Advance online publication. https://doi.org/10.3390/nu9111274

Dodd, A., Lockwood, E., Mansell, W., & Palmier-Claus, J. (2019). Emotion regulation strategies in bipolar disorder: A systematic and critical review. *Journal of Affective Disorders, 246*, 262–284. https://doi.org/10.1016/j.jad.2018.12.026

Donges, U. S., Zeitschel, F., Kersting, A., & Suslow, T. (2015). Adult attachment orientation and automatic processing of emotional information on a semantic level: A masked affective priming study. *Psychiatry Research, 229*(1–2), 174–180. https://doi.org/10.1016/j.psychres.2015.07.045

Drayer, C. S., Cameron, D. C., Woodward, W. D., & Glass, A. J. (1954). Psychological first aid in community disaster. *Journal of the American Medical Association, 156*(1), 36–41.

Dryman, M. T., & Heimberg, R. G. (2018). Emotion regulation in social anxiety and depression: A systematic review of expressive suppression and cognitive reappraisal. *Clinical Psychology Review, 65*, 17–42. https://doi.org/10.1016/j.cpr.2018.07.004

Du, M., Wang, X., Yin, S., Shu, W., Hao, R., Zhao, S., Rao, H., Yeung, W. L., Jayaram, M. B., & Xia, J. (2017). De-escalation techniques for psychosis-induced aggression or agitation. *Cochrane Database of Systematic Reviews.* https://doi.org/10.1002/14651858.CD009922.pub2

D'Zurilla, T. J., & Goldfried, M. R. (1971). Problem solving and behavior modification. *Journal of Abnormal Psychology, 78*(1), 107–126. https://doi.org/10.1037/h0031360

Ellenbogen, M. A., Carson, R. J., & Pishva, R. (2010). Automatic emotional information processing and the cortisol response to acute psychosocial stress. *Cognitive, Affective, & Behavioral Neuroscience, 10*(1), 71–82. https://doi.org/10.3758/CABN.10.1.71

Elliott, R., Bohart, A. C., Watson, J. C., & Murphy, D. (2018). Therapist empathy and client outcome: An updated meta-analysis. *Psychotherapy, 55*(4), 399–410. https://doi.org/10.1037/pst0000175

Erickson, M. H. (1959). Further clinical techniques of hypnosis: Utilization techniques. *The American Journal of Clinical Hypnosis, 2*(1), 3–21. https://doi.org/10.1080/00029157.1959.10401792

Erickson, M. H. (1964). An hypnotic technique for resistant patients: The patient, the technique and its rationale and field experiments. *The American Journal of Clinical Hypnosis, 7*(1), 8–32. https://doi.org/10.1080/00029157.1964.10402387

Erickson, M. H., & Rossi, E. L. (1976). Two level communication and the microdynamics of trance and suggestion. *The American Journal of Clinical Hypnosis, 18*(3), 153–171. https://doi.org/10.1080/00029157.1976.10403794

Eubanks, C. F., Burckell, L. A., & Goldfried, M. R. (2018). Clinical consensus strategies to repair ruptures in the therapeutic alliance. *Journal of Psychotherapy Integration, 28*(1), 60–76. https://doi.org/10.1037/int0000097

Eubanks, C. F., Muran, J. C., & Safran, J. D. (2018). Alliance rupture repair: A meta-analysis. *Psychotherapy, 55*(4), 508–519. https://doi.org/10.1037/pst0000185

Evans, C. A., & Porter, C. L. (2009). The emergence of mother–infant co-regulation during the first year: Links to infants' developmental status and attachment. *Infant Behavior and Development, 32*(2), 147–158. https://doi.org/10.1016/j.infbeh.2008.12.005

Everly, G. S., Jr., Flannery, R. B., Jr., & Eyler, V. A. (2002). Critical incident stress management (CISM): A statistical review of the literature. *Psychiatric Quarterly, 73*(3), 171–182. https://doi.org/10.1023/A:1016068003615

Everly, G. S., Jr., & Flynn, B. W. (2006). Principles and practical procedures for acute psychological first aid training for personnel without mental health experience. *International Journal of Emergency Mental Health, 8*(2), 93–100.

Everly, G. S., Jr., & Mitchell, J. T. (2000). The debriefing "controversy" and crisis intervention: A review of lexical and substantive issues. *International Journal of Emergency Mental Health, 2*(4), 211–225.

Fang, Y., Scott, L., Song, P., Burmeister, M., & Sen, S. (2020). Genomic prediction of depression risk and resilience under stress. *Nature Human Behaviour, 4*(1), 111–118. https://doi.org/10.1038/s41562-019-0759-3

Fani, N., Tone, E. B., Phifer, J., Norrholm, S. D., Bradley, B., Ressler, K. J., Kamkwalala, A., & Jovanovic, T. (2012). Attention bias toward threat is associated with exaggerated fear expression and impaired extinction in PTSD. *Psychological Medicine, 42*(3), 533–543. https://doi.org/10.1017/S0033291711001565

Farber, B. A., Suzuki, J. Y., & Lynch, D. A. (2018). Positive regard and psychotherapy outcome: A meta-analytic review. *Psychotherapy, 55*(4), 411–423. https://doi.org/10.1037/pst0000171

Fareri, D. S., Gabard-Durnam, L., Goff, B., Flannery, J., Gee, D. G., Lumian, D. S., Caldera, C., & Tottenham, N. (2015). Normative development of ventral striatal resting state connectivity in humans. *NeuroImage, 118*, 422–437. https://doi.org/10.1016/j.neuroimage.2015.06.022

Feldman, P. J., Cohen, S., Lepore, S. J., Matthews, K. A., Kamarck, T. W., & Marsland, A. L. (1999). Negative emotions and acute physiological responses to stress. *Annals of Behavioral Medicine, 21*(3), 216–222. https://doi.org/10.1007/BF02884836

Felmingham, K. L., Rennie, C., Manor, B., & Bryant, R. A. (2011). Eye tracking and physiological reactivity to threatening stimuli in posttraumatic stress disorder. *Journal of Anxiety Disorders, 25*(5), 668–673. https://doi.org/10.1016/j.janxdis.2011.02.010

Fisher, J. (2020). Experiential approaches. In J. D. Ford & C. A. Courtois (Eds.), *Treating complex traumatic stress disorders in adults: Scientific foundations and therapeutic models* (2nd ed., pp. 533–549). Guilford Press.

Flannery, R. B., Jr., & Everly, G. S., Jr. (2000). Crisis intervention: A review. *International Journal of Emergency Mental Health, 2*(2), 119–125.

Flückiger, C., Del Re, A. C., Wampold, B. E., & Horvath, A. O. (2018). The alliance in adult psychotherapy: A meta-analytic synthesis. *Psychotherapy, 55*(4), 316–340. https://doi.org/10.1037/pst0000172

Follette, V., Iverson, K. M., & Ford, J. D. (2009). Contextual behavior trauma therapy. In C. A. Courtois & J. D. Ford (Eds.), *Treating complex traumatic stress disorders: An evidence-based guide* (pp. 264–285). Guilford Press.

Fonagy, P., & Campbell, C. (2017). Mentalizing, attachment and epistemic trust: How psychotherapy can promote resilience. *Psychiatria Hungarica, 32*(3), 283–287.

Ford, J. D. (1984). Questioning and answering in psychotherapy. *Voices, 19*(1), 26–35.

Ford, J. D. (2001). *Trauma Affect Regulation: Guide for Educational Therapy (TARGET) Manual—Adult/Adolescent Individual.* Advanced Trauma Solutions: Farmington, CT.

Ford, J. D. (2009a). Dissociation in complex posttraumatic stress disorder or disorders of extreme stress not otherwise specified (DESNOS). In P. F. Dell, J. A. O'Neill, & E. Somer (Eds.), *Dissociation and the dissociative disorders: DSM-V and beyond* (pp. 471–485). Routledge.

Ford, J. D. (2009b). Neurobiological and developmental research: Clinical implications. In C. A. Courtois & J. D. Ford (Eds.), *Treating complex traumatic stress disorders: An evidence-based guide* (pp. 31–58). Guilford Press.

Ford, J. D. (2013). How can self-regulation enhance our understanding of trauma and dissociation? *Journal of Trauma & Dissociation, 14*(3), 237–250. https://doi.org/10.1080/15299732.2013.769398

Ford, J. D. (2017a). Complex trauma and complex PTSD. In S. Gold, S., J. Cook, & C. Dalenberg (Eds.), *Handbook of trauma psychology* (Vol. 1, pp. 322–349). American Psychological Association.

Ford, J. D. (2017b). Emotion regulation and skills-based interventions. In S. Gold (Ed.-in-Chief), *Handbook of trauma psychology* (Vol. 2, pp. 227–252). American Psychological Association.

Ford, J. D. (2018). Trauma memory processing in posttraumatic stress disorder psychotherapy: A unifying framework. *Journal of Traumatic Stress, 31*(6), 933–942. https://doi.org/10.1002/jts.22344

Ford, J. D. (2020a). Developmental neurobiology of complex traumatic stress disorders. In J. D. Ford & C. A. Courtois (Eds.), *Treating complex traumatic stress disorders in adults: Scientific foundations and therapeutic models* (2nd ed., pp. 35–61). Guilford Press.

Ford, J. D. (2020b). Family systems therapy. In J. D. Ford & C. A. Courtois (Eds.), *Treating complex traumatic stress disorders in adults: Scientific foundations and therapeutic models* (2nd ed., pp. 459–486). Guilford Press.

Ford, J. D. (2020c). Trauma affect regulation: Guide for education and therapy for complex traumatic stress disorders. In J. D. Ford & C. A. Courtois (Eds.), *Treating complex traumatic stress disorders in adults: Scientific foundations and therapeutic models* (2nd ed., pp. 390–412). Guilford Press.

Ford, J. D., Chang, R., Levine, J., & Zhang, W. (2013). Randomized clinical trial comparing affect regulation and supportive group therapies for victimization-related PTSD with incarcerated women. *Behavior Therapy, 44*(2), 262–276. https://doi.org/10.1016/j.beth.2012.10.003

Ford, J. D., & Courtois, C. A. (Eds.). (2020). *Treating complex traumatic stress disorders: Scientific foundations and therapeutic models* (2nd ed.). Guilford Press.

Ford, J. D., Courtois, C. A., Steele, K., van der Hart, O., & Nijenhuis, E. R. S. (2005). Treatment of complex posttraumatic self-dysregulation. *Journal of Traumatic Stress, 18*(5), 437–447. https://doi.org/10.1002/jts.20051

Ford, J. D., Grasso, D. J., Greene, C. A., Slivinsky, M., & DeViva, J. C. (2018). Randomized clinical trial pilot study of prolonged exposure versus present centred affect regulation therapy for PTSD and anger problems with male military combat veterans. *Clinical Psychology & Psychotherapy, 25*(5), 641–649. https://doi.org/10.1002/cpp.2194

Ford, J. D., Grasso, D. J., Levine, J., & Tennen, H. (2018). Affect regulation enhancement of cognitive behavior therapy for college problem drinkers: A pilot randomized controlled trial study. *Journal of Child & Adolescent Substance Abuse, 27*(1), 47–58. https://doi.org/10.1080/1067828X.2017.1400484

Ford, J. D., & Hawke, J. (2012). Trauma affect regulation psychoeducation group and milieu intervention outcomes in juvenile detention facilities. *Journal of Aggression, Maltreatment & Trauma, 21*(4), 365–384. https://doi.org/10.1080/10926771.2012.673538

Ford, J. D., Steinberg, K. L., Hawke, J., Levine, J., & Zhang, W. (2012). Randomized trial comparison of emotion regulation and relational psychotherapies for PTSD with girls involved in delinquency. *Journal of Clinical Child & Adolescent Psychology, 41*(1), 27–37. https://doi.org/10.1080/15374416.2012.632343

Ford, J. D., Steinberg, K. L., & Zhang, W. (2011). A randomized clinical trial comparing affect regulation and social problem-solving psychotherapies for mothers with victimization-related PTSD. *Behavior Therapy, 42*(4), 560–578. https://doi.org/10.1016/j.beth.2010.12.005

Ford, J. D., & Wortmann, J. (2013). *Hijacked by your brain: How to free yourself when stress takes over.* Sourcebooks.

Fosha, D., Paivio, S., Gleiser, K., & Ford, J. D. (2009). Experiential and emotion-focused therapy. In C. A. Courtois & J. D. Ford (Eds.), *Treating complex traumatic stress disorders: An evidence-based guide* (pp. 286–314). Guilford Press.

Fossati, A., Acquarini, E., Feeney, J. A., Borroni, S., Grazioli, F., Giarolli, L. E., Franciosi, G., & Maffei, C. (2009). Alexithymia and attachment insecurities in impulsive aggression. *Attachment & Human Development, 11*(2), 165–182. https://doi.org/10.1080/14616730802625235

Foulkes, L., & Blakemore, S. J. (2018). Studying individual differences in human adolescent brain development. *Nature Neuroscience, 21*(3), 315–323. https://doi.org/10.1038/s41593-018-0078-4

Frank, J. D. (1961). *Persuasion and healing: A comparative study of psychotherapy.* Johns Hopkins University Press.

Frank, J. D. (1968). The role of hope in psychotherapy. *International Journal of Psychiatry, 5*(5), 383–395.

Frank, J. D. (1971). Eleventh Emil A. Gutheil memorial conference. Therapeutic factors in psychotherapy. *American Journal of Psychotherapy, 25*(3), 350–361. https://doi.org/10.1176/appi.psychotherapy.1971.25.3.350

Frank, J. D. (1974). Psychotherapy: The restoration of morale. *The American Journal of Psychiatry, 131*(3), 271–274. https://doi.org/10.1176/ajp.131.3.271

Freud, S. (1953). Fragment of an analysis of a case of hysteria. In J. Strachey (Ed. & Trans.), *The standard edition of the complete psychological works of Sigmund Freud* (Vol. 7, pp. 1–122). Hogarth Press. (Original work published 1905)

Freud, S. (1957). Five lectures on psycho-analysis. In J. Strachey (Ed. & Trans.), *The standard edition of the complete psychological works of Sigmund Freud* (Vol. 11, pp. 9–589). Hogarth Press. (Original work published 1910)

Freud, S. (1964). Analysis terminable and interminable. In J. Strachey (Ed. & Trans.), *The standard edition of the complete psychological works of Sigmund Freud* (Vol. 23, pp. 209–254). Hogarth Press. (Original work published 1937)

Freyd, J. J. (1994). Betrayal trauma: Traumatic amnesia as an adaptive response to childhood abuse. *Ethics & Behavior, 4*(4), 307–329. https://doi.org/10.1207/s15327019eb0404_1

Friedlander, M. L., Escudero, V., Welmers-van de Poll, M. J., & Heatherington, L. (2018). Meta-analysis of the alliance-outcome relation in couple and family therapy. *Psychotherapy, 55*(4), 356–371. https://doi.org/10.1037/pst0000161

Friedlander, M. L., Lee, H. H., Shaffer, K. S., & Cabrera, P. (2014). Negotiating therapeutic alliances with a family at impasse. *Psychotherapy, 51*(1), 41–52. https://doi.org/10.1037/a0032524

Frisman, L., Ford, J., Lin, H.-J., Mallon, S., & Chang, R. (2008). Outcomes of trauma treatment using the TARGET model. *Journal of Groups in Addiction & Recovery, 3*(3–4), 285–303. https://doi.org/10.1080/15560350802424910

Gabbard, G. O. (Ed.). (1999). *Countertransference issues in psychiatric treatment.* American Psychiatric Association.

Gaddini, R. (1975). The concept of transitional object. *Journal of the American Academy of Child Psychiatry, 14*(4), 731–736. https://doi.org/10.1016/S0002-7138(09)61469-2

Gagne, J. R., & Saudino, K. J. (2016). The development of inhibitory control in early childhood: A twin study from 2–3 years. *Developmental Psychology, 52*(3), 391–399. https://doi.org/10.1037/dev0000090

Geltner, P. (2013). *Emotional communication: Countertransference analysis and the use of feeling in psychoanalytic technique.* Routledge.

Geva, R., & Feldman, R. (2008). A neurobiological model for the effects of early brainstem functioning on the development of behavior and emotion regulation in infants: Implications for prenatal and perinatal risk. *Journal of Child Psychology and Psychiatry, and Allied Disciplines, 49*(10), 1031–1041. https://doi.org/10.1111/j.1469-7610.2008.01918.x

Giacomo, D., & Weissmark, M. (1987). Toward a generative theory of the therapeutic field. *Family Process, 26*(4), 437–459. https://doi.org/10.1111/j.1545-5300.1987.00437.x

Glenn, J. (1986). Freud, Dora, and the maid: A study of countertransference. *Journal of the American Psychoanalytic Association, 34*(3), 591–606. https://doi.org/10.1177/000306518603400304

Glickauf-Hughes, C., Wells, M., & Chance, S. (1996). Techniques for strengthening clients' observing ego. *Psychotherapy, 33*(3), 431–440. https://doi.org/10.1037/0033-3204.33.3.431

Goldenberg, I., Stanton, M., & Goldenberg, H. (2017). *Family therapy: An overview* (9th ed.). Cengage Learning.

Golombek, K., Lidle, L., Tuschen-Caffier, B., Schmitz, J., & Vierrath, V. (2019). The role of emotion regulation in socially anxious children and adolescents: A systematic review. *European Child & Adolescent Psychiatry.* Advance online publication. https://doi.org/10.1007/s00787-019-01359-9

Gould, M. S., Kalafat, J., Harrismunfakh, J. L., & Kleinman, M. (2007). An evaluation of crisis hotline outcomes. Part 2: Suicidal callers. *Suicide & Life-Threatening Behavior, 37*(3), 338–352. https://doi.org/10.1521/suli.2007.37.3.338

Graham, J., Nosek, B. A., Haidt, J., Iyer, R., Koleva, S., & Ditto, P. H. (2011). Mapping the moral domain. *Journal of Personality and Social Psychology, 101*(2), 366–385. https://doi.org/10.1037/a0021847

Granqvist, P., Sroufe, L. A., Dozier, M., Hesse, E., Steele, M., van IJzendoorn, M., Solomon, J., Schuengel, C., Fearon, P., Bakermans-Kranenburg, M., Steele, H., Cassidy, J., Carlson, E., Madigan, S., Jacobvitz, D., Foster, S., Behrens, K., Rifkin-Graboi, A., Gribneau, N., . . . Duschinsky, R. (2017). Disorganized attachment in infancy: A review of the phenomenon and its implications for clinicians and policy-makers. *Attachment & Human Development, 19*(6), 534–558. https://doi.org/10.1080/14616734.2017.1354040

Greenberg, L. S., & Pascual-Leone, A. (2006). Emotion in psychotherapy: A practice-friendly research review. *Journal of Clinical Psychology, 62*(5), 611–630. https://doi.org/10.1002/jclp.20252

Gross, J. J. (2013). Emotion regulation: Taking stock and moving forward. *Emotion, 13*(3), 359–365. https://doi.org/10.1037/a0032135

Gross, J. J., Uusberg, H., & Uusberg, A. (2019). Mental illness and well-being: An affect regulation perspective. *World Psychiatry, 18*(2), 130–139. https://doi.org/10.1002/wps.20618

Groves, J. E. (1978). Taking care of the hateful patient. *The New England Journal of Medicine, 298*(16), 883–887. https://doi.org/10.1056/NEJM197804202981605

Gumz, A., Brähler, E., Geyer, M., & Erices, R. (2012). Crisis-repair sequences—Considerations on the classification and assessment of breaches in the therapeutic relationship. *BMC Medical Research Methodology, 12*(1), Article 10. https://doi.org/10.1186/1471-2288-12-10

Gunderson, J. G., Bateman, A., & Kernberg, O. (2007). Alternative perspectives on psychodynamic psychotherapy of borderline personality disorder: The case of "Ellen." *The American Journal of Psychiatry, 164*(9), 1333–1339. https://doi.org/10.1176/appi.ajp.2007.07050727

Hallion, L. S., Steinman, S. A., Tolin, D. F., & Diefenbach, G. J. (2018). Psychometric properties of the Difficulties in Emotion Regulation Scale (DERS) and its short forms in adults with emotional disorders. *Frontiers in Psychology, 9,* Article 539. https://doi.org/10.3389/fpsyg.2018.00539

Hamm, J. A., & Lysaker, P. H. (2018). Application of integrative metacognitive psychotherapy for serious mental illness. *American Journal of Psychotherapy, 71*(4), 122–127. https://doi.org/10.1176/appi.psychotherapy.20180033

Hamm, M. P., Osmond, M., Curran, J., Scott, S., Ali, S., Hartling, L., Gokiert, R., Cappelli, M., Hnatko, G., & Newton, A. S. (2010). A systematic review of crisis interventions used in the emergency department: Recommendations for pediatric care and research. *Pediatric Emergency Care, 26*(12), 952–962. https://doi.org/10.1097/PEC.0b013e3181fe9211

Hanna, K. M., Kaiser, K. L., Brown, S. G., Campbell-Grossman, C., Fial, A., Ford, A., Hudson, D. B., Keating-Lefler, R., Keeler, H., Moore, T. A., Nelson, A. E., Pelish, P., & Wilhelm, S. (2018). A scoping review of transitions, stress, and adaptation among emerging adults. *Advances in Nursing Science, 41*(3), 203–215. https://doi.org/10.1097/ANS.0000000000000214

Hansen, N. S., Thayer, R. E., Feldstein Ewing, S. W., Sabbineni, A., & Bryan, A. D. (2018). Neural correlates of risky sex and response inhibition in high-risk adolescents. *Journal of Research on Adolescence, 28*(1), 56–69. https://doi.org/10.1111/jora.12344

Harding, I. H., Yücel, M., Harrison, B. J., Pantelis, C., & Breakspear, M. (2015). Effective connectivity within the frontoparietal control network differentiates cognitive control and working memory. *NeuroImage, 106,* 144–153. https://doi.org/10.1016/j.neuroimage.2014.11.039

Harkness, A. R., Reynolds, S. M., & Lilienfeld, S. O. (2014). A review of systems for psychology and psychiatry: Adaptive systems, personality psychopathology five (PSY-5), and the *DSM-5. Journal of Personality Assessment, 96*(2), 121–139. https://doi.org/10.1080/00223891.2013.823438

Harrison, A., Tchanturia, K., Naumann, U., & Treasure, J. (2012). Social emotional functioning and cognitive styles in eating disorders. *British Journal of Clinical Psychology, 51*(3), 261–279. https://doi.org/10.1111/j.2044-8260.2011.02026.x

Hartnett, D., Carr, A., Hamilton, E., & O'Reilly, G. (2017). The effectiveness of functional family therapy for adolescent behavioral and substance misuse problems: A meta-analysis. *Family Process, 56*(3), 607–619. https://doi.org/10.1111/famp.12256

Harvey, M. R. (1996). An ecological view of psychological trauma and trauma recovery. *Journal of Traumatic Stress, 9*(1), 3–23. https://doi.org/10.1002/jts.2490090103

Hayes, J. A., Gelso, C. J., Goldberg, S., & Kivlighan, D. M. (2018). Countertransference management and effective psychotherapy: Meta-analytic findings. *Psychotherapy, 55*(4), 496–507. https://doi.org/10.1037/pst0000189

Hayes, S. C., Luoma, J. B., Bond, F. W., Masuda, A., & Lillis, J. (2006). Acceptance and commitment therapy: Model, processes and outcomes. *Behaviour Research and Therapy, 44*(1), 1–25. https://doi.org/10.1016/j.brat.2005.06.006

Heimann, P. (1960). Counter-transference. *The British Journal of Medical Psychology, 33*(1), 9–15. https://doi.org/10.1111/j.2044-8341.1960.tb01219.x

Herendeen, P. A., Blevins, R., Anson, E., & Smith, J. (2014). Barriers to and consequences of mandated reporting of child abuse by nurse practitioners. *Journal of Pediatric Health Care, 28*(1), e1–e7. https://doi.org/10.1016/j.pedhc.2013.06.004

Higa-McMillan, C. K., Francis, S. E., Rith-Najarian, L., & Chorpita, B. F. (2016). Evidence base update: 50 years of research on treatment for child and adolescent anxiety. *Journal of Clinical Child & Adolescent Psychology, 45*(2), 91–113. https://doi.org/10.1080/15374416.2015.1046177

Hill, C. E., Knox, S., & Pinto-Coelho, K. G. (2018). Therapist self-disclosure and immediacy: A qualitative meta-analysis. *Psychotherapy, 55*(4), 445–460. https://doi.org/10.1037/pst0000182

Holmes, J. (1993). Attachment theory: A biological basis for psychotherapy? *The British Journal of Psychiatry, 163*(4), 430–438. https://doi.org/10.1192/bjp.163.4.430

Holmes, J. (2017). Roots and routes to resilience and its role in psychotherapy: A selective, attachment-informed review. *Attachment & Human Development, 19*(4), 364–381. https://doi.org/10.1080/14616734.2017.1306087

Hora, T. (1951). The problem of negative countertransference. *American Journal of Psychotherapy, 5*(4), 560–567. https://doi.org/10.1176/appi.psychotherapy.1951.5.4.560

Horowitz, M. J. (2014). Clarifying values in psychotherapy. *Psychodynamic Psychiatry, 42*(4), 671–679. https://doi.org/10.1521/pdps.2014.42.4.671

Hunt, M., Pal, N. E., Schwartz, L., & O'Mathúna, D. (2018). Ethical challenges in the provision of mental health services for children and families during disasters. *Current Psychiatry Reports, 20*(8), Article 60. https://doi.org/10.1007/s11920-018-0917-8

Hunt, T., Wilson, C. J., Woodward, A., Caputi, P., & Wilson, I. (2018). Intervention among suicidal men: Future directions for telephone crisis support research. *Frontiers in Public Health, 6*, Article 1. https://doi.org/10.3389/fpubh.2018.00001

Hunter, V. (1998). Symbolic enactments in countertransference. *Psychoanalytic Review, 85*(5), 747–760.

Iacoviello, B. M., Wu, G., Abend, R., Murrough, J. W., Feder, A., Fruchter, E., Levinstein, Y., Wald, I., Bailey, C. R., Pine, D. S., Neumeister, A., Bar-Haim, Y., & Charney, D. S. (2014). Attention bias variability and symptoms of posttraumatic stress disorder. *Journal of Traumatic Stress, 27*(2), 232–239. https://doi.org/10.1002/jts.21899

Ijaz, S., Davies, P., Williams, C. J., Kessler, D., Lewis, G., & Wiles, N. (2018). Psychological therapies for treatment-resistant depression in adults. *Cochrane Database of Systematic Reviews.* https://doi.org/10.1002/14651858.CD010558.pub2

Jackson, C., Nissenson, K., & Cloitre, M. (2020). Cognitive behavioral therapy. In J. D. Ford & C. A. Courtois (Eds.), *Treating complex traumatic stress disorders in adults: Scientific foundations and therapeutic models* (2nd ed., pp. 369–389). Guilford Press.

Jacobs, T. J. (1986). On countertransference enactments. *Journal of the American Psychoanalytic Association, 34*(2), 289–307. https://doi.org/10.1177/000306518603400203

Jacobs, T. J. (1999). Countertransference past and present: A review of the concept. *International Journal of Psychoanalysis, 80*(Part 3), 575–594.

James, R. K., & Gilliland, B. E. (2017). *Crisis intervention strategies* (8th ed.). Cengage Learning.

Johnson, R., Persad, G., & Sisti, D. (2014). The Tarasoff rule: The implications of interstate variation and gaps in professional training. *The Journal of the American Academy of Psychiatry and the Law, 42*(4), 469–477.

Kächele, H., Albani, C., Pokorny, D., Blaser, G., Grüninger, S., König, S., Marschke, F., Geissler, I., Koerner, A., & Geyer, M. (2002). Reformulation of the core conflictual relationship theme (CCRT) Categories: The CCRT-LU category system. *Psychotherapy Research, 12*(3), 319–338. https://doi.org/10.1093/ptr/12.3.319

Kalaf, J., Vilete, L. M., Volchan, E., Fiszman, A., Coutinho, E. S., Andreoli, S. B., Quintana, M. I., de Jesus Mari, J., & Figueira, I. (2015). Peritraumatic tonic immobility in a large representative sample of the general population: Association with posttraumatic stress disorder and female gender. *Comprehensive Psychiatry, 60*, 68–72. https://doi.org/10.1016/j.comppsych.2015.04.001

Kalafat, J., Gould, M. S., Munfakh, J. L., & Kleinman, M. (2007). An evaluation of crisis hotline outcomes. Part 1: Nonsuicidal crisis callers. *Suicide & Life-Threatening Behavior, 37*(3), 322–337. https://doi.org/10.1521/suli.2007.37.3.322

Kanel, K. (2018). *A guide to crisis intervention* (6th ed.). Cengage.

Kantor, D., & Neal, J. H. (1985). Integrative shifts for the theory and practice of family systems therapy. *Family Process, 24*(1), 13–30. https://doi.org/10.1111/j.1545-5300.1985.00013.x

Kapoor, R., & Zonana, H. (2010). Forensic evaluations and mandated reporting of child abuse. *The Journal of the American Academy of Psychiatry and the Law, 38*(1), 49–56.

Karatsoreos, I. N., & McEwen, B. S. (2011). Psychobiological allostasis: Resistance, resilience and vulnerability. *Trends in Cognitive Sciences, 15*(12), 576–584. https://doi.org/10.1016/j.tics.2011.10.005

Karver, M. S., De Nadai, A. S., Monahan, M., & Shirk, S. R. (2018). Meta-analysis of the prospective relation between alliance and outcome in child and adolescent psychotherapy. *Psychotherapy, 55*(4), 341–355. https://doi.org/10.1037/pst0000176

Kaunhoven, R. J., & Dorjee, D. (2017). How does mindfulness modulate self-regulation in pre-adolescent children? An integrative neurocognitive review. *Neuroscience & Biobehavioral Reviews, 74*(Part A), 163–184. https://doi.org/10.1016/j.neubiorev.2017.01.007

Kelly, C. M., Jorm, A. F., & Kitchener, B. A. (2009). Development of mental health first aid guidelines for panic attacks: A Delphi study. *BMC Psychiatry, 9*(1), Article 49. https://doi.org/10.1186/1471-244X-9-49

Kernberg, O. F. (1979). Some implications of object relations theory for psychoanalytic technique. *Journal of the American Psychoanalytic Association, 27*(Suppl.), 207–239.

Klein, M. (1955). On identification. In M. Klein, P. Heimann, & R. E. Money-Kyrle (Eds.), *New directions in psycho-analysis: The significance of infant conflict in the pattern of adult behaviour* (pp. 309–345). Basic Books.

Kobylińska, D., & Kusev, P. (2019). Flexible emotion regulation: How situational demands and individual differences influence the effectiveness of regulatory strategies. *Frontiers in Psychology, 10*, Article 72. https://doi.org/10.3389/fpsyg.2019.00072

Kocsel, N., Köteles, F., Szemenyei, E., Szabó, E., Galambos, A., & Kökönyei, G. (2019). The association between perseverative cognition and resting heart rate variability: A focus on state ruminative thoughts. *Biological Psychology, 145*, 124–133. https://doi.org/10.1016/j.biopsycho.2019.04.004

Koechlin, H., Coakley, R., Schechter, N., Werner, C., & Kossowsky, J. (2018). The role of emotion regulation in chronic pain: A systematic literature review. *Journal of Psychosomatic Research, 107*, 38–45. https://doi.org/10.1016/j.jpsychores.2018.02.002

Kohrt, B. A., Blasingame, E., Compton, M. T., Dakana, S. F., Dossen, B., Lang, F., Strode, P., & Cooper, J. (2015). Adapting the crisis intervention team (CIT) model of police-mental health collaboration in a low-income, post-conflict country: Curriculum development in Liberia, West Africa. *American Journal of Public Health, 105*(3), e73–e80. https://doi.org/10.2105/AJPH.2014.302394

Kohut, H. (1965). Autonomy and integration. *Journal of the American Psychoanalytic Association, 13*(4), 851–856. https://doi.org/10.1177/000306516501300408

Kohut, H., & Wolf, E. S. (1978). The disorders of the self and their treatment: An outline. *The International Journal of Psycho-Analysis, 59*, 413–425.

Kolden, G. G., Wang, C. C., Austin, S. B., Chang, Y., & Klein, M. H. (2018). Congruence/genuineness: A meta-analysis. *Psychotherapy, 55*(4), 424–433. https://doi.org/10.1037/pst0000162

Korner, I. N. (1963). Values—A stepchild of psychology. *The International Journal of Social Psychiatry, 9*(3), 224–229. https://doi.org/10.1177/002076406300900309

Koweszko, T., Gierus, J., Więdłocha, M., Mosiołek, A., & Szulc, A. (2017). An introduction to the model of crisis intervention procedure for borderline patients (CIP-BP): A case study. *Archives of Psychiatric Nursing, 31*(3), 324–328. https://doi.org/10.1016/j.apnu.2016.11.002

Kramer, U., de Roten, Y., Perry, J. C., & Despland, J. N. (2013). Change in defense mechanisms and coping patterns during the course of 2-year-long psychotherapy and psychoanalysis for recurrent depression: A pilot study of a randomized controlled trial. *Journal of Nervous and Mental Disease, 201*(7), 614–620. https://doi.org/10.1097/NMD.0b013e3182982982

Krentzman, A. R. (2013). Review of the application of positive psychology to substance use, addiction, and recovery research. *Psychology of Addictive Behaviors, 27*(1), 151–165. https://doi.org/10.1037/a0029897

Lahav, Y., & Elklit, A. (2016). The cycle of healing—Dissociation and attachment during treatment of CSA survivors. *Child Abuse & Neglect, 60*, 67–76. https://doi.org/10.1016/j.chiabu.2016.09.009

Lanius, R. A., Rabellino, D., Boyd, J. E., Harricharan, S., Frewen, P. A., & McKinnon, M. C. (2017). The innate alarm system in PTSD: Conscious and subconscious processing of threat. *Current Opinion in Psychology, 14*, 109–115. https://doi.org/10.1016/j.copsyc.2016.11.006

Lating, J. M., & Bono, S. F. (2008). Crisis intervention and fostering resiliency. *International Journal of Emergency Mental Health, 10*(2), 87–93.

Lavelli, M., Carra, C., Rossi, G., & Keller, H. (2019). Culture-specific development of early mother-infant emotional co-regulation: Italian, Cameroonian, and West African immigrant dyads. *Developmental Psychology, 55*(9), 1850–1867. https://doi.org/10.1037/dev0000696

Leahy, R. L. (2001). *Overcoming resistance in cognitive therapy*. Guilford Press.

Lederer, W., & Jackson, D. (1968). *Mirages of marriage*. W. W. Norton.

Lee, E. B., An, W., Levin, M. E., & Twohig, M. P. (2015). An initial meta-analysis of acceptance and commitment therapy for treating substance use disorders. *Drug and Alcohol Dependence, 155*, 1–7. https://doi.org/10.1016/j.drugalcdep.2015.08.004

Leibovich, L., Nof, A., Auerbach-Barber, S., & Zilcha-Mano, S. (2018). A practical clinical suggestion for strengthening the alliance based on a supportive-expressive framework. *Psychotherapy, 55*(3), 231–240. https://doi.org/10.1037/pst0000195

Levi, B. H., & Crowell, K. (2011). Child abuse experts disagree about the threshold for mandated reporting. *Clinical Pediatrics, 50*(4), 321–329. https://doi.org/10.1177/0009922810389170

Levy, K. N. (2013). Introduction: Attachment theory and psychotherapy. *Journal of Clinical Psychology, 69*(11), 1133–1135. https://doi.org/10.1002/jclp.22040

Levy, K. N., Kivity, Y., Johnson, B. N., & Gooch, C. V. (2018). Adult attachment as a predictor and moderator of psychotherapy outcome: A meta-analysis. *Journal of Clinical Psychology, 74*(11), 1996–2013. https://doi.org/10.1002/jclp.22685

Lieberman, A. F., Padron, E., Van Horn, P., & Harris, W. W. (2005). Angels in the nursery: The intergenerational transmission of benevolent parental influences. *Infant Mental Health Journal, 26*(6), 504–520. https://doi.org/10.1002/imhj.20071

Lieberman, A. F., & Zeanah, C. H. (1999). Contributions of attachment theory to infant–parent psychotherapy and other interventions with infants and young children. In J. Cassidy & P. R. Shaver (Eds.), *Handbook of attachment: Theory, research, and clinical applications* (pp. 555–574). Guilford Press.

Liggett, J., & Sellbom, M. (2018). Examining the *DSM-5* alternative model of personality disorders operationalization of obsessive-compulsive personality disorder in a mental health sample. *Personality Disorders, 9*(5), 397–407. https://doi.org/10.1037/per0000285

Liggett, J., Sellbom, M., & Carmichael, K. L. C. (2017). Examining the *DSM-5* section III criteria for obsessive-compulsive personality disorder in a community sample. *Journal of Personality Disorders, 31*(6), 790–809. https://doi.org/10.1521/pedi_2017_31_281

Lincoln, A. (1861). *Inauguration of Mr. Lincoln. His address!* Library of Congress. https://www.loc.gov/resource/lprbscsm.scsm0728/?r=-0.259,-0.133,1.421,0.873,0

Lindemann, E. (1944). Symptomatology and management of acute grief. *The American Journal of Psychiatry, 101*(2), 141–148. https://doi.org/10.1176/ajp.101.2.141

Lindsay, E. K., & Creswell, J. D. (2017). Mechanisms of mindfulness training: Monitor and acceptance theory (MAT). *Clinical Psychology Review, 51*, 48–59. https://doi.org/10.1016/j.cpr.2016.10.011

Linehan, M. M. (1993). *Cognitive behavioral treatment of borderline personality disorder*. Guilford Press.

Liu, D. Y., & Thompson, R. J. (2017). Selection and implementation of emotion regulation strategies in major depressive disorder: An integrative review. *Clinical Psychology Review, 57,* 183–194. https://doi.org/10.1016/j.cpr.2017.07.004

Loewenstein, R. J. (2006). DID 101: A hands-on clinical guide to the stabilization phase of dissociative identity disorder treatment. *Psychiatric Clinics of North America, 29*(1), 305–332. https://doi.org/10.1016/j.psc.2005.10.005

Loizzo, J. (2009). Optimizing learning and quality of life throughout the lifespan: A global framework for research and application. *Annals of the New York Academy of Sciences, 1172*(1), 186–198. https://doi.org/10.1196/annals.1393.006

Lopes, P. N., Nezlek, J. B., Extremera, N., Hertel, J., Fernández-Berrocal, P., Schütz, A., & Salovey, P. (2011). Emotion regulation and the quality of social interaction: Does the ability to evaluate emotional situations and identify effective responses matter? *Journal of Personality, 79*(2), 429–467. https://doi.org/10.1111/j.1467-6494.2010.00689.x

Loughead, J. W., Luborsky, L., Weingarten, C. P., Krause, E. D., German, R. E., Kirk, D., & Gur, R. C. (2010). Brain activation during autobiographical relationship episode narratives: A core conflictual relationship theme approach. *Journal of Psychotherapy Research, 20*(3), 321–336. https://doi.org/10.1080/10503300903470735

Luborsky, L., & Crits-Christoph, P. (1989). A relationship pattern measure: The core conflictual relationship theme. *Psychiatry, 52*(3), 250–259. https://doi.org/10.1080/00332747.1989.11024448

Lückmann, H. C., Jacobs, H. I., & Sack, A. T. (2014). The cross-functional role of frontoparietal regions in cognition: Internal attention as the overarching mechanism. *Progress in Neurobiology, 116,* 66–86. https://doi.org/10.1016/j.pneurobio.2014.02.002

Ludwig, L., Werner, D., & Lincoln, T. M. (2019). The relevance of cognitive emotion regulation to psychotic symptoms—A systematic review and meta-analysis. *Clinical Psychology Review, 72,* Article 101746. https://doi.org/10.1016/j.cpr.2019.101746

Lyon, A. R., Lau, A. S., McCauley, E., Stoep, A. V., & Chorpita, B. F. (2014). A case for modular design: Implications for implementing evidence-based interventions with culturally-diverse youth. *Professional Psychology: Research and Practice, 45*(1), 57–66. https://doi.org/10.1037/a0035301

Lyons-Ruth, K., & Spielman, E. (2004). Disorganized infant attachment strategies and helpless-fearful profiles of parenting: Integrating attachment research with clinical intervention. *Infant Mental Health Journal, 25*(4), 318–335. https://doi.org/10.1002/imhj.20008

Maas, J., Hietbrink, L., Rinck, M., & Keijsers, G. P. (2013). Changing automatic behavior through self-monitoring: Does overt change also imply implicit change? *Journal of Behavior Therapy and Experimental Psychiatry, 44*(3), 279–284. https://doi.org/10.1016/j.jbtep.2012.12.002

Madigan, S., Benoit, D., & Boucher, C. (2011). Exploration of the links among fathers' unresolved states of mind with respect to attachment, atypical paternal behavior, and disorganized infant–father attachment. *Infant Mental Health Journal, 32*(3), 286–304. https://doi.org/10.1002/imhj.20297

Madigan, S., Moran, G., Schuengel, C., Pederson, D. R., & Otten, R. (2007). Unresolved maternal attachment representations, disrupted maternal behavior and disorganized attachment in infancy: Links to toddler behavior problems. *Journal of Child Psychology and Psychiatry, and Allied Disciplines, 48*(10), 1042–1050. https://doi.org/10.1111/j.1469-7610.2007.01805.x

Mahony, P. J. (1996). *Freud's Dora: A psychoanalytic, historical, and textual study.* Yale University Press.

Main, M. (2000). The organized categories of infant, child, and adult attachment: Flexible vs. inflexible attention under attachment-related stress. *Journal of the American Psychoanalytic Association, 48*(4), 1055–1096. https://doi.org/10.1177/00030651000480041801

Marchand, W. R. (2014). Neural mechanisms of mindfulness and meditation: Evidence from neuroimaging studies. *World Journal of Radiology, 6*(7), 471–479. https://doi.org/10.4329/wjr.v6.i7.471

March-Llanes, J., Marqués-Feixa, L., Mezquita, L., Fañanás, L., & Moya-Higueras, J. (2017). Stressful life events during adolescence and risk for externalizing and internalizing psychopathology: A meta-analysis. *European Child & Adolescent Psychiatry, 26*(12), 1409–1422. https://doi.org/10.1007/s00787-017-0996-9

Markowitz, J. C., Lowell, A., Milrod, B. L., Lopez-Yianilos, A., & Neria, Y. (2020). Symptom-specific reflective function as a potential mechanism of interpersonal psychotherapy outcome: A case report. *American Journal of Psychotherapy, 73*(1), 35–40. https://doi.org/10.1176/appi.psychotherapy.20190026

Marmarosh, C. L. (2014). Empirical research on attachment in group psychotherapy: Moving the field forward. *Psychotherapy, 51*(1), 88–92. https://doi.org/10.1037/a0032523

Marrow, M. T., Knudsen, K. J., Olafson, E., & Bucher, S. E. (2012). The value of implementing TARGET within a trauma-informed juvenile justice setting. *Journal of Child & Adolescent Trauma, 5,* 257–270. https://doi.org/10.1080/19361521.2012.697105

Marsland, A. L., Bachen, E. A., Cohen, S., Rabin, B., & Manuck, S. B. (2002). Stress, immune reactivity and susceptibility to infectious disease. *Physiology & Behavior, 77*(4–5), 711–716. https://doi.org/10.1016/S0031-9384(02)00923-X

Marsland, A. L., Walsh, C., Lockwood, K., & John-Henderson, N. A. (2017). The effects of acute psychological stress on circulating and stimulated inflammatory markers: A systematic review and meta-analysis. *Brain, Behavior, and Immunity, 64,* 208–219. https://doi.org/10.1016/j.bbi.2017.01.011

Marusak, H. A., Elrahal, F., Peters, C. A., Kundu, P., Lombardo, M. V., Calhoun, V. D., Goldberg, E. K., Cohen, C., Taub, J. W., & Rabinak, C. A. (2018).

Mindfulness and dynamic functional neural connectivity in children and adolescents. *Behavioural Brain Research, 336,* 211–218. https://doi.org/10.1016/j.bbr.2017.09.010

Marx, B. P., Forsyth, J. P., Gallup, G. G., Fuse, T., & Lexington, J. M. (2008). Tonic immobility as an evolved predator defense: Implications for sexual assault survivors. *Clinical Psychology: Science and Practice, 15*(1), 74–90. https://doi.org/10.1111/j.1468-2850.2008.00112.x

Mason, T. B., Smith, K. E., Engwall, A., Lass, A., Mead, M., Sorby, M., Bjorlie, K., Strauman, T. J., & Wonderlich, S. (2019). Self-discrepancy theory as a transdiagnostic framework: A meta-analysis of self-discrepancy and psychopathology. *Psychological Bulletin, 145*(4), 372–389. https://doi.org/10.1037/bul0000186

Masten, A. S. (2019). Resilience from a developmental systems perspective. *World Psychiatry, 18*(1), 101–102. https://doi.org/10.1002/wps.20591

Maxwell, H., Tasca, G. A., Grenon, R., Faye, M., Ritchie, K., Bissada, H., & Balfour, L. (2018). Change in attachment dimensions in women with binge-eating disorder following group psychodynamic interpersonal psychotherapy. *Psychotherapy Research, 28*(6), 887–901. https://doi.org/10.1080/10503307.2017.1278804

McClelland, M. M., & Cameron, C. E. (2011). Self-regulation and academic achievement in elementary school children. *New Directions for Child and Adolescent Development, 2011*(133), 29–44. https://doi.org/10.1002/cd.302

McEwen, B. S. (2017). Allostasis and the epigenetics of brain and body health over the life course: The brain on stress. *JAMA Psychiatry, 74*(6), 551–552. https://doi.org/10.1001/jamapsychiatry.2017.0270

McLaughlin, K. A., Rith-Najarian, L., Dirks, M. A., & Sheridan, M. A. (2015). Low vagal tone magnifies the association between psychosocial stress exposure and internalizing psychopathology in adolescents. *Journal of Clinical Child & Adolescent Psychology, 44*(2), 314–328. https://doi.org/10.1080/15374416.2013.843464

Meeten, F., & Davey, G. C. (2011). Mood-as-input hypothesis and perseverative psychopathologies. *Clinical Psychology Review, 31*(8), 1259–1275. https://doi.org/10.1016/j.cpr.2011.08.002

Meeten, F., Davey, G. C., Makovac, E., Watson, D. R., Garfinkel, S. N., Critchley, H. D., & Ottaviani, C. (2016). Goal directed worry rules are associated with distinct patterns of amygdala functional connectivity and vagal modulation during perseverative cognition. *Frontiers in Human Neuroscience, 10,* Article 553. https://doi.org/10.3389/fnhum.2016.00553

Merriam-Webster. (n.d.). Crisis. In *Merriam-Webster.com dictionary.* Retrieved May 12, 2020, from https://www.merriam-webster.com/dictionary/crisis

Mickleburgh, W. E. (1992). Clarification of values in counselling and psychotherapy. *The Australian and New Zealand Journal of Psychiatry, 26*(3), 391–398. https://doi.org/10.3109/00048679209072061

Mikulincer, M., & Shaver, P. R. (2012). An attachment perspective on psychopathology. *World Psychiatry, 11*(1), 11–15. https://doi.org/10.1016/j.wpsyc.2012.01.003

Miljkovitch, R., Moss, E., Bernier, A., Pascuzzo, K., & Sander, E. (2015). Refining the assessment of internal working models: The attachment multiple model interview. *Attachment & Human Development, 17*(5), 492–521. https://doi.org/10.1080/14616734.2015.1075561

Miller, A. (1981). *Prisoners of childhood.* Basic Books.

Miller, A. (1983). *For your own good.* Farrar, Straus & Giroux.

Miller, A. A., Isaacs, K. S., & Haggard, E. A. (1965). On the nature of the observing function of the ego. *The British Journal of Medical Psychology, 38*(2), 161–169. https://doi.org/10.1111/j.2044-8341.1965.tb00537.x

Miller, W. R., & National Institute on Alcohol Abuse and Alcoholism. (1995). *Motivational enhancement therapy manual: A clinical research guide for therapists treating individuals with alcohol abuse and dependence.* U.S. Department of Health and Human Services, Public Health Service, National Institutes of Health, National Institute on Alcohol Abuse and Alcoholism.

Miller, W. R., & Rollnick, S. (2002). *Motivational interviewing: Preparing people for change* (2nd ed.). Guilford Press.

Minuchin, S. (1982). Reflections on boundaries. *American Journal of Orthopsychiatry, 52*(4), 655–663. https://doi.org/10.1111/j.1939-0025.1982.tb01455.x

Minuchin, S. (1999). Retelling, reimagining, and re-searching: A continuing conversation. *Journal of Marital and Family Therapy, 25*(1), 9–14. https://doi.org/10.1111/j.1752-0606.1999.tb01106.x

Mishara, B. L., Chagnon, F., Daigle, M., Balan, B., Raymond, S., Marcoux, I., Bardon, C., Campbell, J. K., & Berman, A. (2007). Comparing models of helper behavior to actual practice in telephone crisis intervention: A silent monitoring study of calls to the U.S. 1-800-SUICIDE network. *Suicide & Life-Threatening Behavior, 37*(3), 291–307. https://doi.org/10.1521/suli.2007.37.3.291

Modell, A. H. (1976). "The holding environment" and the therapeutic action of psychoanalysis. *Journal of the American Psychoanalytic Association, 24*(2), 285–307. https://doi.org/10.1177/000306517602400202

Mor, N., & Winquist, J. (2002). Self-focused attention and negative affect: A meta-analysis. *Psychological Bulletin, 128*(4), 638–662. https://doi.org/10.1037/0033-2909.128.4.638

Moran, K. E., Ommerborn, M. J., Blackshear, C. T., Sims, M., & Clark, C. R. (2019). Financial stress and risk of coronary heart disease in the Jackson Heart Study. *American Journal of Preventive Medicine, 56*(2), 224–231. https://doi.org/10.1016/j.amepre.2018.09.022

Morris, A. S., Squeglia, L. M., Jacobus, J., & Silk, J. S. (2018). Adolescent brain development: Implications for understanding risk and resilience processes through neuroimaging research. *Journal of Research on Adolescence, 28*(1), 4–9. https://doi.org/10.1111/jora.12379

Mueller, S. C., Cromheeke, S., Siugzdaite, R., & Boehler, C. N. (2017). Evidence for the triadic model of adolescent brain development: Cognitive load and task-relevance of emotion differentially affect adolescents and adults. *Developmental Cognitive Neuroscience, 26*, 91–100. https://doi.org/10.1016/j.dcn.2017.06.004

Mullen, S. P., & Hall, P. A. (2015). Editorial: Physical activity, self-regulation, and executive control across the lifespan. *Frontiers in Human Neuroscience, 9*, Article 614. https://doi.org/10.3389/fnhum.2015.00614

Murphy, S. M., Irving, C. B., Adams, C. E., & Waqar, M. (2015). Crisis intervention for people with severe mental illnesses. *Cochrane Database of Systematic Reviews*. https://doi.org/10.1002/14651858.CD001087.pub5

Musicaro, R. M., Spinazzola, J., Arvidson, J., Swaroop, S. R., Goldblatt Grace, L., Yarrow, A., Suvak, M. K., & Ford, J. D. (2019). The complexity of adaptation to childhood polyvictimization in youth and young adults: Recommendations for multidisciplinary responders. *Trauma, Violence & Abuse, 20*(1), 81–98. https://doi.org/10.1177/1524838017692365

Myer, R. A., & James, R. K. (2005). *Workbook for crisis intervention.* Thomson Brooks/Cole.

Myrick, A. C., Chasson, G. S., Lanius, R. A., Leventhal, B., & Brand, B. L. (2015). Treatment of complex dissociative disorders: A comparison of interventions reported by community therapists versus those recommended by experts. *Journal of Trauma & Dissociation, 16*(1), 51–67. https://doi.org/10.1080/15299732.2014.949020

Newman, C. F. (2002). A case illustration of resistance from a cognitive perspective. *Journal of Clinical Psychology, 58*(2), 145–149. https://doi.org/10.1002/jclp.1137

Ng, V., Cao, M., Marsh, H. W., Tay, L., & Seligman, M. E. P. (2017). The factor structure of the Values in Action Inventory of Strengths (VIA-IS): An item-level exploratory structural equation modeling (ESEM) bifactor analysis. *Psychological Assessment, 29*(8), 1053–1058. https://doi.org/10.1037/pas0000396

Nichols, M. P., & Davis, S. D. (2020). *The essentials of family therapy* (7th ed.). Pearson Education.

Nienhuis, J. B., Owen, J., Valentine, J. C., Winkeljohn Black, S., Halford, T. C., Parazak, S. E., Budge, S., & Hilsenroth, M. (2018). Therapeutic alliance, empathy, and genuineness in individual adult psychotherapy: A meta-analytic review. *Psychotherapy Research, 28*(4), 593–605. https://doi.org/10.1080/10503307.2016.1204023

Niles, B. L., Williston, S. K., & Mori, D. L. (2020). Mindfulness approaches. In J. D. Ford & C. A. Courtois (Eds.), *Treating complex traumatic stress disorders in adults: Scientific foundations and therapeutic models* (2nd ed., pp. 550–568). Guilford Press.

Norcross, J. C., & Lambert, M. J. (2018). Psychotherapy relationships that work III. *Psychotherapy, 55*(4), 303–315. https://doi.org/10.1037/pst0000193

Noyce, G. (2016). Crisis intervention for people with severe mental illness. *Issues in Mental Health Nursing, 37*(11), 881–882. https://doi.org/10.1080/01612840.2016.1249237

O'Connell, B. (2012). *Solution-focused therapy* (3rd ed.). SAGE. https://doi.org/10.4135/9781473957794

Ogden, P. (2020). Sensorimotor psychotherapy. In J. D. Ford & C. A. Courtois (Eds.), *Treating complex traumatic stress disorders in adults: Scientific foundations and therapeutic models* (2nd ed., pp. 509–532). Guilford Press.

O'Hanlon, B. (2003). *Inclusive therapy: 26 methods of respectful, resistance-dissolving therapy.* W. W. Norton.

Okur Güney, Z. E., Sattel, H., Witthöft, M., & Henningsen, P. (2019). Emotion regulation in patients with somatic symptom and related disorders: A systematic review. *PLOS ONE, 14*(6), Article e0217277. https://doi.org/10.1371/journal.pone.0217277

Oldershaw, A., Lavender, T., Sallis, H., Stahl, D., & Schmidt, U. (2015). Emotion generation and regulation in anorexia nervosa: A systematic review and meta-analysis of self-report data. *Clinical Psychology Review, 39*, 83–95. https://doi.org/10.1016/j.cpr.2015.04.005

Ottaviani, C., Thayer, J. F., Verkuil, B., Lonigro, A., Medea, B., Couyoumdjian, A., & Brosschot, J. F. (2016). Physiological concomitants of perseverative cognition: A systematic review and meta-analysis. *Psychological Bulletin, 142*(3), 231–259. https://doi.org/10.1037/bul0000036

Paivio, S. C. (2013). Essential processes in emotion-focused therapy. *Psychotherapy, 50*(3), 341–345. https://doi.org/10.1037/a0032810

Pallini, S., Chirumbolo, A., Morelli, M., Baiocco, R., Laghi, F., & Eisenberg, N. (2018). The relation of attachment security status to effortful self-regulation: A meta-analysis. *Psychological Bulletin, 144*(5), 501–531. https://doi.org/10.1037/bul0000134

Pam, A., & Pearson, J. (1994). The geometry of the eternal triangle. *Family Process, 33*(2), 175–190. https://doi.org/10.1111/j.1545-5300.1994.00175.x

Parker, C. L., Everly, G. S., Jr., Barnett, D. J., & Links, J. M. (2006). Establishing evidence-informed core intervention competencies in psychological first aid for public health personnel. *International Journal of Emergency Mental Health, 8*(2), 83–92.

Parmentier, F. B. R., García-Toro, M., García-Campayo, J., Yañez, A. M., Andrés, P., & Gili, M. (2019). Mindfulness and symptoms of depression and anxiety in the general population: The mediating roles of worry, rumination, reappraisal and suppression. *Frontiers in Psychology, 10*, Article 506. https://doi.org/10.3389/fpsyg.2019.00506

Peale, N. V. (1952). *Power of positive thinking.* Prentice-Hall.

Peluso, P. R., & Freund, R. R. (2018). Therapist and client emotional expression and psychotherapy outcomes: A meta-analysis. *Psychotherapy*, *55*(4), 461–472. https://doi.org/10.1037/pst0000165

Penela, E. C., Walker, O. L., Degnan, K. A., Fox, N. A., & Henderson, H. A. (2015). Early behavioral inhibition and emotion regulation: Pathways toward social competence in middle childhood. *Child Development*, *86*(4), 1227–1240. https://doi.org/10.1111/cdev.12384

Pérez-Rojas, A. E., Palma, B., Bhatia, A., Jackson, J., Norwood, E., Hayes, J. A., & Gelso, C. J. (2017). The development and initial validation of the Counter-transference Management Scale. *Psychotherapy*, *54*(3), 307–319. https://doi.org/10.1037/pst0000126

Perry, J. C., & Bond, M. (2012). Change in defense mechanisms during long-term dynamic psychotherapy and five-year outcome. *The American Journal of Psychiatry*, *169*(9), 916–925. https://doi.org/10.1176/appi.ajp.2012.11091403

Perry, J. C., Bond, M., & Presniak, M. D. (2013). Alliance, reactions to treatment, and counter-transference in the process of recovery from suicidal phenomena in long-term dynamic psychotherapy. *Psychotherapy Research*, *23*(5), 592–605. https://doi.org/10.1080/10503307.2013.809560

Petraglia, J., Bhatia, M., de Roten, Y., Despland, J. N., & Drapeau, M. (2015). An empirical investigation of defense interpretation depth, defensive functioning, and alliance strength in psychodynamic psychotherapy. *American Journal of Psychotherapy*, *69*(1), 1–17. https://doi.org/10.1176/appi.psychotherapy.2015.69.1.1

Pittel, S. M., & Mendelsohn, G. A. (1966). Measurement of moral values: A review and critique. *Psychological Bulletin*, *66*(1), 22–35. https://doi.org/10.1037/h0023425

Plakun, E. M. (2019). Psychotherapy with suicidal patients part 2: An alliance based intervention for suicide. *Journal of Psychiatric Practice*, *25*(1), 41–45. https://doi.org/10.1097/PRA.0000000000000355

Plutchik, R., Conte, H. R., & Karasu, T. B. (1994). Critical incidents in psychotherapy. *American Journal of Psychotherapy*, *48*(1), 75–84. https://doi.org/10.1176/appi.psychotherapy.1994.48.1.75

Porges, S. W. (2007). The polyvagal perspective. *Biological Psychology*, *74*(2), 116–143. https://doi.org/10.1016/j.biopsycho.2006.06.009

Porges, S. W. (2009). The polyvagal theory: New insights into adaptive reactions of the autonomic nervous system. *Cleveland Clinic Journal of Medicine*, *76*(4 Suppl. 2), S86–S90. https://doi.org/10.3949/ccjm.76.s2.17

Porter, E., & Chambless, D. L. (2015). A systematic review of predictors and moderators of improvement in cognitive-behavioral therapy for panic disorder and agoraphobia. *Clinical Psychology Review*, *42*, 179–192. https://doi.org/10.1016/j.cpr.2015.09.004

Price, O., & Baker, J. (2012). Key components of de-escalation techniques: A thematic synthesis. *International Journal of Mental Health Nursing*, *21*(4), 310–319. https://doi.org/10.1111/j.1447-0349.2011.00793.x

Price, O., Baker, J., Bee, P., & Lovell, K. (2015). Learning and performance outcomes of mental health staff training in de-escalation techniques for the management of violence and aggression. *The British Journal of Psychiatry*, *206*(6), 447–455. https://doi.org/10.1192/bjp.bp.114.144576

Racker, H. (2007). The meanings and uses of countertransference. *The Psychoanalytic Quarterly*, *76*(3), 725–777. https://doi.org/10.1002/j.2167-4086. 2007.tb00277.x (Original work published 1957)

Radkovsky, A., McArdle, J. J., Bockting, C. L., & Berking, M. (2014). Successful emotion regulation skills application predicts subsequent reduction of symptom severity during treatment of major depressive disorder. *Journal of Consulting and Clinical Psychology*, *82*(2), 248–262. https://doi.org/10.1037/a0035828

Redish, A. D., Jensen, S., & Johnson, A. (2008). A unified framework for addiction: Vulnerabilities in the decision process. *Behavioral and Brain Sciences*, *31*(4), 415–437. https://doi.org/10.1017/S0140525X0800472X

Robbins, O. S. (1978). Crisis theory and its relation to psychotherapy. *Psychotherapy and Psychosomatics*, *29*(1–4), 288–292. https://doi.org/10.1159/000287143

Roberts, A. R. (2002). Assessment, crisis intervention, and trauma treatment: The integrative ACT intervention model. *Brief Treatment and Crisis Intervention*, *2*(1), 1–21. https://doi.org/10.1093/brief-treatment/2.1.1

Roberts, A. R. (Ed.). (2005). *Crisis intervention handbook: Assessment, treatment, and research*. Oxford University Press.

Roberts, A. R., & Everly, G. S., Jr. (2006). A meta-analysis of 36 crisis intervention studies. *Brief Treatment and Crisis Intervention*, *6*(1), 10–21. https://doi.org/10.1093/brief-treatment/mhj006

Rodrigo, M. J., Padrón, I., de Vega, M., & Ferstl, E. (2018). Neural substrates of counterfactual emotions after risky decisions in late adolescents and young adults. *Journal of Research on Adolescence*, *28*(1), 70–86. https://doi.org/10.1111/jora.12342

Roes, N. A. (2002). *Solutions for the "treatment resistant" addicted client: Therapeutic techniques for engaging challenging clients*. Haworth Press.

Rogers, C. R. (1951). *Client-centered therapy*. Houghton-Mifflin.

Rogers, C. R. (1957). The necessary and sufficient conditions of therapeutic personality change. *Journal of Consulting Psychology*, *21*(2), 95–103. http://www.ncbi.nlm.nih.gov/pubmed/13416422. https://doi.org/10.1037/h0045357

Rogers, C. R. (1964). Toward a modern approach to values: The valuing process in the mature person. *Journal of Abnormal Psychology*, *68*(2), 160–167. https://doi.org/10.1037/h0046419

Roth, L. H., & Meisel, A. (1977). Dangerousness, confidentiality, and the duty to warn. *The American Journal of Psychiatry*, *134*(5), 508–511. https://doi.org/10.1176/ajp.134.5.508

Rubin, S. S. (2001). Ethical dilemmas, good intentions, and the road to hell: A clinical-ethical perspective on Yalom's depiction of Trotter's therapy. *Psychiatry, 64*(2), 146–157. https://doi.org/10.1521/psyc.64.2.146.18620

Ruchlewska, A., Kamperman, A. M., van der Gaag, M., Wierdsma, A. I., & Mulder, N. C. (2016). Working alliance in patients with severe mental illness who need a crisis intervention plan. *Community Mental Health Journal, 52*(1), 102–108. https://doi.org/10.1007/s10597-015-9839-7

Sable, P. (2004). Attachment, ethology and adult psychotherapy. *Attachment & Human Development, 6*(1), 3–19. https://doi.org/10.1080/14616730410001663498

Sagui-Henson, S. J., Levens, S. M., & Blevins, C. L. (2018). Examining the psychological and emotional mechanisms of mindfulness that reduce stress to enhance healthy behaviours. *Stress and Health, 34*(3), 379–390. Advance online publication https://doi.org/10.1002/smi.2797

Satten, W. (2002). A case illustration of resistance from a psychodynamic perspective. *Journal of Clinical Psychology, 58*(2), 139–144. https://doi.org/10.1002/jclp.1136

Sauer, C., Sheppes, G., Lackner, H. K., Arens, E. A., Tarrasch, R., & Barnow, S. (2016). Emotion regulation choice in female patients with borderline personality disorder: Findings from self-reports and experimental measures. *Psychiatry Research, 242*, 375–384. https://doi.org/10.1016/j.psychres.2016.04.113

Schäfer, J. O., Naumann, E., Holmes, E. A., Tuschen-Caffier, B., & Samson, A. C. (2017). Emotion regulation strategies in depressive and anxiety symptoms in youth: A meta-analytic review. *Journal of Youth and Adolescence, 46*(2), 261–276. https://doi.org/10.1007/s10964-016-0585-0

Schmideberg, M. (1958). Values and goals in psychotherapy. *Psychiatric Quarterly, 32*(2), 233–265. https://doi.org/10.1007/BF01561631

Schwaber, E. A. (1992). Countertransference: The analyst's retreat from the patient's vantage point. *The International Journal of Psycho-Analysis, 73*(Part 2), 349–361.

Schwartz, S. L. (1971). A review of crisis intervention programs. *Psychiatric Quarterly, 45*(4), 498–508. https://doi.org/10.1007/BF01563211

Selye, H. (1951). The general adaptation syndrome and the diseases of adaptation. *The American Journal of Medicine, 10*(5), 549–555. https://doi.org/10.1016/0002-9343(51)90327-0

Sheppes, G., & Gross, J. J. (2011). Is timing everything? Temporal considerations in emotion regulation. *Personality and Social Psychology Review, 15*(4), 319–331. https://doi.org/10.1177/1088868310395778

Sheppes, G., Scheibe, S., Suri, G., Radu, P., Blechert, J., & Gross, J. J. (2014). Emotion regulation choice: A conceptual framework and supporting evidence. *Journal of Experimental Psychology: General, 143*(1), 163–181. https://doi.org/10.1037/a0030831

Shields, G. S. (2017). Response: Commentary: The effects of acute stress on core executive functions: A meta-analysis and comparison with cortisol. *Frontiers in Psychology, 8*, Article 2090. https://doi.org/10.3389/fpsyg.2017.02090

Shimoji, A., & Miyakawa, T. (2000). Culture-bound syndrome and a culturally sensitive approach: From a viewpoint of medical anthropology. *Psychiatry and Clinical Neurosciences, 54*(4), 461–466. https://doi.org/10.1046/j.1440-1819.2000.00737.x

Shing, Y. L., Lindenberger, U., Diamond, A., Li, S. C., & Davidson, M. C. (2010). Memory maintenance and inhibitory control differentiate from early childhood to adolescence. *Developmental Neuropsychology, 35*(6), 679–697. https://doi.org/10.1080/87565641.2010.508546

Silverman, M. H., Jedd, K., & Luciana, M. (2015). Neural networks involved in adolescent reward processing: An activation likelihood estimation meta-analysis of functional neuroimaging studies. *NeuroImage, 122*, 427–439. https://doi.org/10.1016/j.neuroimage.2015.07.083

Simpson, S. A. (2019). A single-session crisis intervention therapy model for emergency psychiatry. *Clinical Practice and Cases in Emergency Medicine, 3*(1), 27–32. https://doi.org/10.5811/cpcem.2018.10.40443

Sisk, C. L. (2017). Development: Pubertal hormones meet the adolescent brain. *Current Biology, 27*(14), R706–R708. https://doi.org/10.1016/j.cub.2017.05.092

Skodol, A. E., Kass, F., & Charles, E. (1979). Crisis in psychotherapy: Principles of emergency consultation and intervention. *American Journal of Orthopsychiatry, 49*(4), 585–597. https://doi.org/10.1111/j.1939-0025.1979.tb02644.x

Slade, A. (2009). Review of attachment in psychotherapy. *Psychotherapy, 46*(2), 270–271. https://doi.org/10.1037/a0016079

Slade, A., & Holmes, J. (2019). Attachment and psychotherapy. *Current Opinion in Psychology, 25*, 152–156. https://doi.org/10.1016/j.copsyc.2018.06.008

Sloan, E., Hall, K., Moulding, R., Bryce, S., Mildred, H., & Staiger, P. K. (2017). Emotion regulation as a transdiagnostic treatment construct across anxiety, depression, substance, eating and borderline personality disorders: A systematic review. *Clinical Psychology Review, 57*, 141–163. https://doi.org/10.1016/j.cpr.2017.09.002

Smith, M. B. (2000). Values, politics, and psychology. *American Psychologist, 55*(10), 1151–1152. https://doi.org/10.1037/0003-066X.55.10.1151

Smith, S., & Ford, J. D. (2020). Complementary and healing therapies. In J. D. Ford & C. A. Courtois (Eds.), *Treating complex traumatic stress disorders in adults: Scientific foundations and therapeutic models* (2nd ed., pp. 569–590). Guilford Press.

Spencer, S., Johnson, P., & Smith, I. C. (2018). De-escalation techniques for managing non-psychosis induced aggression in adults. *Cochrane Database of Systematic Reviews.* https://doi.org/10.1002/14651858.CD012034.pub2

Spiegel, E. B. (2016). Attachment-focused psychotherapy and the wounded self. *The American Journal of Clinical Hypnosis, 59*(1), 47–68. https://doi.org/10.1080/00029157.2016.1163658

Spinazzola, J., van der Kolk, B., & Ford, J. D. (2018). When nowhere is safe: Interpersonal trauma and attachment adversity as antecedents of post-traumatic stress disorder and developmental trauma disorder. *Journal of Traumatic Stress, 31*(5), 631–642. https://doi.org/10.1002/jts.22320

Steele, K., & van der Hart, O. (2020). Assessing and treating complex dissociative disorders. In J. D. Ford & C. A. Courtois (Eds.), *Treating complex traumatic stress disorders in adults: Scientific foundations and therapeutic models* (2nd ed.; pp. 149–167). Guilford Press.

Stein, D. M., & Lambert, M. J. (1984). Telephone counseling and crisis intervention: A review. *American Journal of Community Psychology, 12*(1), 101–126. https://doi.org/10.1007/BF00896931

Steinbeis, N., Engert, V., Linz, R., & Singer, T. (2015). The effects of stress and affiliation on social decision-making: Investigating the tend-and-befriend pattern. *Psychoneuroendocrinology, 62*, 138–148. https://doi.org/10.1016/j.psyneuen.2015.08.003

Steinberg, K. L., Levine, M., & Doueck, H. J. (1997). Effects of legally mandated child-abuse reports on the therapeutic relationship: A survey of psychotherapists. *American Journal of Orthopsychiatry, 67*(1), 112–122. https://doi.org/10.1037/h0080216

Stern, D. N., Bruschweiler-Stern, N., Harrison, A. M., Lyons-Ruth, K., Morgan, A. C., Nahum, J. P., Sander, L., & Tronick, E. Z. (2001). Die Rolle des impliziten Wissens bei der therapeutischen Veränderung [The role of implicit knowledge in therapeutic change: Some implications of developmental observations for adult psychotherapy]. *Psychotherapie, Psychosomatik, Medizinische Psychologie, 51*(3/4), 147–152. https://doi.org/10.1055/s-2001-12386

Strauß, B., Altmann, U., Manes, S., Tholl, A., Koranyi, S., Nolte, T., Beutel, M. E., Wiltink, J., Herpertz, S., Hiller, W., Hoyer, J., Joraschky, P., Nolting, B., Ritter, V., Stangier, U., Willutzki, U., Salzer, S., Leibing, E., Leichsenring, F., & Kirchmann, H. (2018). Changes of attachment characteristics during psychotherapy of patients with social anxiety disorder: Results from the SOPHO-Net trial. *PLOS ONE, 13*(3), Article e0192802. https://doi.org/10.1371/journal.pone.0192802

Studer, R. K., Nielsen, C., Klumb, P. L., Hildebrandt, H., Nater, U. M., Wild, P., Heinzer, R., Haba-Rubio, J., Danuser, B., & Gomez, P. (2019). The mediating role of mood in the relationship between perseverative cognition, sleep and subjective health complaints in music students. *Psychology & Health, 34*(6), 754–770. https://doi.org/10.1080/08870446.2019.1574014

Suri, G., Sheppes, G., Young, G., Abraham, D., McRae, K., & Gross, J. J. (2018). Emotion regulation choice: The role of environmental affordances. *Cognition and Emotion, 32*(5), 963–971. https://doi.org/10.1080/02699931.2017.1371003

Szabo, Y. Z., Slavish, D. C., & Graham-Engeland, J. E. (in press). The effect of acute stress on salivary markers of inflammation: A systematic review and meta-analysis [Corrected proof]. *Brain, Behavior, and Immunity.* https://doi.org/10.1016/j.bbi.2020.04.078

Talia, A., Muzi, L., Lingiardi, V., & Taubner, S. (2020). How to be a secure base: Therapists' attachment representations and their link to attunement in psychotherapy. *Attachment & Human Development, 22*(2), 189–206. https://doi.org/10.1080/14616734.2018.1534247

Tamir, M. (2016). Why do people regulate their emotions? A taxonomy of motives in emotion regulation. *Personality and Social Psychology Review, 20*(3), 199–222. https://doi.org/10.1177/1088868315586325

Tamnes, C. K., Bos, M. G. N., van de Kamp, F. C., Peters, S., & Crone, E. A. (2018). Longitudinal development of hippocampal subregions from childhood to adulthood. *Developmental Cognitive Neuroscience, 30*, 212–222. https://doi.org/10.1016/j.dcn.2018.03.009

Taylor, S. E., Klein, L. C., Lewis, B. P., Gruenewald, T. L., Gurung, R. A., & Updegraff, J. A. (2000). Biobehavioral responses to stress in females: Tend-and-befriend, not fight-or-flight. *Psychological Review, 107*(3), 411–429. https://doi.org/10.1037/0033-295X.107.3.411

Teckchandani, S., & Barad, M. (2017). Treatment strategies for the opioid-dependent patient. *Current Pain and Headache Reports, 21*, Article 45. https://doi.org/10.1007/s11916-017-0644-6

Thayer, J. F., Yamamoto, S. S., & Brosschot, J. F. (2010). The relationship of autonomic imbalance, heart rate variability and cardiovascular disease risk factors. *International Journal of Cardiology, 141*(2), 122–131. https://doi.org/10.1016/j.ijcard.2009.09.543

Tortella-Feliu, M., Morillas-Romero, A., Balle, M., Bornas, X., Llabrés, J., & Pacheco-Unguetti, A. P. (2014). Attentional control, attentional network functioning, and emotion regulation styles. *Cognition and Emotion, 28*(5), 769–780. https://doi.org/10.1080/02699931.2013.860889

Trick, L., Watkins, E., Windeatt, S., & Dickens, C. (2016). The association of perseverative negative thinking with depression, anxiety and emotional distress in people with long term conditions: A systematic review. *Journal of Psychosomatic Research, 91*, 89–101. https://doi.org/10.1016/j.jpsychores.2016.11.004

Tronick, E., Als, H., Adamson, L., Wise, S., & Brazelton, T. B. (1978). The infant's response to entrapment between contradictory messages in face-to-face interaction. *Journal of the American Academy of Child Psychiatry, 17*(1), 1–13. https://doi.org/10.1016/S0002-7138(09)62273-1

Tryon, G. S., Birch, S. E., & Verkuilen, J. (2018). Meta-analyses of the relation of goal consensus and collaboration to psychotherapy outcome. *Psychotherapy, 55*(4), 372–383. https://doi.org/10.1037/pst0000170

Ulberg, R., Høglend, P., Marble, A., & Sørbye, Ø. (2009). From submission to autonomy: Approaching independent decision making. A single-case study in a randomized, controlled study of long-term effects of dynamic psychotherapy. *American Journal of Psychotherapy*, *63*(3), 227–243. https://doi.org/10.1176/appi.psychotherapy.2009.63.3.227

Ungar, M. (2015). Social ecological complexity and resilience processes. *Behavioral and Brain Sciences*, *38*, Article e124. https://doi.org/10.1017/S0140525X14001721

van der Feltz-Cornelis, C. M., Sarchiapone, M., Postuvan, V., Volker, D., Roskar, S., Grum, A. T., Carli, V., McDaid, D., O'Connor, R., Maxwell, M., Ibelshäuser, A., Van Audenhove, C., Scheerder, G., Sisask, M., Gusmão, R., & Hegerl, U. (2011). Best practice elements of multilevel suicide prevention strategies: A review of systematic reviews. *Crisis*, *32*(6), 319–333. https://doi.org/10.1027/0227-5910/a000109

van der Kolk, B. A. (2014). *The body keeps the score*. Penguin.

van der Pol, T. M., Hoeve, M., Noom, M. J., Stams, G. J. J. M., Doreleijers, T. A. H., van Domburgh, L., & Vermeiren, R. R. J. M. (2017). Research review: The effectiveness of multidimensional family therapy in treating adolescents with multiple behavior problems—A meta-analysis. *Journal of Child Psychology and Psychiatry*, *58*(5), 532–545. https://doi.org/10.1111/jcpp.12685

van Hoof, M. J., Riem, M. M. E., Garrett, A. S., van der Wee, N. J. A., van IJzendoorn, M. H., & Vermeiren, R. R. J. M. (2019). Unresolved-disorganized attachment adjusted for a general psychopathology factor associated with atypical amygdala resting-state functional connectivity. *European Journal of Psychotraumatology*, *10*(1), Article 1583525. https://doi.org/10.1080/20008198.2019.1583525

Vilhelmsson, A., Svensson, T., & Meeuwisse, A. (2013). A pill for the ill? Patients' reports of their experience of the medical encounter in the treatment of depression. *PLOS ONE*, *8*(6), Article e66338. https://doi.org/10.1371/journal.pone.0066338

Villalta, L., Smith, P., Hickin, N., & Stringaris, A. (2018). Emotion regulation difficulties in traumatized youth: A meta-analysis and conceptual review. *European Child & Adolescent Psychiatry*, *27*(4), 527–544. https://doi.org/10.1007/s00787-018-1105-4

Visted, E., Vøllestad, J., Nielsen, M. B., & Schanche, E. (2018). Emotion regulation in current and remitted depression: A systematic review and meta-analysis. *Frontiers in Psychology*, *9*, Article 756. https://doi.org/10.3389/fpsyg.2018.00756

Vohs, J. L., Leonhardt, B. L., James, A. V., Francis, M. M., Breier, A., Mehdiyoun, N., Visco, A. C., & Lysaker, P. H. (2018). Metacognitive reflection and insight therapy for early psychosis: A preliminary study of a novel integrative psychotherapy. *Schizophrenia Research*, *195*, 428–433. https://doi.org/10.1016/j.schres.2017.10.041

Volchan, E., Souza, G. G., Franklin, C. M., Norte, C. E., Rocha-Rego, V., Oliveira, J. M., David, I. A., Mendlowicz, M. V., Coutinho, E. S., Fiszman, A., Berger, W., Marques-Portella, C., & Figueira, I. (2011). Is there tonic immobility in humans? Biological evidence from victims of traumatic stress. *Biological Psychology, 88*(1), 13–19. https://doi.org/10.1016/j.biopsycho.2011.06.002

Wang, Y. Y., Li, X. H., Zheng, W., Xu, Z. Y., Ng, C. H., Ungvari, G. S., Yuan, Z., & Xiang, Y. T. (2018). Mindfulness-based interventions for major depressive disorder: A comprehensive meta-analysis of randomized controlled trials. *Journal of Affective Disorders, 229,* 429–436. https://doi.org/10.1016/j.jad.2017.12.093

Waters, H. S., & Waters, E. (2006). The attachment working models concept: Among other things, we build script-like representations of secure base experiences. *Attachment & Human Development, 8*(3), 185–197. https://doi.org/10.1080/14616730600856016

Watson, H., & Levine, M. (1989). Psychotherapy and mandated reporting of child abuse. *American Journal of Orthopsychiatry, 59*(2), 246–256. https://doi.org/10.1111/j.1939-0025.1989.tb01656.x

Watzlawick, P., Weakland, J., & Fisch, R. (1974). *Change: Principles of problem formation and problem resolution.* W. W. Norton.

Webb, T. L., Miles, E., & Sheeran, P. (2012). Dealing with feeling: A meta-analysis of the effectiveness of strategies derived from the process model of emotion regulation. *Psychological Bulletin, 138*(4), 775–808. https://doi.org/10.1037/a0027600

Weick, K. E. (1984). Small wins: Redefining the scale of social problems. *American Psychologist, 39*(1), 40–49. https://doi.org/10.1037/0003-066X.39.1.40

Weiner, I. B. (1975). *Principles of psychotherapy.* John Wiley & Sons.

Weisz, J. R., Chorpita, B. F., Palinkas, L. A., Schoenwald, S. K., Miranda, J., Bearman, S. K., Daleiden, E. L., Ugueto, A. M., Ho, A., Martin, J., Gray, J., Alleyne, A., Langer, D. A., Southam-Gerow, M. A., Gibbons, R. D., & the Research Network on Youth Mental Health. (2012). Testing standard and modular designs for psychotherapy treating depression, anxiety, and conduct problems in youth: A randomized effectiveness trial. *Archives of General Psychiatry, 69*(3), 274–282. https://doi.org/10.1001/archgenpsychiatry.2011.147

Westra, H. A., Aviram, A., Connors, L., Kertes, A., & Ahmed, M. (2012). Therapist emotional reactions and client resistance in cognitive behavioral therapy. *Psychotherapy, 49*(2), 163–172. https://doi.org/10.1037/a0023200

Wheelock, M. D., Rangaprakash, D., Harnett, N. G., Wood, K. H., Orem, T. R., Mrug, S., Granger, D. A., Deshpande, G., & Knight, D. C. (2018). Psychosocial stress reactivity is associated with decreased whole-brain network efficiency and increased amygdala centrality. *Behavioral Neuroscience, 132*(6), 561–572. https://doi.org/10.1037/bne0000276

Wierenga, L., Langen, M., Ambrosino, S., van Dijk, S., Oranje, B., & Durston, S. (2014). Typical development of basal ganglia, hippocampus, amygdala and cerebellum from age 7 to 24. *NeuroImage, 96*, 67–72. https://doi.org/10.1016/j.neuroimage.2014.03.072

Winnicott, D. W. (1945). Primitive emotional development. *The International Journal of Psycho-Analysis, 26*(3–4), 137–143.

Winnicott, D. W. (1949). Hate in the counter-transference. *The International Journal of Psycho-Analysis, 30*, 69–74.

Winnicott, D. W. (1955). Metapsychological and clinical aspects of regression within the psycho-analytical set-up. *The International Journal of Psycho-Analysis, 36*(1), 16–26.

Winnicott, D. W. (1963). Dependence in infant care, in child care, and in the psycho-analytic setting. *The International Journal of Psycho-Analysis, 44*, 339–344.

Wolf, E. S. (1976). Recent advances in the psychology of the self: An outline of basic concepts. *Comprehensive Psychiatry, 17*(1), 37–46. https://doi.org/10.1016/0010-440X(76)90055-9

Wolf, E. S. (1979). Transferences and countertransferences in the analysis of disorders of the self. *Contemporary Psychoanalysis, 15*(4), 577–594. https://doi.org/10.1080/00107530.1979.10745599

Wolf, E. S. (1993). Disruptions of the therapeutic relationship in psychoanalysis: A view from self psychology. *The International Journal of Psycho-Analysis, 74*(Part 4), 675–687.

Yaple, Z., & Arsalidou, M. (2018). *N*-back working memory task: Meta-analysis of normative fMRI studies with children. *Child Development, 89*(6), 2010–2022. Advance online publication. https://doi.org/10.1111/cdev.13080

Zhang, Q., Ma, J., & Nater, U. M. (2019). How cortisol reactivity influences prosocial decision-making: The moderating role of sex and empathic concern. *Frontiers in Human Neuroscience, 13*, Article 415. https://doi.org/10.3389/fnhum.2019.00415

Zimmermann, P. (1999). Structure and functions of internal working models of attachment and their role for emotion regulation. *Attachment & Human Development, 1*(3), 291–306. https://doi.org/10.1080/14616739900134161

Index

About the Author

Julian D. Ford, PhD, ABPP, is a board-certified clinical psychologist and professor of psychiatry and law at the University of Connecticut, where he directs two Treatment and Services Adaptation Centers in The National Child Traumatic Stress Network: the Center for Trauma Recovery and Juvenile Justice and the Center for the Treatment of Developmental Trauma Disorders. Dr. Ford is past president of the International Society for Traumatic Stress Studies, a fellow of the American Psychological Association, and associate editor of both the *European Journal of Psychotraumatology* and the *Journal of Trauma and Dissociation.* He has published more than 250 articles and book chapters. He also is the author or editor of 10 books, including the second edition of *Treating Complex Traumatic Stress Disorders in Adults: Scientific Foundations and Therapeutic Models*, published in 2020 by Guilford Press.